MOTHER-TO-BE

....

A GUIDE TO PREGNANCY AND BIRTH FOR WOMEN WITH DISABILITIES

Judi Rogers, OTR, ACCE

Occupational Therapist
Berkeley, California

Molleen Matsumura
Alin Foundation
Berkeley, California

$\mathcal{D}$*emos*

Demos Publications, 156 Fifth Avenue, New York, NY 10010

Made in the United States of America.

ISBN: 0-939957-30-2 (HC)
      0-939957-29-9 (SC)

LC: 91-073256 (HC)
    91-073256 (SC)

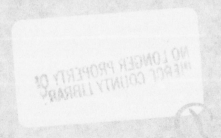

DEDICATION

To Nancy Kaye—
who provided me with the necessary second push to write this book

Judi Rogers

To my grandfather, Nachman Rightman—
Slowing my steps to match his pace gave me time to look
and listen. I never knew he was disabled—only that he loved me

Molleen Matsumura

CONTENTS

FOREWORD

"That's it, that's it, that's what it feels like!" As a childbirth educator who had myself given birth to four children, I had been searching for an image that could communicate the intense experience of childbirth. One night, watching TV with my husband, I saw a group of exhausted mountain climbers reach their summit. In spite of their exhaustion, several leaped up, arms outspread, shouting into the sky, "We did it!" As I watched and felt their joy, I knew that I had found what I had been looking for... an analogy of the entire birth process.

Shortly thereafter, I received a call from Jan, who had attended my sexuality classes when hospitalized for a spinal cord injury. Paralyzed from the shoulders down, she now found herself pregnant despite her precautions. Frightened and confused, she poured out her dilemma.

When Jan had first felt nauseated and began gaining weight, the idea that she might be pregnant never entered her mind. Neither did it occur to her physician, who dismissed her by saying that the weight gain was due to sitting in a wheelchair. Weeks later, when she finally learned she was indeed pregnant, it was too late to consider an abortion. "What should I do?" she asked in a shaky voice.

At that moment, feeling this woman's desperation and determined to help her, I recognized all the themes of my work coming together—a deep respect for the needs of pregnant women and those close to them, a commitment to holistic rehabilitation, and the recognition that persons with disabilities are fully sexual human beings. I said, "You can do it and you can do it with dignity." And so a new adventure began with the safety of both mother-to-be and child-to-be-born being the prime goal.

Mountain climbers have manuals and other resources, ways in which they can benefit from the knowledge and experiences of others throughout the planning, preparation, and actual stages of the climbing experience. And, after their goal is reached and they return, a support system exists to meet their physical and emotional needs. In 1979, when Jan was starting on her childbearing experience, there were no books or articles to be found. What we would have given for a copy of this book!

As I read this Guide, I wondered at the comprehensive yet sensitive resource I had in my hands. The book is based in the childbirth experiences of 36 women with a wide variety of disabilities. Each of their pregnancy histories is detailed in Chapter I, and throughout the book there are pertinent quotations describing their experiences. Like mountain climbers who benefit from the experiences of their peers, women with disabilities can now learn from others with similar concerns.

Just as important, health professionals have a practical approach to what, not too many years ago, was seen as next to impossible. The book rightly emphasizes the value of all health professionals having supportive attitudes and behaviors. Sasha, a woman with spina bifida, did not seek medical care until her fifth month because she "didn't want a big hassle." Such unwise decisions might be avoided when women have therapists, nurses, childbirth educators, and physicians with positive approaches. And Celeste's advice to "be aware that a disabled woman may need more time and more involvement than other new mothers" may be followed by first asking if help is wanted, as Clara suggests. Acknowledging the woman's expertise on her own disability may reward the health care provided with remarks such as Sibyl's, "The nurse in the recovery room was excited for me and made me feel good."

Birth is one of the greatest events in life. This Guide lets us all know that every woman, able-bodied or with a disability, has a right to knowledge of her body and its biological capacity. Every woman has the right to weigh the consequences of childbearing and to decide on her own risk-taking capabilities. Not every mountain climbing experience lives up to expectations; for example, weather conditions may cause plans to be delayed or altered. Likewise, problems related to disability or obstetrical complications cannot always be avoided and may result in disappointment or more. The book's attention to complications respects the intelligence and maturity of the mother-to-be and her professional team by being realistic without being threatening.

Like mountain climbing, childbirth is both a physical and emotional event. By using a wellness approach, this book encourages replacing passivity with responsibility. The authors clearly recognize that women who are disabled have the right to know their options and to choose their own route to a healthy outcome through good nutrition, exercise, stress reduction, and attention to their environment. Significant others, including life partners, family, friends, and peers will find this important book supportive of their roles. The information and attention to significant details will provide a measure of confidence to all.

Jan, her 12-year-old son Aaron, and I congratulate you, Judi and Molleen. This is a resource to be treasured.

Wilma Asrael, OTR/L, MHDL
Childbirth Educator (ASPO);
Sexuality Counselor and Educator (AASECT);
Consultant at the Mercy Hospital Rehabilitation Center
and The Rehab Center in Charlotte, North Carolina

PREFACE

Judi Rogers has been disabled since birth. Being disabled meant being without a role model. There was no person or book she could turn to for information about crucial issues. Most writing about disabilities focused on disabled children, and that continues to be true today. Yet the disabled child grows into a disabled adult, with questions of her own. In recent years, there has been greater acceptance of disabled people's sexuality, and more attention paid to their needs. The next step has to be validation of disabled women's reproductive capacity. Giving this validation is especially important now that social services and special adaptive equipment offer new solutions to the problems of pregnancy, labor, delivery, and child-rearing.

When Judi became pregnant, she again found that there was hardly any literature concerning her particular needs. She searched through the abundant literature on pregnancy, labor, and delivery, but found little that was relevant to the concerns of the disabled. Most of this was limited to single examples in technical journals, personal accounts, and vague generalizations.

At that time, she was working at the Center for Independent Living, an organization run for and by disabled people. Finally, she had role models and peers to share her concern with, including one co-worker who had been pregnant. At the same time, she was receiving calls from other pregnant, disabled women with unanswered questions. Judi began to see that the best way for women with disabilities to find answers to their questions would be to share their experiences. To make sure she would gather as much useful information as possible, she compiled a questionnaire in a series of intense conferences with friends and colleagues. She posted notices in pediatric clinics, centers for the disabled, and at conferences about disability. Some people heard about the project by word of mouth. Finally, thirty-six women answered the questionnaires in personal interviews. Their responses are the heart of this book.

While Judi was conducting these interviews, she supplemented her knowledge about disability by learning more about pregnancy. She trained as a birthing instructor, and taught for four years. She added to her practical knowledge of pregnancy by questioning her students about their experiences, and attending numerous births. After the interviews of mothers with disabilities were completed, Judi and her coauthor conducted formal research on pregnancy, disability, and the interaction of pregnancy and disability. They extensively reviewed the literature on these subjects, and interviewed professionals in the fields of obstetrics, genetic counseling, physical therapy, nutrition, nursing, psychiatry, neurology, emergency medicine, anesthesiology, and rehabilitation.

All the women Judi interviewed were physically disabled. They were a true cross section of the community. There were married, divorced, and single mothers; some full-time homemakers; professionals, white-collar workers, and women needing public assistance; lesbian and heterosexual women; and women of different races and religions. Some women had had their children thirty years before, some were new mothers. While some had given birth in other regions, most gave birth in the San Francisco Bay area, where Judi lives and works. She was careful to include women with a variety of disabilities. Among those with the same diagnosis, the degree of disability varied. It is interesting that there was more similarity among women with the same *degree* of disability than among women with the same *type* of disability.

The most important lesson to be learned from this study is that disabled mothers-to-be have much the same concerns as *all* pregnant women. This became even clearer when Judi invited Molleen Matsumura to join the project, and Molleen, who is able-bodied, kept commenting as she read the material Judi had gathered, "That's exactly how I felt when I was pregnant!"

Although this book has much information that is important to women with disabilities, it can be useful to any pregnant woman. Anyone can benefit from the problem-solving approaches and specific solutions suggested here. (A personal favorite is sleeping on satin sheets to prevent leg cramps.)

Much attention is given to differentiating between changes and discomforts which are common in pregnancy, and those which are disability-related. In general, disabled women experience many of the same changes as able-bodied women, but they are often unsure whether what they are feeling is disability-related, which can be a major source of anxiety.

Health professionals should also find this book valuable, as they will learn about problems that students and patients have been hesitant to express. Some of the information presented here may also suggest new directions for research. Often, simply sharing this book with patients will be helpful.

The opening chapter describes the pregnancy experiences of the women who were interviewed for this book, and underscores how much women with different disabilities have common. This chapter includes simple explanations of different types of disability, since readers may be unfamiliar with some of the problems of people with different disabilities. It describes the physical changes each woman experienced during each of her pregnancies. Finally, it includes the insights women shared about pregnancy and disability, including their ideas for building cooperation between the pregnant woman and her health care team, and their insistence that a pregnant woman with disabilities be seen primarily as a mother-to-be.

The next chapter discusses the many questions that must be answered by a woman who is considering having children. It examines not only the effects on the health of mother and child, but other practical and emotional concerns such as, "What do I do when different doctors give different advice?" "How would I feel about giving birth to a disabled child?" and "How will having children affect my marriage?" Just as important as the medical information covered in this chapter are the suggestions for questions that women can ask themselves, their doctors, and their counselors, so that each woman can make the decision that is best for her.

The chapter on obtaining the best health care possible contains advice on how to select a doctor and hospital, what specialists might need to be consulted, and how to assure cooperation and communication among care providers. Again, questions are presented that women can ask, and techniques they can use, so that they can be sure all their needs will be met.

A pregnant woman can easily feel that there is little she can do to affect the course of the pregnancy, but the suggestions in the chapters on prenatal nutrition and exercise can help her maintain her own health and comfort, and further ensure her baby's well-being. Besides explaining the role of various nutrients, the chapter on nutrition gives attention to special concerns of disabled women, including an explanation of why it is important to gain weight, even though weight gain may interfere with mobility. The chapter on exercise contains exercises adapted for varying levels of disability, so that even severely disabled women can maintain flexibility and good circulation.

The chapter that follows deals comprehensively with every aspect of pregnancy. It is divided into three sections, one for each trimester of pregnancy, and each section contains discussions of the physical changes of pregnancy, what to expect during office visits, pregnancy discomforts and ways of coping with them, fetal development, routine and special medical procedures, possible complications, and emotional concerns. Each section also includes a discussion of special concerns of that trimester; for example, the section on the second trimester includes suggestions for choosing a good birthing class. Throughout the chapter, the special concerns of disabled women are addressed; for example, it describes the different ways interviewees managed to measure their weight, and explains how to instruct a doctor's office staff in assisting a transfer from wheelchair to examining table. Again, there are lists of questions that women can ask to help them understand what is happening, get the information they need to choose appropriate treatment, and make sure they are given appropriate care.

The chapter on labor describes the normal course of labor and delivery, ways of coping with labor discomfort, and possible complications and how they might be treated. It begins by explaining how to recognize that labor has begun, including a description of labor symptoms that may be experienced by women who have reduced sensation. The special information that is provided for women with disabilities includes suggestions for relieving muscle spasms and finding alternate positions for giving birth.

Cesarean birth is covered in a separate chapter, and it may be reassuring reading for many women with disabilities, who often assume that they will have to give birth surgically. It begins with an explanation of the reasons for cesarean delivery, including a discussion of the concerns of disabled women who are considering this procedure. Next is a description of what happens during cesarean delivery, including what the mother can expect to feel, what happens in the recovery room just after surgery, and recovery and self-care during the weeks following cesarean birth. Special attention is given to the effect of cesarean delivery on mobility and other disability symptoms. The chapter closes with a discussion of vaginal birth after cesarean section, including the comments of two interviewees who gave birth in this way.

The closing chapter describes what women experience during the postpartum period, the six weeks after birth during which their bodies return (more or less) to a pre-pregnant state. It discusses the usual physical changes, variations experienced by women with disabilities, signs and symptoms of infection and other problems, suggestions for good self-care, and information about birth control methods. Some of the most important changes at this time are psychological, and there is considerable discussion of these issues, including changes in the sexual relationship. This chapter also contains information that will help women decide whether to breast- or bottle-feed their babies, and suggestions for breast care and breastfeeding. It ends with some ideas for making the new tasks of childcare easier for mothers with disabilities.

While *Mother-to-Be* is meant to be a practical guide to pregnancy, we hope, most of all, that it will encourage women with disabilities to enjoy their pregnancies. Most of the interviewees, whether or not they would choose to become pregnant again, were glad they had their children. Pregnancy is an exciting time. If this book helps you feel that you know what to expect, if it leads you to try other people's ideas and inspires you to try some of your own, if it can be like a friend who's sharing your excitement—then it's doing what it's meant to do.

Judi Rogers
Molleen Matsumura

ACKNOWLEDGMENTS

Writing this book has sometimes felt more like conducting an orchestra than composing a sonata—we could not have done it without the help and support of more people than it is possible to mention here. We are grateful to all of them and hope they will feel that the good this book can do is some reward for their efforts.

Special recognition is due to Frank Osborne Brown, M.D., and Hope Ewing, M.D. Between them they read our entire draft. Several chapters were read by both. They contributed clinical insights gained from years of obstetric experience, information on the latest research, and even their proofreading skills. They were more than generous with their time and thoughtfulness. They improved the book significantly, and it is certainly true that any remaining inaccuracies are the authors' responsibility.

We are also grateful to Barbara Abrams, R.D., Dr. P.H., for reviewing the nutrition chapter; Liane Abrams, M.S., for suggesting resources and reviewing the information on genetic counseling; Alexandra Enders, O.T., for giving personal support, locating many useful resources, and assisting with compilation of the resource directory; Ira Janowitz, R.P.T., for reviewing the exercise chapter; Mary Catherine O'Keeffe, M.D., for reviewing the sections on anesthesia; and Kathe Rogers, for her sensitive and accurate illustrations. Their suggestions contributed to both accuracy and readability.

Others who provided information and support in ways too numerous to list include: Jane Carpenter Bittle, M.S.W.; Ann Canty, P.T.; Martha Casselman; Rita Davis, M.A.; April Devine, R.N.; Carol Fewell, Elinor Freedman, M.D.; Peter Freedman, M.D.; Nancy Kaye; Diana Lee, M.P.H., R.D.A.; Shiu Li; Kenneth Matsumura, M.D.; Betty McMuldren; Vicky Newman, M.S., R.D.; Bill Rogers, R.N.; Janet Sach, L.C.S.W.; Suzi Scott; Robin Stephens; and Walter Verduyn, M.D.

We are grateful to our publisher, Diana Schneider, Ph.D., for recognizing the need for a book on this subject, and for her enthusiasm and practical support. We also wish to thank Sandra Thorn for her editorial contributions, Lori Thorn for her elegant design, and Nancy Berliner for her editorial insight and managerial assistance in producing this book.

In thanking our families and friends, we are not simply following tradition. They were willing to listen to our ideas at all hours of the day and night, uncomplaining when we gave all our time to our work, ever generous with their enthusiasm and support. (Judi's children point out that if she hadn't given birth to them, she never would have been inspired to write this book.) We can never thank them enough.

Finally, our heartfelt gratitude to the 36 women whose sharing of their experiences and insights made this book possible... including Judith Dadak, who did not wish to be anonymous!

1 EXPERT OPINIONS— EXPERIENCES AND ADVICE OF 36 WOMEN

This chapter introduces the women who were interviewed for *Mother-to-Be*. Because the interviews were confidential, we have given each woman a pseudonym that has the same initial as her disability. For example, Clara has Cerebral palsy, and Samantha has a Spinal cord dysfunction. Thus, when you read the women's comments in later chapters, you will be able to identify their disabilities from the first letter of their names.

This chapter contains tables that list the physical changes each woman experienced during pregnancy. As a group, they reveal a broad range of possible reactions to pregnancy. The tables cannot be used to predict what any one woman *will* experience—rather, they show the kinds of changes she *might* experience. Experiences will differ even for women with the same type of disability. For example, some arthritic women experienced an increase in joint pain during pregnancy, while others experienced a decrease. Variations such as these are the subject of continuing research, and in the future there may be information that will help women predict what they are likely to experience during pregnancy.

During their interviews women were asked to describe positive changes as well as discomforts, yet the tables and the comments following them appear to emphasize discomforts. While it is true that many such symptoms were reported, it should be pointed out that women tended to answer questions about problems by describing physical changes, and questions about positive experiences by describing emotional changes. Like able-bodied women, our interviewees often mentioned feeling happy about normal pregnancy changes, even the discomforts. Many women enjoyed looking pregnant, or having larger breasts, or being able to feel fetal movement, or being able to carry a baby to term. Many women were delighted by the idea that, "For once my body is working right."

During the interviews, each woman was asked, "What advice would you give to other disabled women about pregnancy, labor, and delivery?" and "What advice would you give to obstetricians and hospital obstetric departments about the care of disabled women?" Their replies to these questions constitute an important contribution to this book, and we include their specific suggestions throughout. In this chapter, we summarize the main themes of their responses.

The pregnancy histories record the physical changes each woman experienced during each trimester of pregnancy. These tables also indicate whether a physical change was likely to have been due to disability, to pregnancy (including both normal pregnancy changes and complications), or to the interaction of disability and pregnancy. In some cases, it is very difficult to judge the cause of a symptom; for example, one cannot be certain whether some women's pregnancy-associated edema would have been milder if they had been able to exercise. A question mark (?) in the table indicates that it was difficult to judge the cause of a physical change.

Key to Tables:
D   Disability-related physical change
P   Pregnancy-related changes
PD   Changes related to interaction between pregnancy and disability
?   Difficult to judge cause of physical change

ARLENE
. . . .

Arthrogryposis

Arthrogryposis is a rare disability. Approximately 30% of cases of arthrogryposis are known to be genetically caused. The causes of the remaining 70% of cases vary greatly. For example, if the fetus is in a position that makes movement difficult, or the mother has myasthenia gravis, the fetus may develop arthrogryposis.

There are two types of arthrogryposis: in *neuropathic* arthrogryposis, nerve function is affected and, because the nerves cannot stimulate the muscles properly, muscle function is indirectly affected. In *myopathic* arthrogryposis, the muscles are directly affected. In either case, arthrogryposis is characterized by multiple muscle contractures which limit movement of the joints. In some individuals, only a few joints are affected. In the most severe cases, nearly every joint is involved, including those of the spine and the jaw. The degree to which the range of motion is limited in the affected joints also varies among individuals. The affected muscles cannot develop normally, instead they *atrophy* (decrease in mass and strength).

Arlene's myopathic arthrogryposis, which is not hereditary, affects all of her limbs. Her arm and leg muscles have atrophied, and she has *lordosis* (swayback). Arlene uses a wheelchair. Her usual disability-related problems include heartburn, poor circulation in the legs, and a persistent *decubitus ulcer* (pressure sore) on her thigh.

ARLENE'S PREGNANCY HISTORY

Pregnancy: Age 36; miscarriage[a]

Pregnancy: Age 36; miscarriage[a]

Pregnancy: Age 37

Trimester	Cause	Physical Change
1st	D	Light-headed after hot baths[a]
	PD	Swollen feet
	P	More constipation than usual; urinating frequently
2nd	PD	Swollen feet
	PD	Transferring became difficult
	P	Constipation; increased frequency of urination
3rd	PD	Swollen feet worst
	PD	Transferring still harder, often avoided
	P	Constipation worst
	P	Further increase in frequency of urination
All	P	Never felt cold

Comments
[a]Arlene's doctor thought poor circulation may have contributed to her miscarriages. She advised Arlene to spend as much time as possible lying down with her legs raised, in an attempt to improve circulation to the uterus. Her light-headedness may also have been related to her circulatory problems.

After-Effects
Occasional swollen feet ever since the pregnancy.

ATHINA

. . . .

Spinal Muscular Atrophy

Spinal muscular atrophy (SMA) is not one condition but a group of eight similar conditions. All SMAs are genetically caused, but not all are familial. (As we explain in Chapter 2, a genetic disorder can result from a new mutation.) Spinal muscular atrophies involve degeneration of neurons in the spinal cord, medulla, and midbrain. Dysfunction of these nerves leads to degeneration of the nerves in the muscles, which, in turn, leads to muscle atrophy and progressive paralysis. In some individuals, one set of opposing muscles is weakened more than the opposite set, causing scoliosis. The mode of inheritance, age of onset, severity, and progression of the condition vary among the different types of SMA.

Athina is able to move all parts of her body, though she has little strength in her limbs. She can move her arms more easily than her legs. Athina's condition has caused a scoliosis so severe that her hips are *subluxed* (the heads of her femurs do not rest properly in the sockets). A surgically implanted Harrington rod helps her maintain an erect posture. On various occasions, Athina has broken her knees and each of her ankles. Her inability to use her lower limbs has also contributed to *osteoporosis* (bone thinning).

ATHINA'S PREGNANCY HISTORY

Pregnancy: Age 22; elective abortion

Pregnancy: Age 24

Trimester	Cause	Physical Change
1st	PD	Fatigue (end of trimester)
2nd	PD	Bronchitis (three times)
	PD	Difficulty transferring, especially in shower, by end of trimester; lower back pain
3rd	P	Bladder infection
	PD	Continued difficulty transferring
	PD	Lower back pain continued; lower back stiff
	PD	Difficulty balancing, used arms for stabilizing
Unknown	PD?	Breathing more difficult
	PD	Back pain worse

After-Effects
Two years after she gave birth, Athina's breathing difficulties and back pain remained worse than they had been before pregnancy.

CARLA, CELESTE, CHERYL, CHRISTINA, CLARA, AND CORRINE

Cerebral Palsy

Cerebral palsy is a group of disorders caused by damage to the motor area of the brain. Damage can occur prenatally, or as a result of birth trauma, or during childhood. Symptoms vary, depending on just where the injury occurred. From one to four limbs may be affected, and head control may be affected as well. The different types of cerebral palsy are distinguished by the muscle tone and pattern of movement of the affected limb(s). A person may have more than one type of cerebral palsy. The three most common types are:

Spastic Cerebral Palsy. This disorder involves increased muscle tone which results in the affected limb being stiffly held. In spastic paraplegia only the legs are involved. The legs are *adducted* (held close together), and when the person walks the legs tend to cross in a manner called "scissors gait." In spastic hemiplegia the leg and arm on one side are involved. The arm is held rigidly in a *semiflexed* (bent) position.

Athetoid Cerebral Palsy. The major characteristic of this disorder is involuntary, irregular, slow movements of the affected body part. In the mildest forms, the person simply appears rather fidgety.

Ataxic Cerebral Palsy. This disorder involves a wide-based, unsteady gait and, often, reduced manual dexterity.

Carla

When this book was nearly completed, Carla learned that she does not have cerebral palsy but an extremely rare inherited disorder, *familial spastic paresis.* The two disorders have the same symptoms, and Carla was diagnosed as having cerebral palsy until some of her relatives developed similar symptoms and the genetic basis of their condition was identified. Carla commented, "I'm so glad this information will be included in your book, so that other people will know they might have an inherited problem." Her symptoms are those of spastic paraplegia. She can walk two to five blocks, and never used a wheelchair before pregnancy. Her usual disability-related problems include her limited walking range, back problems, difficulty in lifting and carrying, and muscle cramps ("charley horses").

Carla felt that, on the whole, her second pregnancy was easier than her first, because she had a better idea of what to expect, and took a more flexible approach to her problems. She also said, "Taking care of a little kid had gotten me into better shape." Looking back on her pregnancies, Carla commented, "I would have been more comfortable if I had started using a wheelchair in the second trimester."

CARLA'S PREGNANCY HISTORY

Pregnancy: Age 21

Trimester	Cause	Physical Change
1st	PD	Abdominal muscle cramps
	PD	Tight feeling in groin[a]
	PD	Sciatica
	P	Morning sickness
2nd	P	Heartburn
	PD	Leg cramps more intense
	PD	Walking and standing difficult
3rd	PD	Mobility generally a problem: difficulty getting out of bed, chairs, bathtub
	PD	Walking increasingly difficult
	P	Edema
	P	Hemorrhoids
Unknown		Miscarriage[b]

Pregnancy: Age 27

Trimester	Cause	Physical Change
1st	P	Same as first pregnancy, but morning sickness and sciatica worse
2nd		Same as first pregnancy
3rd		None reported

Comments

[a] It is difficult to say whether the tight feeling described by Carla and other women was due to their disabilities or to pregnancy. This sensation may have been a result of *round ligament syndrome,* which is very common among able-bodied pregnant women. There are two round ligaments—one on the right and one on the left of the uterus. The uterus is suspended from the upper ends of the round ligaments, like a tent from tent ropes. On each side of the uterus, the pelvic bones act like tent pegs, anchoring the uterus to the ligaments. The lower ends of the ligaments are attached to the pelvic rami. As the uterus grows, it stretches the ligaments. Sometimes, when the weight of the uterus is shifted, a woman feels a sharp pain due to the stretching of the ligaments. This stretching, and the consequent pain, can be caused by a movement such as rolling over in bed. These pains are known as round ligament syndrome. There is another possible explanation for Carla's groin discomfort. If a woman's disability causes *hypertonicity* in the muscles of the abdominal wall, these muscles might spasm when stressed by an increasingly heavy uterus.

[b] Carla's miscarriage was not caused by her disability, and it was not a pregnancy complication; it was caused by an unusual accident which injured her uterus.

Celeste

All four of Celeste's limbs are affected with spasticity. Her hand movements are somewhat awkward and she walks with a scissors gait. She had used crutches before and during pregnancy, but now uses a wheelchair. Celeste's usual disability-related problems include edema of her ankles and feet, and muscle cramps in her hips.

CELESTE'S PREGNANCY HISTORY

Pregnancy: Age 29

Trimester	Cause	Physical Change
1st	?	Edema[a]
	P	Nausea
	P	Fatigue
2nd	PD	Edema
	P	Felt "great" during 2nd trimester!
3rd	D	Anxiety[b]
	PD?	Edema

Pregnancy: Age 32

Trimester	Cause	Physical Change
1st	P	Same as previous pregnancy
2nd	P	Same as previous pregnancy

Comments

[a]Edema in the first trimester is unusual, and probably resulted from disability; in later trimesters, increased edema may have resulted from pregnancy alone.

[b]Celeste said, "I was so afraid I would have a disabled child, it blocked everything else. I don't remember any other problems."

Cheryl

All four of Cheryl's limbs are slightly affected, somewhat more on the left than on the right. Because she has both ataxia and athetosis, her balance is poor. Cheryl's usual disability-related problems include hand tension and tension in the abdominal muscles.

CHERYL'S PREGNANCY HISTORY

Pregnancy: Age 28

Trimester	Cause	Physical Change
1st	P	Nausea
	P	Mood swings
	PD	Abdominal muscle cramps worse than usual
	P	Fatigue
	P	Cervical bleeding[a]
2nd	PD	Muscle spasms in back, thighs, and groin
	PD	Balance and walking more difficult
	P	Fatigue worse
3rd	PD	Muscle spasms in groin
	PD	Balance and walking still difficult
	P	Heartburn
	PD?	Shortness of breath[b]
	P	Urinating frequently
All		General health was excellent

Comments

[a]The bleeding caused concern that Cheryl was going to have a miscarriage. After a sonogram showed a normal pregnancy, it was found that a local irritation was causing bleeding from the cervical tissue.

[b]If her cerebral palsy affected her chest muscles, then her breathing capacity may have been diminished, making her more susceptible to shortness of breath during pregnancy.

Christina

Christina has spastic paraplegia but is able to walk. Her usual disability-related problems are muscle spasms and backaches.

CHRISTINA'S PREGNANCY HISTORY

Pregnancy: Age 32

Trimester	Cause	Physical Change
1st	PD	Backaches
	PD	Muscle spasms
	P	Nausea
2nd	PD	Backaches
	PD	Muscle spasms
	P	Shortness of breath[a]
	P	Threatened miscarriage[b]
3rd	PD	Backaches
	PD	Muscle spasms
	PD?	Shortness of breath
	PD	Balancing, transferring, and daily activities such as bathing and dressing became more difficult
Unknown	P	Edema
	P	Tired more easily

Comments

[a]If her cerebral palsy affected her chest muscles, then her breathing capacity may have been diminished, making her more susceptible to shortness of breath during pregnancy.

[b]Christina's threatened miscarriage was caused by *placenta previa,* a pregnancy complication in which the placenta implants too low in the uterus (see *Chapter 6*). Placenta previa has nothing to do with disability. Christina was advised to try to prevent miscarriage by resting in bed as much as possible. Lack of exercise caused some muscle atrophy and increased stiffness in the second and third trimesters.

Clara

Clara has a combination of athetosis and spasticity on her left side. Her left arm is slightly affected and can be used as a helper. She walks with a limp and often twists her ankle, sometimes falling. Clara's usual disability-related problems include infrequent muscle spasms, edema of her ankles if she walks too far in hot weather, and infrequent backaches.

CLARA'S PREGNANCY HISTORY

Pregnancy: Age 30

Trimester	Cause	Physical Change
1st	P	Nausea
	P	Fatigue
2nd	PD	Muscle spasms
3rd	PD	Balance difficult: fell once, difficulty getting out of tub
All	P	Felt comfortably warm

Pregnancy: Age 34

Trimester	Cause	Physical Change
1st	P	Nausea
	P	Fatigue
2nd	PD	Muscle spasms
3rd	PD	Baby was low in pelvis, causing cramps in groin area that made walking difficult
	PD?	Edema
All	P	Felt warmer than usual

Corrine

Corrine has spastic cerebral palsy on her left side. Her usual disability-related problems include aching in her upper back and difficulty walking. She has problems walking because it is hard for her to maintain balance, and she frequently trips and falls. For long distances, she rides a bicycle rather than walks.

CORRINE'S PREGNANCY HISTORY

Pregnancy: Age 30

Trimester	Cause	Physical Change
1st	P	Nausea
	PD	Abdominal wall muscle cramps
2nd	PD	None recalled
3rd	PD	Physically awkward (had to to take showers because getting in and out of tub was difficult)
	PD	Constant backaches
All	PD	Over course of pregnancy, posture became gradually more hunched over, and movement slower and more awkward

Pregnancy: Age 32
Same problems as first pregnancy, only more severe

DAWN
. . . .

Dystonia

Dawn has a *dystonia*—a disorder involving *hypertonicity* (increased tone) of some muscles. There are various causes for dystonias, including hormone abnormality, brain injury, and genetic factors. Hereditary dystonia first becomes apparent when the affected person is between 5 and 15 years old.

Dawn has a type of dystonia which, like athetoid cerebral palsy, is caused by damage to the basal ganglia in the brain. Her symptoms include involuntary twisting movements of the trunk. All four limbs are involved, and most of the time they are moving. Her speech is also affected. Dawn can walk short distances, but for long distances she uses an electric wheelchair. Her disability also causes bladder and kidney problems.

DAWN'S PREGNANCY HISTORY

Pregnancy: Age Unknown[a]

Pregnancy: Age 27

Trimester	Cause	Physical Change
1st	P	Nausea
	P	Fatigue
2nd	PD	No specific changes recalled
3rd	PD	Urinating frequently
	PD	Hospitalized for kidney infections (problems persisted despite drinking plenty of water)
	P	Gastric ulcer
	PD	Backaches
	PD	Frequent muscle spasm
	P	Anemia
All		Dawn tripped so often she really could not walk at all. Transferring was not a problem, but getting out of the tub, and sitting up, from a lying down position, were difficult.

Comments

[a]Dawn did not discuss this pregnancy because the baby died, and the memory was very painful.

FAITH

. . . .

Friedreich's Ataxia

Faith has *Friedreich's ataxia,* an inherited, progressive disorder characterized by degeneration of portions of the brain and spinal cord. The disorder progresses slowly, usually causing death by the time the individual is 30 years old. The earliest manifestations are a wide-based gait in which the feet slap the ground as they land, and difficulty sensing where the limbs are located in space. Scoliosis and club feet are also commonly associated with this disorder.

Faith had been walking with the aid of Canadian crutches, but started using an electric wheelchair a month before she became pregnant. Her other disability-related problems included leg cramps, stress incontinence, back problems caused by her scoliosis, and some difficulty breathing. Four years after her pregnancy, her ataxia had progressed so that Faith could only stand, supported, for half a minute.

FAITH'S PREGNANCY HISTORY

Pregnancy: Age 25

Trimester	Cause	Physical Change
1st		No specific changes recalled
2nd	P	Shortness of breath after large meals
	PD	Sharp pains with fetal movement[a]
3rd	P	Heartburn
	PD	Increased scoliosis and backache
	PD	Stress incontinence worsened
	P	Constipation
All	D	Disability symptoms slowly worsened throughout pregnancy; bladder problems increased; leg cramps became more frequent;[b] increased mobility difficulties

Comments

[a]Faith attributed this pain—a normal, if uncommon, pregnancy discomfort—to her disability.

[b]Faith retained enough leg strength to transfer, but needed support when standing or getting in and out of the shower.

After-Effects

During the 6 months after childbirth, Faith's disability symptoms returned to what they had been before pregnancy. Later worsening of symptoms can be attributed to the usual progression of her disorder.

During a conversation, several years after her interview, Faith had had a second child, and was pregnant for the third time. Her first child was delivered surgically and her second was born vaginally. Faith commented, "I often wonder whether I really needed to have that C-section the first time." She also commented that she recovered much more quickly after vaginal delivery.

HEATHER
· ·

Hip Dysplegia

Heather has *hip dysplegia* (a developmental abnormality), *scoliosis,* (S-shaped curvature of the spine) and an amputation. Her *acetabulum* (a cup-shaped cavity in the pelvis which receives the head of the femur) and *femoral head* (knob at the end of the thigh bone) never developed—she has no hip joint. Her dysplegia may have caused her scoliosis. Her right leg did not develop normally and was amputated above the knee when she was 14 years old. Heather has not been able to find a comfortable prosthesis and uses crutches. She moves so skillfully that she has even learned to ski.

Heather's usual disability-related problems include muscle spasms in the stump, phantom pain when she is tired, and a constant, mild lower back ache.

HEATHER'S PREGNANCY HISTORY

Pregnancy: Age 27

Trimester	Cause	Physical Change
1st	P	Heartburn
2nd	PD	Difficulty keeping balance
	P	Bladder control worse for remainder of pregnancy
	PD	Back pain and phantom pain worse
	P	Threatened miscarriage: bleeding, passing clots, and cervix dilating at 6 months (bed rest prescribed)
	P	Heartburn
3rd	PD	Balance worse: difficulty getting in and out of tub, began to use wheelchair outside of house
All	P	Heartburn
	PD	Muscle spasms in amputated leg more frequent
	P	Hair and nails healthier during pregnancy

Comments
Heather was interviewed during her second pregnancy and mentioned that she was much more comfortable than during her first pregnancy. She attributes feeling better to being more relaxed, because she knew what to expect. She comments, "I knew what my body would do; I knew my back would not be seriously affected."

After-Effects
Heather's bladder control continues to be worse than before pregnancy; she urinates more frequently and has to go to the bathroom more frequently when she feels the urge.

HILARY

. . . .

Congenital Hip Deformity

Hilary has *femoral hypoplasia syndrome,* a congenital hip deformity. Characteristics of the syndrome are malformation of the lower spine and short *femoral* (thigh) bones with missing knee joints. Hilary's uterus is a normal size but has two chambers.

Hilary has difficulty walking. She uses artificial legs that are similar to stilts, and Canadian crutches. She falls about once a month and has difficulty climbing stairs. Another disability-related problem is stress incontinence.

HILARY'S PREGNANCY HISTORY

Pregnancy: Age 27

Trimester	Cause	Physical Change
1st	PD	Vertebrae slipped when lying down (had to realign joints before rising or movement was painful)[a]
2nd	PD	Balance became difficult
3rd	P	Edema
	PD?	Shortness of breath
	PD	Continued difficulty balancing
All	PD	Stress incontinence worse than usual

Pregnancy: Age 29

Symptoms were the same as with the first pregnancy, except that exacerbation of stress incontinence (PD) was even worse. In this pregnancy, Hilary decided to use a wheelchair.

Comments

[a]This problem may have resulted from an interaction between Hilary's disability and the usual increase of joint mobility caused by pregnancy hormones.

After-Effects

Hilary's back condition improved after the birth, but did not return to its original state.

JENNIFER AND JULIE

· ·

Juvenile Rheumatoid Arthritis

Other names for j*uvenile rheumatoid arthritis* (JRA) include Still's disease, juvenile chronic polyarthritis, and chronic childhood arthritis. Juvenile rheumatoid arthritis refers to a group of disorders which, like adult-onset arthritis, all involve inflammation of the joints. About a quarter of a million children in the United States have JRA; most of them are girls. In JRA, joint inflammation often takes longer to lead to permanent damage than the inflammation of adult arthritis, and many individuals do not suffer permanent joint damage. However, systemic symptoms, including eye and skin problems, are more common with JRA. Juvenile rheumatoid arthritis may also cause growth disturbances. The exact combination of symptoms depends on the type of JRA an individual has; which type of JRA a person has cannot be predicted at the onset of the disease.

Jennifer
Jennifer's joints and skin are affected by JRA. Different joints are affected at different times; every joint is symptomatic at some time. Pain, swelling, or limitation of range of motion are more severe at some times than others. The skin over her whole body usually feels sore and sensitive. Her skin and joint symptoms are worse when she is feeling tired or weak.

JENNIFER'S PREGNANCY HISTORY

Pregnancy: Age 30

Trimester	Cause	Physical Change
1st	P	Hungry all the time, felt sick when not eating enough
	PD	Started to enjoy walking[a]
2nd	P	Nasal congestion
	P	Leg cramps
	PD	Walked longer distances[b]
	P	Dropped objects often
3rd	P	Nasal congestion
	PD	Uncomfortable when sitting
	PD	Back pain
	PD	Increased skin sensitivity
	P	Feet swollen[c]
	P	Toe nails hurt[c]
	P	Edema
	P	Vaginal infection

Comments

[a]She used a wheelchair while at school, but walked more at other times.

[b]By the second trimester, the increase in how much she walked was dramatic: "I took walks for the first time in my life. Usually I complained when I needed to walk across the room."

[c]The pain of her swollen feet reminded Jennifer of the arthritic pain she often felt in her ankles, but was most likely due to edema. The pain in her toe nails was probably another side effect of the swelling in her feet.

Julie

Julie's arthritis affects all her joints. Her usual disability-related problems are difficulty walking and stiffness of the joints. Joint stiffness is especially severe in her ankles, which have become deformed; in her hands; and in her knees. She usually uses an electric wheelchair. Despite her joint discomfort, Julie commented, "I felt better than some of my able-bodied friends did when they were pregnant."

JULIE'S PREGNANCY HISTORY

Pregnancy: Age 27

Trimester	Cause	Physical Change
1st		No specific changes recalled
2nd	PD	As weight increased, ankle pain became more severe than usual
	PD	As pregnancy progressed, some movements became more awkward and she had to change her way of getting in and out of cars
	P	Feet began to swell
3rd	PD	Ankles still more painful Eighth month, fell and tore leg muscle[a]
	PD	Hips more painful after fall
	P	Increased heartburn
	PD	Swollen feet
	PD	Pain in hips and tailbone
	PD	Standing and sitting difficult[b]
All		The level of arthritic pain in general remained unchanged

Comments

[a]Julie's arthritis did not cause her fall—she tripped on a throw rug. However, the fall did cause a worsening of arthritic pain.

[b]Julie adapted by sitting in different types of chairs at different times; for example, she sat on a high stool when she was washing dishes.

After-Effects

After she gave birth, Julie's ankles bothered her more than they had before she was pregnant.

LAURA AND LESLIE

. . . .

Systemic Lupus Erythematosus ("Lupus")

Systemic lupus erythematosus (SLE)—often referred to simply as lupus—is a disease resembling rheumatoid arthritis. It is an autoimmune disorder, which means that the immune system attacks other body tissues in the same way it would attack invading bacteria and viruses. Unlike the lupus disorder which affects only the skin, SLE is a *systemic* disease, because many organ systems may be affected.

Systemic lupus erythematosus causes a variety of symptoms, and different individuals have different combinations of symptoms. The most common problems are pain and swelling in the joints, and kidney damage. Other problems include fever, fatigue, weakness, skin rashes, sensitivity to sunlight, headaches, and muscle aches. If the brain is affected, seizures, personality changes, or emotional depression may result. No cure has been found for SLE, but the symptoms may be controlled with proper treatment. Many people experience remissions of symptoms.

Laura

Laura's usual problems before pregnancy were aching joints, fatigue, high blood pressure, loss of vision in one eye (probably as a result of high blood pressure), and confusion.

Leslie

Leslie's SLE was not diagnosed until she had had one premature baby and one miscarriage. She now realizes that she had been experiencing SLE symptoms for approximately 13 years before the disease was diagnosed. When working in hot weather that did not affect her co-workers, Leslie experienced severe rashes, vomiting, and hair loss. She had a constantly recurring streptococcal infection of the vagina, and later realized that the infection kept recurring because her immune system was too weakened by SLE to resist reinfection. The effects of SLE on her pregnancies led to diagnosis of the disease.

Since the time of the diagnosis, Leslie has had continuous problems with psoriasis. Her shoulders, hips, knees, feet, and hands have become arthritic.

LAURA'S PREGNANCY HISTORY

Pregnancy: Age 37

Trimester	Cause	Physical Change
1st	P	Lupus mask darkened[a]
	D	Unpredictable joint pains
	P	Constipation
	P	Urinary infection
2nd	D	Joint pains continued
	P	Frequent bladder infections
	D?	Several mild seizures
3rd	D?	Food sensitivities developed
All	PD	Fatigue; mobility[b] lessened; blood pressure labile (extremely variable)[c]

Comments

[a]"Lupus mask" is a reddish rash found on the faces of some people who have lupus. *Chloasma*, known as the "mask of pregnancy," occurs in some pregnant women and consists of a darkening of areas of facial skin (with the same brown pigment found in a sun-tan or freckles). What seems to have happened is that chloasma darkened the same area of Laura's face which is affected by lupus mask.

[b]Laura could not get around much because she needed to move slowly and stop for rest even after walking short distances.

[c]In the third trimester she was hospitalized for pre-eclampsia (see *Chapter 2*) and treated with medication for blood pressure.

After-Effects

After she gave birth, Laura suffered a severe depression. She had two or three seizures, and continued to have problems with fatigue and high blood pressure. Nine years later, when Laura was interviewed, her problems were fatigue; arthritis in her hands, shoulders, and knees; episodes of confusion; and frequent seizures.

LESLIE'S PREGNANCY HISTORY

First Pregnancy: Age 26

Trimester	Cause	Physical Change
1st	P	Nausea
	D	Occasional blood spotting
2nd	D	Continued spotting (bed rest prescribed)
3rd	D	Premature birth with placental abruption[a]
All	PD	Psoriasis cleared up for duration of pregnancy
	D	Temperature fluctuations between 96° and 101°F
	PD	Remission of arthritic symptoms

Second Pregnancy: Age 29

Trimester	Cause	Physical Change
1st	P	Nausea
	D	Blood spotting
2nd	D	Felt pelvic pressure 4th month, miscarriage 5th month
All	PD	Psoriasis cleared up for duration of pregnancy
	D	Temperature fluctuations worse than during first pregnancy
	PD	Remission of arthritic symptoms

Third Pregnancy: Age 31

Trimester	Cause	Physical Change
1st	D	Temperature fluctuations (controlled with medication)
	D	Blood spotting
	P	Nausea
	PD	Partial miscarrige, one twin died (bed rest to end of term)
	P	Anemia after miscarriage to end of term
	P	Diabetes from 3rd month to end of term[b]
2nd	P	Yeast infection at end of trimester
	D	Less spotting with medication
	D	High blood pressure[c]

(continued)

LESLIE'S PREGNANCY HISTORY *(continued)*

Third Pregnancy *(continued)*

Trimester	Cause	Physical Change
3rd	D	Temporary loss of vision in one eye[c]
	D	High blood pressure[c]
	D	Short-term memory impaired[c]
	D	Proteinuria[c]
	PD	Birth in 7th month
All	PD	Psoriasis cleared up for duration of pregnancy
	D	Temperature fluctuations in first trimester controlled by medication
	PD	Remission of arthritic symptoms

Comments

[a]The presence of lupus antibodies led to placental rejection.

[b]This appears to have been diabetes of pregnancy. Leslie did not need to use medication to control her diabetes, as she was able to do so with diet.

[c]Leslie said she had pre-eclampsia during her third pregnancy. However, these symptoms are also symptoms of SLE exacerbation, so it can be difficult to determine whether a woman is experiencing pre-eclampsia or SLE exacerbation. Since pre-eclampsia typically occurs in a first pregnancy, it seems likely that Leslie's problems were related to SLE.

After-Effects

At the end of each pregnancy, Leslie's psoriasis returned. After the third pregnancy, her vision began to return gradually. However, there was a flare-up of many other symptoms just after the third pregnancy: she had difficulty walking and the arthritis in her shoulders became so severe it was hard for her to pick up her baby. She was bothered by fevers, nausea, and fatigue. At the time of her interview, when her daughter was 5 months old, she had only slight difficulty walking and the arthritis in her shoulders and hands had improved.

MARGIE, MARSHA, MARY, AND MICHELLE
. . . .

MULTIPLE SCLEROSIS

Multiple sclerosis (MS) is difficult to describe. Not only do people have different sets of symptoms, but one person's symptoms will vary over time. These variations are due to the nature of the disorder. In medical terms, the symptoms of MS are caused by demyelinization of the axon sheaths at various locations, followed by glial scar formation at some sites. Think of your nervous system as a set of telephone wires connecting a central switchboard (your brain) and the various parts of your body. With MS, the insulation of the wires wears away at various points, disrupting communications. If the damage occurs in the nerve connecting the eye to the brain, blurring of vision may result; if damage occurs in the nerves connecting the bladder to the brain, urinary difficulties may result. If a worn patch is repaired, remission of symptoms will result, but *demyelinization* (loss of insulation) of a different part of the nerve could cause a symptom to reappear.

Multiple sclerosis most often appears in individuals between the ages of 20 and 40 years. However, because MS symptoms are so variable and confusing, the disorder may not be diagnosed until years after the first symptoms appear. The causes of MS are not completely understood. It is an *autoimmune disorder;* that is, a disorder in which a person's antibodies attack her own body tissues. It is possible that a combination of inherited and environmental factors are involved. The reasons the rate of progression varies among individuals are also not understood. While there are no medications for treating the disease itself, some symptoms can be treated.

Margie

Margie had MS before she became pregnant. Her symptoms before pregnancy were weakness in the arm and leg on one side, and occasional bladder problems. Margie commented about her first pregnancy, "I felt great while I was pregnant! I enjoyed feeling so healthy, and I had a positive outlook on life."

MARGIE'S PREGNANCY HISTORY

Pregnancy: Age 27

Trimester	Cause	Physical Change
All	PD	Walking difficult, one leg dragged; bladder problems disappeared

Pregnancy: Age 30

Physical changes same as previous pregnancy

After-Effects
After her first pregnancy, Margie's MS worsened slightly. Her main problem was blurred vision. After her second pregnancy, she made sure she had extra help, and there was no exacerbation of MS.

Marsha

Before her pregnancy, Marsha walked with a limp and used a cane.

MARSHA'S PREGNANCY HISTORY

Pregnancy: Age Unknown; miscarriage

Pregnancy: Age 32

Trimester	Cause	Physical Change
All	D	Impaired mobility (needed to use two canes)
	PD	Bladder problems: alternated between urgency and incontinence

After-Effects
Three years later, Marsha needed to use a wheelchair almost all the time.

Mary

Before pregnancy, Mary tired easily. She could walk short distances unassisted but used a walker for longer distances, especially for getting up and down stairs. Her bladder control was slightly affected.

MARY'S PREGNANCY HISTORY

Pregnancy: Age Unknown; miscarriage (caused by placenta previa)

Pregnancy: Age 31

Trimester	Cause	Physical Change
All	PD	Fatigue[a]
Unknown	PD	Poor bladder control[c]

Comments
[a]Mary said, "I went on using my walker, but sometimes I was so tired I thought of using a wheelchair."
[b]Bladder control was so poor that she stayed close to home much of the time.

After-Effects
Ten years later, Mary still tired very easily, and had considered using a wheelchair. She also had some muscle spasms.

Michelle

Michelle's MS symptoms were mild. The problems that led to her diagnosis were urgency and occasional incontinence, and blurred vision. Later, she had problems with muscle spasms, and tired easily.

MICHELLE'S PREGNANCY HISTORY

Pregnancy: Age 35

Trimester	Cause	Physical Change
1st	PD	Tired more easily than usual
	P	Nausea
2nd	P	Lower back pain
3rd	PD	Tired more easily than usual
	D	Vision more blurred
	D	Pins-and-needles sensation on right arm, leg, and scalp
	PD	Frequent muscle spasms for one week
All	PD	Increased urgency to urinate, but no incontinence
Unknown	P	Trouble sleeping

After-Effects

Two years after she gave birth, Michelle's hand and feet were somewhat numb.

PAM, PATRICIA, PAULA, PORTIA, AND PRISCILLA
. . . .

POSTPOLIO SYNDROME

Poliomyelitis is a viral illness which affects the central nervous system. Postpolio syndrome refers to problems remaining after the viral infection has ended. The virus attacks anterior horn cells in the spinal cord. When these nerve cells have been destroyed, the muscles they serve become paralyzed, although sensation remains. Different muscles are affected in different individuals, depending on which nerves were damaged. One person may have difficulty breathing, whereas another may be unable to move her legs. Sometimes surgery is helpful: the surgeon may move a functioning muscle into the position of a nonfunctional muscle, making movement possible.

Pam

Pam's arms and hands were weakened by polio; she describes them as "60% functional." She can write, cook, and hold a glass of water, but heavy tasks are difficult. Her legs are completely paralyzed and she uses an electric wheelchair. Pam's abdominal muscles are weak. In order to give her trunk enough support for sitting up, a muscle fascia was transplanted from her right thigh, with one end attached to her ribs and the other to her pelvis. Also, Pam's left shoulder was surgically fused, and she has a sway back. Before she became pregnant, Pam had pulmonary function tests and was assured that she would not have too much difficulty breathing.

Patricia

Patricia's polio affects all four limbs, and she has a scoliosis. She can walk with the aid of braces and crutches, but she usually prefers to use a wheelchair. Her arms are somewhat weak, but she is able to use them to propel a light-weight manual wheelchair. Patricia's comment about her pregnancy was, "I had a better pregnancy than most of my able-bodied friends."

Paula

Paula's arms, legs, abdominal muscles, and back are all affected by postpolio syndrome. Her usual disability-related problems include difficulty in carrying large loads such as grocery bags, tiring easily, hip pain, poor circulation in the legs, and occasional muscle spasms. She walks with Canadian crutches. During her second pregnancy, Paula contracted polio and the illness caused a miscarriage. She felt that, on the whole, her later, postpolio pregnancies were similar to the first.

PAM'S PREGNANCY HISTORY

Pregnancy: Age 26

Trimester	Cause	Physical Change
1st	P	Fatigue
	P	Nausea
2nd	P	Continued nausea
	PD	Weight of pregnancy caused stretching of implanted fascia, burning pain in fascia
3rd	P	Badly swollen feet
	PD	Pain in fascia increased
	P	Urinating frequently
	PD	Constant aching in right hip[a]
	PD	Some decrease in mobility (rolling over became more difficult, could not sit up in tub)
All	P	Fewer bladder problems than usual, but continuous problems with edema

Comments

[a]Pam could not lie on her left side because of her scoliosis and shoulder fusion. Her baby was positioned to the right, so while she was pregnant, there was more pressure when she lay on her right side. The extra weight led to the aching in her hip.

PATRICIA'S PREGNANCY HISTORY

Pregnancy: Age 20

Trimester	Cause	Physical Change
1st	P	Fatigue
2nd		No specific changes recalled
3rd	P	Heartburn
All	P	Occasional hemorrhoids

PAULA'S PREGNANCY HISTORY

Pregnancy: Age 25

Trimester	Cause	Physical Change
1st	P	Morning sickness
2nd	P	Morning sickness continued
3rd	P	Urinating frequently

Pregnancy: Age 27; miscarriage due to polio infection (first trimester)

Pregnancy: Age 29

Trimester	Cause	Physical Change
1st	P	Morning sickness
2nd	P	Morning sickness
	PD	Difficulty balancing (getting in and out of car)
	PD	Swollen legs
	PD	Aching in hips and back
	PD	Muscle spasms
3rd	P	Urinating frequently
	PD	Problems with balance

Pregnancy: Age 31

Symptoms same as previous pregnancy

Portia

Portia's polio affected her legs, left arm and hand, neck, abdominal and low back muscles, and diaphragm. Her usual disability-related problems include occasional bladder infections, difficulty breathing and coughing, and anemia. Portia uses a wheelchair. Because Portia had had five children, with the last pregnancy occurring several years before her interview, she simply summarized her pregnancy symptoms as follows:

Portia contracted polio when she was 19 years old. Two years later, she had her first child. Her fifth child was born when she was 34 years old. Portia's anemia PD continued to be a problem during all her pregnancies. She also had morning sickness P with all of her pregnancies, and bladder infections PD during three pregnancies. Pregnancy also exacerbated her disability-related problems with constipation. PD Portia said that it was easier for her to cough PD when she was pregnant, explaining, "I didn't need a corset when I was pregnant. The baby did the same job." By the second trimester of each pregnancy, transferring was getting difficult; PD Portia was able to adapt, except that by the third trimester using a bathtub was impossible, and she avoided going out alone. Portia said, "I stopped driving when I stopped fitting behind the steering wheel." All of Portia's babies were delivered surgically. PD

Priscilla

Priscilla's polio affected only her right leg. When she was nine years old, a muscle transplant was performed so she would be able to use her right leg. When she was eleven, a pin was implanted in her left leg to slow its growth to a rate consistent with that of the right leg. Now, her right leg is somewhat thinner than her left, and she walks with a slight limp. Before Priscilla's first pregnancy, her right leg and hip often ached after she carried groceries up a steep hill to her house.

PRISCILLA'S PREGNANCY HISTORY

Pregnancy: Age 27

Trimester	Cause	Physical Change
1st	P	Fatigue
2nd		No specific changes recalled
3rd	P	Anemia

Pregnancy: Age 37

Trimester	Cause	Physical Change
1st	P	Fatigue
2nd		No specific changes recalled
3rd	P	Heartburn

Comments
Pregnancy did not seem to impair Priscilla's mobility.

After-Effects
She feels she has gotten much stronger since her second child was born, and she started taking yoga classes.

RENEE AND ROBERTA

Rheumatoid Arthritis

There are a number of types of arthritis, all characterized by swelling, pain, and stiffness of the joints. *Rheumatoid arthritis* (RA), which affects about 1% of the population, is one of the more common forms of arthritis. People who have rheumatoid arthritis may experience other symptoms, including anemia, eye inflammation, and pleurisy. Rheumatoid nodules occur in about 20% of rheumatoid arthritis patients, in areas subject to pressure or trauma (often just under the skin), in the lungs, and in the heart. The causes of rheumatoid arthritis are still not completely understood, but inherited susceptibility, viral infection, and autoimmune response all seem to play roles in this disease. (Autoimmunity is discussed above in the section on SLE.)

Renee

Renee's rheumatoid arthritis was diagnosed when she was 6 months pregnant with her first child. Most of Renee's symptoms were in remission between her first and second pregnancies. A month after the birth of her second child, Renee's feet and hands were constantly painful. The pain and swelling in her hands was so severe that she could hardly use them.

Roberta

Roberta's usual disability-related symptoms before her pregnancy included aching and weakness in her hands, aching shoulders and knees, morning stiffness, and susceptibility to bladder infections.

RENEE'S PREGNANCY HISTORY

Pregnancy: Age 22

Trimester	Cause	Physical Change
1st	D	Leg became stiff and sore [a]
2nd	D	Increased difficulty walking
	D	Arthritis diagnosed: unable to move one leg
	PD	Difficulty getting in and out of tub
3rd	D	Increased difficulty walking
	P	Occasional dizziness in afternoon (improved with iron tablets)
	PD	Difficulty sitting (driving became difficult)

Pregnancy: Age 26

Trimester	Cause	Physical Change
1st	D	No arthritic pain
2nd	D	Increased difficulty walking
	D	Arthritic pain increased
	PD	More difficulty getting in and out of tub than in previous pregnancy
3rd	D	Increased difficulty walking
	D	Arthritic pain increased

Comments
[a]First symptoms of arthritis occurred: leg became increasingly sore and stiff throughout pregnancy. Arthritic pain was worse at times of emotional stress.

After-Effects
After Renee's first child was born, her leg improved somewhat but was still stiff and painful.

ROBERTA'S PREGNANCY HISTORY

Pregnancy: Age 28

Trimester	Cause	Physical Change
1st	D	Worst arthritic pain: stiffness in hands, shoulders, and knees in morning[a]
2nd	PD	Pain and stiffness improved
3rd	PD	Further improvement in arthritic pain
All	PD	Continuous problems with bladder and urinary tract infections
Unknown	P	Experienced muscle cramps about five times

Comments

[a]Roberta said, "My arthritis improved about 95%. I felt as if I could walk forever. I felt better than usual and I had lots of energy."

SAMANTHA, SHARON, SHEILA, STACY, STEPHANIE, AND SYLVIA

. . . .

Spinal Cord Injuries

Spinal cord injury refers to irreversible mechanical damage to the spinal cord. The damage results from the kind of injury that might be sustained in a driving or diving accident, or a fall. This damage can cause loss of movement, loss of sensation, or both.

The spinal cord is a bundle of nerves that carries messages between the brain and the rest of the body, in much the same way that a cable carries messages between a central switchboard and several houses. If a storm occurs, damaging several wires in the cable, not all the houses will lose telephone service, but only those connected to the damaged wires. Similarly, the particular disabilities that a person experiences will depend on just which nerves in the spinal cord bundle were damaged. Significant in determining the type of disability is the level, or area, of the spinal cord, that is injured, as well as the extent of damage that occurred at that level. The level of injury is defined by referring to the *vertebrae* (spinal bones) closest to the injury site. Starting from the top, the neck vertebrae are numbered from C1 to C-7; the vertebrae in the upper and midback are numbered from T1 to T12; and the vertebrae in the lower back are numbered from L1 to L5.

If the spinal cord injury occurs in the neck, all four limbs will be affected. This condition is called *quadriplegia.* Injuries closer to the skull cause *high quadriplegia.* (Injuries above the C-3 vertebra are almost always fatal, injuries at C-3 are often fatal; injuries from C-3 to C-5 cause high quadriplegia, and quadriplegics with injuries from C-5 to C-7 have limited hand use.) Injury to the thoracic spine (the part of the spine behind the breastbone) causes *high paraplegia.* Injury to the lumbar (low back) spine causes *paraplegia.* The muscles in the limbs are not the only ones affected. In both quadriplegics and high paraplegics, the abdominal muscles, and some back muscles, are also affected. Bowel and bladder control are also affected to varying degrees. Quadriplegics have difficulty coughing, and may have other breathing difficulties.

Women whose injuries are above T-6 sometimes experience autonomic *dysreflexia,* also called *hyperreflexia.* Dysreflexia is a reflexive response to specific types of stimuli including distension of the bladder, cervix, or rectum, uterine contractions, excessive deep breathing, and immersion of the feet in cold water. Normally, this spinal reflex to these stimuli is modulated by higher nerve centers, but cord injury makes such modulation impossible. Because the unmodulated reaction to stimuli can become dangerous, it is appropriately called *dys*reflexia. Symptoms of dysreflexia include hypertension (increased blood pressure), heavy perspiration, goose bumps and flushing above the level of injury, feelings of anxiety or fear, dilation of the pupils (sometimes asymmetrical), nasal stuffiness, and changes in heart rhythm. Very severe hypertension is accompanied by a pounding headache. On any one occasion, an individual might experience any combination of possible symptoms. A common term for episodes involving relatively mild symptoms is "quad sweats." Episodes involving prolonged, sustained hypertension can be life-threatening. Dysreflexia can be stimulated by ordinary events such as bladder fullness or the insertion of a speculum during a pelvic examination. Symptoms may be resolved by removal of the stimulus; for example, by emptying the bladder or removing a speculum.

While some women did not feel labor contractions, all the women we interviewed were able to feel fetal movement.

Samantha

Samantha is paraplegic. Her injury occurred at T-10, T-11, and T-12. She was injured after she had already had two children. Her third child was born ten years after she was injured. Her legs are paralyzed; there is some calicification in her hips, and she has a suprapubic catheter. Samantha felt that, with the exception of specific disability problems like trouble transferring, her last pregnancy was much the same as her first two. She remarked, "It wasn't as bad as I thought it would be."

SAMANTHA'S PREGNANCY HISTORY

Pregnancy: Age 15

Trimester	Cause	Physical Change
1st	P	Bladder infections
2nd		None recalled
3rd	P	Edema

Pregnancy: Age 17

Trimester	Cause	Physical Change
1st	P	Bladder infections
2nd		None recorded
3rd	P	Edema

Pregnancy: Age 27

Trimester	Cause	Physical Change
1st	P	Bladder infections
	P	Morning sickness
2nd	PD	Difficulty transferring into van
	PD	Couldn't bend to reach floor
3rd	PD	Increased difficulty transferring into van; difficulty transferring into bed
	PD	Backaches
	P	Edema not as severe as in previous pregnancies

Sharon

Sharon's injury occurred at the T-6 level. She is a high paraplegic. Her legs, feet, lower abdominal muscles, and some low back muscles are paralyzed. Just after she was injured, she had phlebitis in one leg. Another problem was occasional muscle spasms. She had surgery for bladder spasticity, and before she was pregnant, she catheterized herself.

SHARON'S PREGNANCY HISTORY

Pregnancy: Age 34

Trimester	Cause	Physical Change
1st	P	Tired easily
	P	Stomach aches
	PD	Difficulty inserting catheter[a]
2nd	PD	Difficulty transferring into tub
	PD	Difficulty maneuvering wheelchair into car
	PD	Increased difficulty bending and picking things up
	PD	Urine constantly dripping[b]
	PD	Chronic bladder infection
3rd	P	Hospitalized for premature labor in 7th month (baby was born 6 weeks early)
	D	Muscle stiffness and increased muscle spasms (due to insufficient physical therapy in hospital)
	P	Swollen ankles
	PD	Backaches
	P	Improved circulation in upper body, felt warmer than usual
	PD	Phlebitis in legs reappeared
All		Condition of hair and skin improved

Comments

[a]Pressure from the growing uterus may have compressed the bladder outlet enough to make insertion of the catheter more difficult.

[b]Sharon started using the Foley catheter, which remains in place constantly. When Sharon requested an indwelling catheter, her doctor expressed concern that she would not be able to discontinue its use later. Still, because of the difficulties she was having, Sharon decided to try using the indwelling catheter. After giving birth, she found she had to continue using it. (Her doctor's concern was justified. Surveys have found that spinal-cord-injured women who use indwelling catheters may not be able to discontinue their use afterward.)

Sheila

Sheila is a quadriplegic whose level of injury is at C-5 and C-6. She has limited use of all her limbs. She can lift her arms, has some use of her hands, can stand with support, and can do a pivot transfer with support. Her bladder tends to retain urine, and she knows when she has to urinate because she starts to sweat (a dysreflexia symptom). When she is under stress, she has problems with dysreflexia and constipation.

SHEILA'S PREGNANCY HISTORY

Pregnancy: Age 24

Trimester	Cause	Physical Change
1st		None recorded
2nd	PD	Muscle spasms[a]
	PD	Began having difficulty transferring in and out of bed
	PD	Difficulty breathing
	P	Edema
3rd	P	Anemia
	PD	Muscle spasms
	PD	Difficulty transferring to tub
	PD	Unable to find comfortable position for intercourse
	PD	Difficulty bending when dressing
All	PD	Persistent bladder infections[b]
	P	Nausea

(continued)

SHEILA'S PREGNANCY HISTORY *(continued)*

Pregnancy: Age 29

Trimester	Cause	Physical Change
1st	P	Fatigue[c]
2nd	PD	Muscle spasms
3rd	PD	Episode of premature labor[d]
All	PD	Persistent bladder infections[d]

Comments

[a]During the first pregnancy, a physical therapist did leg stretches which helped reduce Sheila's muscle spasm; she wishes she had had the same therapy during her second pregnancy.

[b]During her first pregnancy, Sheila's bladder infections were recurrent, and she only used antibiotics when she had an active infection. During her second pregnancy, a bladder infection caused uterine contractions in the seventh month, and she was advised to use antibiotics continuously until she gave birth. She later remarked that she was much more comfortable when she used antibiotics continuously, and she wishes she had done so during her first pregnancy.

[c]Sheila thinks that she felt so tired early in her second pregnancy because she was feeling upset; the pregnancy was unplanned and her husband was not as supportive as he had been during the first pregnancy.

[d]Her disability did not directly cause premature labor; the effect was indirect, because her disability made her more susceptible to infections.

Stacy

Stacy's injury was at the C-5 and C-6 level. She has some use of her hands. She uses a walker for short distances and a manual wheelchair for long distances. Her usual problems include scoliosis, an inability to sit up without support from a girdle, dysreflexia when she needs to urinate, and occasional light-headedness.

STACY'S PREGNANCY HISTORY

Pregnancy: Age 24

Trimester	Cause	Physical Change
1st	P	Felt tired[a]
	PD	Back pain
2nd	P	Still tired
	PD	No back pain[b]
	PD	Felt faint at times
	PD	Problems with balance (did not walk for fear of falling)
3rd	PD	Difficulty bending to pick things up
	PD	Back pain
	PD	Difficulty transferring
	PD	Could not stand
	P	Difficulty breathing when lying on back
	PD	Increased constipation
	PD	Bladder never emptied completely
	PD	Urinary bleeding (possibly caused by irritation from catheter)

Comments

[a]It is interesting that while Stacy said she had often felt tired, she also said she had frequently pushed her wheelchair for 60 laps on a 200 meter track!

[b]During the second trimester, Stacy's back pain was alleviated by the use of a maternity girdle.

Stephanie

Stephanie is paraplegic; her injury is at the T-12 level. She has some sensation in the right hip. She has some internal sensation in her lower abdomen. She feels bladder fullness, but needs to use a catheter. She has problems with edema. Sometimes she walks with the help of braces and crutches.

Stephanie's comment about her pregnancy was that it "didn't seem that different from other people's. My cousin has a heart-shaped uterus, too, and she had the same problems as I did."

STEPHANIE'S PREGNANCY HISTORY

Pregnancy: Age Unknown; miscarriage (12th week)

Pregnancy: Age 31

Trimester	Cause	Physical Change
1st	P	Fatigue
	P	Faintness
2nd	P	Hemorrhoids
	P	Vaginal swelling
	P	Continued faintness
	PD	Mobility so reduced that she began using wheelchair all the time)
	PD	Difficulty transferring in and out of car
	PD	Lower back pain
3rd	P	Chest ached from upward pressure of uterus
	D	Urinary bleeding[a]
	P	Urinating more frequently
	P	Increased edema
	PD	Continued lower back pain
	PD	Aching in lower pelvis

Comments
[a]Her doctor suggested that the bleeding was caused by her catheter irritating the urinary tract more than usual.

Sylvia

Sylvia is a high quadriplegic. Her injury is at C-3, C-4, and C-5. Her whole body is affected from the neck and shoulders down. Her bowels often retain feces, and she has no bladder control. She sometimes has muscle spasms so strong that her body thrashes about. She has occasional episodes of dysreflexia, and often has fainting spells just before menstruating.

SYLVIA'S PREGNANCY HISTORY

Pregnancy: Age 23

Trimester	Cause	Physical Change
1st	P	Morning sickness
	P	Mood swings
	P	Anemia
2nd	P	Light-headedness
	PD	Bowels relaxed (unpredictable bowel movements to end of term)
	P	Anemia
3rd	PD	Problems with breathing
	P	Anemia worsened
	PD	Episode of premature labor (6½ months) [a]
All	D	Episodes of dysreflexia, which were often worse when bowel or bladder was full
	PD	Muscle spasms more intense
	PD	Increased mobility difficulties [b]

Comments

[a]Premature labor was precipitated by dysreflexia and bowel problems. Also, the baby was low in the pelvis and the doctor manually changed its position.

[b]Balancing became more difficult as pregnancy progressed, especially since the baby was carried low. Maintaining balance while transferring and sitting became increasingly difficult.

After-Effects

After the baby was born Sylvia needed a blood transfusion.

SARA

. . . .

Spinal Tumor

Sara had a spinal tumor removed when she was a child, and is now paraplegic. She has some sensation and movement in her left leg, but none in her right. She uses crutches. She has never had pressure sores, but does have problems with muscle spasms. She has a scoliosis and frequent back-aches. Her other problems are frequent constipation, susceptibility to bladder infections, and frequent urination.

SARA'S PREGNANCY HISTORY

Pregnancy: Age 22

Trimester	Cause	Physical Change
1st	P	Morning sickness
	P	Frequent urination
2nd	PD	Muscle spasms increased
	PD	Some days urinated frequently, retained urine on others (stayed close to home)
	P	Numbness in hands[a]
	P	Shooting pains in hands and feet[a]
3rd	PD	Began falling (started using wheelchair in 7th month)
	PD	Retained urine

Pregnancy: Age 26

Trimester	Cause	Physical Change
1st	P	Morning sickness
	PD	Frequent urination
	P	Threatened miscarriage
2nd	PD	Muscle spasms less severe than previous pregnancy
	PD	Some days urinated frequently, retained urine on others (stayed close to home)
	P	Numbness in hands[a]
	P	Shooting pains in hands and feet[a]
	PD	Began falling (started using wheelchair in 7th month)

(continued)

SARA'S PREGNANCY HISTORY *(continued)*

Pregnancy: Age 26 *(continued)*

Trimester	Cause	Physical Change
3rd	PD	Bowels became impacted several times
	PD	Retained urine
	PD	Back pain
	PD?	Edema

Comments

[a]Although Sara did not identify them as such, the numbness and/or pain in her extremities are common symptoms of edema. They were probably caused by edema in Sara's case, since she remembers being told late in her second pregancy that she had this problem.

[b]Sara was hospitalized in the 8th month because her doctor did not know what to expect. She saw her doctor every other day.

SASHA AND SYBIL
. . . .

Spina Bifida

These women have *spina bifida,* a deformity of the spine which occurs early in embryonic development. There is definitely a genetic component to spina bifida, and the disorder may result from an interaction of genetic and environmental factors.

As was explained above, the spinal cord contains a bundle of nerves.The bundle is surrounded by a protective covering called the *meningeal membrane.* The spinal cord passes through a column of ring-shaped bones, the vertebrae, which are separated and cushioned by discs of cartilage. The cord occupies the space inside the spinal column, the spinal or vertebral canal. Spina bifida results from a failure of the canal to close properly. Other deformities, such as club feet, may be associated with this defect.

There are three types of spina bifida, differentiated by the severity of the defect. In *spina bifida occulta,* the opening does not extend to the surface of the body (*occulta* means "hidden"). The defect is in the vertebrae. Sometimes there are visible changes in the tissues overlying the defect; sometimes it is found by palpation or by X-ray examination. Spina bifida occulta usually occurs in the lower spine. It is occasionally accompanied by scoliosis or by deformities of the feet. Symptoms will depend on the extent of the lesions. It can be very mild and in some individuals, the only symptoms may be backaches. Others may have more severe symptoms, such as atrophied leg muscles, bowel and bladder disorders, or sensory loss.

More severe types of spina bifida are *meningocele* and *meningomyocele*. In meningocele, some of the meningeal membrane protrudes through the hole in the vertebra to the surface of the body. In meningomyocele, nerve roots and spinal cord are attached to the wall of the meningeal sac. In these forms of spina bifida, symptoms are more severe. As with spinal cord injury, symptoms depend on the location and extent of the lesion.

Sasha

Sasha had a meningocele, and she had the club feet which are sometimes associated with spina bifida. She was able to walk with the aid of Canadian crutches, but used a manual wheelchair more as she grew older. Her bladder control was poor and she had frequent infections of the bladder and kidneys. Her other problems included muscle spasms in her legs, edema of the legs, and frequent pressure sores on her feet.

SASHA'S PREGNANCY HISTORY

Pregnancy: Age 24

Trimester	Cause	Physical Change
1st	P	Fatigue
2nd	P	Heartburn (developed hiatus hernia)
	PD	Difficulty walking (began using crutches)[a]
	PD	Difficulty getting in and out of car
	PD	Problems with pressure sores disappeared for remainder of term[b]
3rd	P	Continued heartburn
	PD	Continued difficulty walking
	P	Edema
	PD	Back pain
All	PD	Bladder problems worse than usual—constant dripping

Comments

[a]When interviewed, Sasha said she wished that during the second trimester she had started using a wheelchair all the time. She thinks she would have been much more comfortable. Sasha had cancer at the time she was interviewed, and died shortly afterward.

[b]This was the first time that Sasha was not troubled by pressure sores.

Sybil

Sybil has meningocele and arthritis of the spine. The arthritis causes backaches in cold weather. Sybil can walk with crutches, but she has no sensation in her legs. She often gets pressure sores on her legs, and muscle spasms are also a problem. She has had a urotomy, which is an operation in which the ureters, the tubes leading from the kidney to the bladder, are detached from the bladder and brought to the surface of the skin. The urine then drains into a collecting bag. Her bowel control is poor.

SYBIL'S PREGNANCY HISTORY

Pregnancy: Age 22

Trimester	Cause	Physical Change
1st	P	Morning sickness
2nd	PD	Back pain
	PD	Kidney infection
3rd	PD	Continued back pain
	P	Edema
	PD	Difficulty transferring from bed to chair and from chair to tub
	PD	Difficulty bending, particularly when putting on shoes
	PD	Difficulty using crutches (began using wheelchair)
All	PD	Muscle spasms in legs worsened
Unknown	P	Sleeplessness

LEARNING FROM THE PREGNANCY EXPERIENCE

· ·

These pregnancy histories summarize the experiences of thirty-six women during sixty-two pregnancies (including a few pregnancies before onset of the disability). When analyzing the charts, we kept two considerations in mind: First, since the charts are based on the women's *memories* of their pregnancies, the information is not as accurate as it would have been if they had been keeping notes on symptoms as they occurred. The reported incidence of some ordinary pregnancy changes, such as stuffy nose or breast soreness, is lower than average, and we suspect that, in many instances, the memory of some symptoms was eclipsed by the memory of other, more noticeable symptoms. Secondly, our sample size is not large enough to answer several questions about specific disabilities. In particular, we cannot say whether women whose symptoms were worse after pregnancy would have experienced the same degree of exacerbation if they had not been pregnant. (More information about the interaction between pregnancy and specific types of disability is included in Chapters 2 and 6.) Still, the conclusions that can be drawn from these histories are confirmed by other studies, and they allow us to make some basic recommendations to disabled women and to the professionals working with them.

Take a Positive Approach

Our first recommendation concerns the importance of taking a positive approach to the pregnancy of a disabled woman.

All the women we interviewed would encourage other disabled women to have children. They did not deny the potential for problems—Sharon spoke for the whole group when she said, "It may take a toll on your body. You will have to decide if you want to make the sacrifice." Yet no one saw the physical problems of pregnancy as an insurmountable obstacle. As Portia commented, "Pregnancy, labor, and delivery are just steps you go through to reach the goal of being a parent." Several women felt they had been too fearful, and stressed the importance of enjoying pregnancy. Others commented that, after they had learned what to expect during a first pregnancy, they worried less during later pregnancies.

It is very clear that when a physically disabled woman says, "I'm pregnant—what happens now?" the likeliest answer will be, "You're going to have a baby!" While there may be problems and discomforts, disability does not necessarily make pregnancy hazardous for the mother or fetus, because treatment is available for many of the problems that do occur. Of course, appropriate treatment depends on the type and severity of the disability; for example, the level of a spinal cord injury.

In general, the women we interviewed said they had expected more problems and discomforts than they actually experienced—some even felt better than usual while they were pregnant. The problems that many of these women experienced were not substantially different from those that able-bodied women experience, although mobility impairment, of course, was worse for disabled women. In Chapter 6 we discuss the normal physical changes that occur during pregnancy, common complications, and the ways that pregnancy affects disabled women in particular.

Make Pregnancy the Primary Concern

Our second recommendation is that the mother with disabilities be seen primarily as a *pregnant* woman—both in her own mind and in the mind of her physician.

In their advice to obstetricians, many of the women we interviewed emphasized their desire to be treated "just like everyone else." For example, Arlene said, "...be open-minded. We are just like everyone else—a woman is having a baby," and Cheryl said, "Treat me like a woman first, and then secondly as a woman with a disability." These statements were not simply expressions of an ideal. Much of the advice our interviewees offered to other disabled women centered on ordinary pregnancy concerns: "Try to have your baby vaginally" (Celeste). "Get two people to go in as labor coaches. That way, one person can be a back-up" (Marsha). "I found the holistic approach helpful" (Samantha). "Find one nurse who will stay with you. I had my baby that way and I loved it" (Heather).

Yet women also expressed the feeling that their pregnancies were different. In Chapter 2 we report some women's feeling of surprise that they had been able to get pregnant, and other women's fears that they could not have a healthy pregnancy or childbirth. Also, some of the advice women offered stressed disability-related concerns: "Consult with other specialists about the woman's disabilities" (Sylvia). "Hold an in-service training for the obstetrics department ... invite some disabled women to come in" (Stacy). "Even if you are only slightly disabled, make sure all the doctors involved know you are disabled" (Priscilla). "Be aware of your limitations and learn about adaptations" (Pam).

The fact is, a woman may need her doctor or hospital to bend the rules in consideration of her disability on one occasion, and "treat her like everyone else" on another occasion. There is no contradiction involved, but a need to maintain a delicate balance. Corinne described the balance well in her advice to health professionals: "Be sensitive to the needs and concerns of the prospective mother." An able-bodied woman may have special needs and concerns, too—perhaps a concern that an older sibling will not welcome a new arrival, or the hope that it will be possible to give birth vaginally after a prior Cesarean surgery. Most disabled women would like their disability concerns to be seen in the same light, as the special concerns of women who are, first and foremost, expectant mothers.

Use a Team Approach

Our third recommendation is that physicians follow the advice of disabled women and concerned professionals by using a team approach to pregnancy and birth.

The pregnant woman, her obstetrician, and the disability specialists must all contribute to planning her care. While disability will not always directly affect pregnancy outcome, indirect effects must always be kept in mind. For example, pregnant women generally avoid using medications; but if a woman's disability makes her vulnerable to urinary infections, she and her doctor will need to weigh the risks of using medication against the risk that a very severe infection could precipitate premature labor. Treatment for pregnancy may affect a woman's disability: for example, when Christina used bed rest to prevent a miscarriage, her muscles atrophied and stiffened. She would have retained better muscle mass and flexibility if physical therapy had been prescribed to alleviate these effects of bed rest.

Cooperation among the obstetrician, disability specialists, and the mother-to-be—who is the most expert on many aspects of her disability—can assure that important decisions take account of both pregnancy and disability concerns. Some women even suggested additional training for hospital personnel. Stacy elaborated, "In the recovery room, they checked my blood pressure just before I had to urinate. The nurse didn't know about dysreflexia and she got really worried when she saw my blood pressure. If she had been given the information beforehand, she would have known what to do."

Cooperation requires flexibility and openness on the part of all concerned. Just as our interviewees emphasized the importance of doctors' listening sensitively to disabled women, they emphasized that women should be patient with questions and be ready to teach others about disability. Chapter 3 contains many of their suggestions for building good working relationships between pregnant women and medical professionals.

Approaches to the Best Possible Outcome

Our last recommendation to the pregnant woman and her health specialists is to use sensitivity, education, and careful planning as the means to achieve the best possible outcome.

Everything we have said above implies the need for great sensitivity. Depending on their experiences, different women emphasized different dimensions of this need. Some addressed their concern to disabled women, as Heather did when she said, "Know what is normal for your body so you can decipher what is a pregnancy symptom and what is a disability symptom." Others addressed their concern to medical professionals, often with very specific, practical comments: "Be aware that a disabled woman may need more time.... I had trouble with nursing, because I was left alone with my baby. Stay around and see if the woman needs extra help...." (Celeste). "*Ask* the woman if she needs help before you give it...." (Clara). "Don't leave a woman alone on the examining table!" (Sharon).

The pregnancy of a woman with disabilities is often a new experience for everyone involved, and no one can anticipate every possibility. Sensitivity must be supplemented by education. Most often patients expect medical personnel to be knowledgeable; expertise is a basis for trust, and an admission of ignorance can be unsettling, to say the least. But women with disabilities are well aware that their problems are the subject of specialized training, and they are most likely to be reassured by a willingness to listen and learn. Paula's straightforward advice to health professionals was, "Ask questions about the disability—don't think you have to seem to know everything. Your patient knows you have something special to offer, and she won't mind if you want to learn more about her." Not only did women advise doctors and nurses to show a willingness to learn about disability, they advised other disabled women to be willing to teach.

However, women who felt that they were "the experts" about their disabilities also wished they had been given more information about pregnancy. Portia, who advised doctors to "Listen to women—they know their own bodies," went on to urge them to "Explain to women what will happen at various stages and prepare them for situations they might not expect." Not only did women conclude that advice and education are an important part of the physician's role, they also felt the mother-to-be should make it her responsibility to learn as much as she can. Julie summed up what many women had expressed in various ways when she said, "Know your body as much as you can. Get information on exercise, rest, diet, and the methods of delivery available for you. Be educated about the birthing process...."

Sensitivity and education, valuable in themselves, are integral to the planning and preparation which are needed to make pregnancy and the first months after birth an enjoyable experience. Whatever practical details they gave as examples, women agreed on the importance of preparing in advance: "Set up a support system *before* your baby is born" (Clara). "Get a physical exam *before* you get pregnant" (Hilary). "Have arrangements made *before* delivery for things like diapers, baby clothes, and furniture. Fill your freezer with enough dinners to last three months" (Stephanie). "Don't wait until you're in labor to find out how a medication could affect you" (Priscilla).

CLOSING COMMENTS

These four recommendations comprise the underlying themes of this book, and are reiterated throughout in the comments of the women whose experiences are recorded here:

- Take a positive approach to pregnancy and disability.
- The disabled mother-to-be should be seen primarily as a pregnant woman, both in her own mind and in the mind of her physician.
- Use a team approach to pregnancy and birth.
- Use sensitivity, education, and careful planning as the means to achieve the best possible outcome.

Pregnancy is an enterprise of uncertainty and hope. While nobody can guarantee an ideal experience, following these recommendations, drawn from the experience and heart-felt advice of thirty-six women, can help assure the best possible pregnancy experience. They can also make it possible to take the advice all the women gave most emphatically—"Enjoy yourself!"

2

THE FIRST STEP—
DECIDING WHETHER
TO HAVE A CHILD

Unlike most women, who experience social and emotional pressures *to have* children, disabled women are under pressure *not to have* children. Yet disabled women feel the same needs for emotionally satisfying relationships as other women. We support their right to choose motherhood. The purpose of this chapter is to provide women with decision-making tools: to provide some basic information, suggest questions women can ask to get information relevant to their individual situations, and help them explore their own feelings.

A great number of books that have been written to help people decide whether to become parents fail to address an important concern of women with disabilities. Because these books are written with the assumption that most women are under considerable pressure to become mothers, their authors make a point of reassuring women that the decision not to have children can be reasonable and acceptable.

Yet women with disabilities are in an unusual situation. The forces of social disapproval and, often, their own fears, work against their having children. Even when they were illegal, abortions were relatively easily obtained by women with physical disabilities. When Sasha, a woman with spina bifida, told of her pregnancy some twenty years ago, she said that she did not seek medical care until her fifth month because she "didn't want a big hassle." Even then, five months pregnant, Sasha had to visit four doctors before she found one who would help her, while "The others all pressured me to have an abortion." Sasha finished her story by commenting, "I hope some changes have come about, that it is not [considered] a cardinal sin for women with

disabilities to have babies." But many disabled women still encounter negative attitudes toward their pregnancies. Sharon, who is paraplegic, says that
when she became pregnant in 1979, her gynecologist's first reaction was "[to
ask whether] I was going to keep it"; such responses are common.

Friends, family, and strangers react to a disabled woman's pregnancy in a
number of ways. In Chapter 6, we describe some reactions women encountered, ranging from approval and support to open surprise and even hostility.

Whatever the external pressures, women with disabilities often have the
same feelings about parenthood as do able-bodied women. They describe the
same hopes for building loving families, and expressing their creativity by
doing a good job of child-rearing. Michelle captured that feeling beautifully
when she said, "I wanted to have a child so I could be part of the flow of history." When a woman's disabilities create obstacles to her contributing to the
world around her in other ways (as when she encounters negative reactions to
her disability), she may attach even more significance to child-bearing.

Disabled women's lives are changing. More and more, they are taking
part in the efforts of all women to increase their freedoms and their responsibilities. They are claiming a right every woman should have—the right to
decide whether and when she will become a mother.

For a woman with disabilities, making this decision involves answering
three questions: How will pregnancy affect her disability? How will her disability affect the course of pregnancy, and the health and development of
the baby? How might her disability influence the way she fulfills the emotional and physical tasks of child-rearing?

As you think about the many issues affecting your decision, it is important to differentiate emotional from realistic and practical aspects of these
questions. Sometimes women's feelings, or even a lack of information, lead
them to make unrealistic assumptions about what will happen during pregnancy. One such assumption is, "My pregnancy will be just like my
mother's." This was so for Celeste, who was afraid she would have a stillborn child. After giving birth to a healthy baby, she discussed why she had
assumed that she would have stillborn children, as her mother had. (Celeste
had been born prematurely.) For example, she should not have assumed
that her vomiting in late pregnancy, like her mother, meant that she would
have a stillborn child, as her mother had (and unlike the vast majority of
people who experience vomiting late in pregnancy). Celeste said, "There
isn't any excuse. It was a neurotic fear. My mother was such a dynamic
woman, and I felt I couldn't do better [than she had]."

Many interviewees mentioned their fears about falling during pregnancy.
Ordinarily they might worry because their disabilities made falling likely, or
because falls could lessen their mobility. Now they worried that falling might
injure the fetus. Ever since Scarlett O'Hara's tumble down the stairs in *Gone
with the Wind*, the idea that falls inevitably cause miscarriages has probably

been the most common misconception about pregnancy in twentieth century America. It is not true, as Celeste discovered when she fell—she said, "It's like landing on a balloon." A variation on the theme was one woman's fear that pressing on her bladder to eliminate urine would cause mental retardation in her child. In fact, the fetus is so well protected by the amnionic sac and amniotic fluid, the uterine wall, and other structures, that falling, or pressing the bladder, present no danger at all. Some women did have mobility problems in late pregnancy, and a concern about being injured by falling can be realistic. But the idea that a fetus will be injured by the mother's falling is an example of the kind of misinformation that can interfere with good decision-making.

As you sort out practical, factual, and emotional concerns, you may also discover feelings you were unaware of. Heather's answers to her questionnaire exemplify the complex emotions we all experience: In explaining why she decided to have children, Heather said, "I always wanted babies. It never occurred to me I couldn't." Yet, when asked, "What was your reaction to learning you were pregnant?" she replied, "Sheer excitement that I could do it." Clearly, it had been difficult for her to recognize her self-doubt. We hope that as you read what other women have to say, you will discover that you are not alone in anything you feel and, perhaps, you will make new discoveries about yourself.

One surprising discovery may be that your desire to have a child is more intense than you realized. Some women, not realizing how much they wanted children, had unplanned pregnancies partly because they were unaware of their own feelings. Not only was Julie's pregnancy unplanned, but the timing was unfortunate, and she became a single parent in a community that frowned on single motherhood. Later, she commented, "It just happened. Probably subconsciously I was ready for it." Stacy's unplanned pregnancy occurred when she discontinued birth control pills because she thought that "having a lot of X-rays for many years" had made her infertile. One wonders why she took birth control pills for several years, then changed her mind. Had she not thought about the X-rays before, or did she, like Julie, unconsciously hope to become pregnant? In either case, the experience shows the importance of carefully exploring your feelings, and learning all the facts—if necessary, by getting medical advice—before making decisions about pregnancy and birth control.

We cannot over-emphasize the importance of examining your own feelings. To aid you in this process of self-examination, this chapter explores the questions and issues involved in the following seven areas:

1. **Self-image:** *How does the effect of disability on a woman's self-image influence the decision-making process?*
2. **Interaction Between Pregnancy and Disability:** *What are the physical*

consequences of pregnancy? How will pregnancy affect you? Will your disability affect your ability to give birth to a healthy, full-term baby?

3. **The Possibility of Having Disabled Children:** *What is the possibility that you will have a disabled child? How likely are you to have a disabled child? How can genetic counseling help answer this question? What are your feelings about having a disabled child?*

4. **Parenting:** *Do people with disabilities have unique experiences in their role as parents? What skills does a good parent need? Are these skills really affected by disability? How do children feel about disabled parents?*

5. **The Cost of Having a Child:** *How can you plan for the expenses of pregnancy, childbirth, and child-rearing?*

6. **Motherhood and Marriage:** *How will having a child affect your other relationships, particularly your relationship with your husband/partner?*

7. **Combining Career and Family:** *What are some of the advantages and disadvantages of combining a career and family? Choosing to be a full-time parent?*

In discussing these questions, we will present general information as well as examples from women's experiences, and suggestions made by women with disabilities.

SELF-IMAGE

Certainly, there is a sense in which any woman considering motherhood feels that her selfhood would be enhanced by having children. She may be seeking self-validation in a broad sense, hoping to join "the flow of history" or to prove her femininity. There may be a more specific motivation, like a desire to "do better a job than my parents did," or to disprove stereotypes about disability.

The unique experiences of women with disabilities lend a special flavor to these concerns. For example, a disabled woman, as she ages, is concerned not only about declining fertility but also about declining physical powers. She may believe (often correctly) that if she is going to have children, she had better hurry. As Julie examined the unconscious reasons for her unplanned pregnancy, she commented, "The older I get, the more limitation I have to deal with, so having children became more important." Even for women whose disability is not progressive, concerns about aging are strengthened by the knowledge that disability adds to the usual stresses of aging. Whether a woman is eager to have children or nervous about the idea, her feelings may be strengthened by fears about aging.

A disabled woman's self-image may have been damaged by negative social attitudes, or by the frustrations of physical limitation. Judi recalls a painful childhood experience: whenever her elementary school had air-raid or fire drills, she was left behind. The principal proudly informed Judi's father that Judi was being "protected"—by excluding Judi from the drills, the principal hoped to prevent her being jostled and knocked down by other children. Her father insisted that she be included in future drills, because she would need to know what to do in a real emergency. But, in the child's mind, the damage had already been done; she felt she was being left behind because children like her were less valuable than others.

Since they know that many people see them as asexual, it is not surprising that some women with disabilities, like many able-bodied women, feel a need to prove their femininity, maturity, or worthiness by having children. The wish to prove oneself may have to do with the physical self-image, or the social self-image. For example, Julie "loved being pregnant because for once my body worked right." Arlene said, "Having a baby made me less handicapped because I was able to fulfill one of the female roles in society and I was really rewarded for it." Heather felt that she was "proving [that she] was as independent and self-reliant as anyone." Faith "loved being associated with the nondisabled population.... It was my only chance," adding that the shared interests and concerns of parenthood offered a basis for friendships with nondisabled people.

If you share the kind of feelings we describe, you have good company, and lots of it. Attaching such hopes and fears to the idea of parenthood is not a problem in itself. But pregnancy and parenthood are full of surprises; the unpleasant surprises will be more unpleasant for people who are unprepared for them, and needless fears can dampen enjoyment of the happy ones. Sasha remembered, "I was afraid.... I wish I'd let myself enjoy it more." The best way to prepare for the surprises is to know the possibilities—and know yourself.

INTERACTION BETWEEN PREGNANCY AND DISABILITY

Several of the women interviewed had feared that their disabilities would cause problems in pregnancy, or that pregnancy would affect their disabilities. Celeste, who was "ecstatic" when she found out she was pregnant, was also "scared.... I knew it was going to be difficult. My first reaction was, 'You'll need a C-section.' I was welcoming that." Sasha had thought she could not get pregnant, then, "I was afraid I would die in pregnancy, because of my disability (spina bifida), or die in childbirth." Sharon was "shocked, not really excited, because of my age, and being paraplegic. I didn't know what to expect."

Celeste and Sasha later felt that they had worried more than necessary. Celeste gave birth vaginally, and had such ordinary pregnancy symptoms as morning sickness. Sasha, looking back at her pregnancy, said, "I'm sorry I didn't enjoy it more."

Most interviewees either experienced remission of symptoms during pregnancy or felt better than usual. Some experienced no change, and a very few experienced temporary exacerbations of their disabilities. But, in interviews given between four weeks and twenty years after giving birth, all the women said they had returned to much the same level of disability as had existed before pregnancy. No one felt that her disability had been permanently worsened or improved. (A few women, in informal conversations a few years after their interviews, wondered aloud whether there had, in fact, been lasting effects. However, it was also possible that aging, or continuing disease processes, were responsible for the new problems these women were experiencing.)

Most often, the problems and discomforts that women described were the same ones able-bodied women experience, such as fatigue or back pain. While existing disability symptoms were sometimes exacerbated, few women developed new symptoms. The symptoms most likely to intensify seem to be those that can also be caused by pregnancy. For example, pregnant women experience an increased frequency of urination and an increased risk of bladder infection, and women who are prone to bladder infections may find that they worsen. Back problems and respiratory difficulties may also worsen during late pregnancy.

The interviews also suggested that often it is the severity of disability, rather than the type, that helps predict how difficult a pregnancy may be. For example, a woman who is quadriplegic because of cerebral palsy may have more in common with a woman who is quadriplegic due to spinal cord injury than with a woman with milder cerebral palsy.

In the following section we describe some pregnancy complications known to occur in connection with specific disabilities. This can be your starting point in learning what the consequences of pregnancy might be for you. The complications described are not always the same as those commonly associated with pregnancy, which are described in Chapter 6. It can be very difficult for a pregnant woman to know whether she is experiencing a *pregnancy*-related problem, or a *disability*-related problem. So, if you are considering pregnancy, it is important to follow Heather's advice: "Try to know your body. Get to be aware of what is normal for *your* body, so that you can decipher what is a pregnancy symptom and what is a disability symptom."

The list describes problems that may occur: for you, the problem described may be severe, it may be mild, or it may not occur at all. For example, pregnant women with spinal cord injuries have an increased risk of developing *decubitus ulcers* (pressure sores) during pregnancy, yet our interviewees found that their skin condition was much better than usual.

Complications Associated with Disabilities

All Disabilities

All women with physical disabilities are likely to have increased mobility problems and associated fatigue in late pregnancy. Any woman may experience ordinary pregnancy discomforts, such as morning sickness, and typical pregnancy complications.

Specific problems sometimes associated with disability, such as kidney dysfunction, can affect pregnancy, and should be evaluated before conception (several examples will be given below). Also, some disability symptoms may be worsened by pregnancy symptoms. For example, a woman with respiratory problems may have more difficulty breathing during late pregnancy, when pressure from the uterus causes many women to become short of breath.

Arthrogryposis

Women who are severely affected may have such poor circulation that there is an increased risk of miscarriage.

Cerebral Palsy

Many women experience increased muscle spasms during pregnancy. Delivery may be complicated by spasms, and the mother may be unable to bear down. Women who are unaware that their chest muscles are mildly affected may be surprised to notice breathing difficulties for the first time with the added stress of pregnancy.

Friedreich's Ataxia

Back problems are likely to worsen, and there is an increased likelihood of incontinence. Respiratory difficulties increase as well.

Multiple Sclerosis

The most important consideration is your current level of disability. Pregnancy does not affect the long-term course of MS, and MS in itself does not affect the course of pregnancy or the health of the fetus. Onset or exacerbation of MS is more likely to occur in the six months after childbirth than during pregnancy; but fewer than half of the women who have MS before becoming pregnant, experience deterioration during or after pregnancy.

Most new mothers are fatigued during the first few months after childbirth, when they must care for a young infant while recovering physically. This fatigue undoubtedly contributes to temporary exacerbations. Our interviewees found that breastfeeding worsened fatigue. For some women, delivery has been complicated by spasms of the hip adductor muscles.

Muscular Dysfunctions

Delivery could be complicated by back and hip deformities, or by an inability to bear down with atrophied muscles. Some women may need surgical delivery.

Myasthenia Gravis

The combination of myasthenia gravis and pregnancy involves serious risks, and decisions should be carefully made. If you want to have a child, it is important to control the disease as much as possible before conception; thymectomy may be necessary. You may have to change medications, since some drugs used to treat myasthenia must be avoided during pregnancy.

Various studies have found that 30%–40% of women experience exacerbations during pregnancy (especially late pregnancy), about 33% experience some improvement, and about 33% experience no change. Symptoms may become life-threatening, and in one study, the maternal mortality rate was 3.4% of live births. New therapies may improve these statistics, and it is important to ask a doctor about the latest research.

Vaginal delivery is usual, but sometimes when the mother lacks strength to push, forceps are necessary.

Myasthenia gravis is associated with increased rates of stillbirth (3%), neonatal death (5%), pre-term birth and intrauterine growth retardation. Between 10% and 20% of newborn infants experience temporary myasthenia symptoms. They must be watched carefully for the development of symptoms, which appear 12–48 hours after birth; they will be treated with medication and, in extreme cases, plasmapheresis.

Postpolio Syndrome

The effects on pregnancy depend on your particular symptoms. Women whose mobility is very limited may be at risk for developing deep vein *thrombosis* (clots) during pregnancy. If back deformities have developed, they might make pregnancy and/or delivery more difficult. Women whose breathing is affected may also experience difficulties during pregnancy and delivery, because they tire more easily, and because pressure from the enlarged uterus in late pregnancy makes breathing even more difficult. If severe chronic respiratory insufficiency occurs, it could affect fetal growth.

Rheumatoid Arthritis and Juvenile Rheumatoid Arthritis

About 70% of women experience some remission of symptoms during pregnancy, while a few suffer exacerbations. While it cannot be predicted which women will experience such changes, it does seem that a woman can expect each of her pregnancies to follow the same pattern. Almost always, women who have remissions have relapses after giving birth. Usually by the end of the first postpartum month, and certainly by the eighth month, symptoms will return to what they were before pregnancy. Otherwise, pregnancy does not seem to affect the long-term course of the arthritis, and arthritis is not known to affect pregnancy symptoms or fetal health.

If arthritis has caused hip or spine deformities, delivery may be complicated and cesarean delivery may be necessary (for example, one of our interviewees needed surgical delivery because she could not spread her legs widely enough.)

Scoliosis

Individual experiences will differ depending on the level and severity of the curvature. Some women under twenty-five may be advised to delay pregnancy so that there is less chance that it will worsen the curvature. There is also some evidence that the more severe the curve, the more likely it is to be exacerbated by pregnancy, especially multiple pregnancies.

For women with severe *kyphoscoliosis* (upper back curvature), respiratory compromise is a concern. Some women have had to be hospitalized in late pregnancy for negative pressure ventilation. Women with such curvatures need to have a pulmonary evaluation.

On the whole, scoliosis does not seem to increase risks of miscarriage, stillbirth, low birth weight, or birth defects. Still, in some individuals, displacement of internal organs may affect fetal growth. In women who experience respiratory problems, the fetus could be affected by lack of oxygen, and preventive care is important.

In some women with hip dysplasia, bladder difficulties may increase.

Short Stature

As uterine growth displaces other organs, respiratory insufficiency and/or back strain may develop. Many women experience pre-term labor. Cesarean delivery is often necessary. Women who have arthritic symptoms may find that they worsen during pregnancy.

Spina Bifida

Back problems, urinary infections, pressure sores, and incontinence may increase during pregnancy. Intestinal obstruction is also common (about 10%). If urinary infection is severe, it may cause premature labor.

Vaginal delivery is common, though some women may need assistance with vacuum extraction or forceps if reduced sensation makes bearing down difficult. Cesarean delivery would be needed only for obstetric reasons such as malpresentation.

Spinal Cord Injuries

Bladder infections are likely to become more frequent, and care must be taken to prevent severe infections which could cause premature labor.

Constipation may also worsen. If the diaphragm is paralyzed, pressure from the uterus or impacted fecal matter could worsen breathing difficulties. Pressure sores may develop more easily because of increased weight, and preventive care is important.

Some surveys suggest that injury during pregnancy increases the risk that infants will be born with deformities or disabilities, while in pregnancies occurring after injury, the risk is greater that the baby will be growth retarded or premature (possibly because of urinary infection).

Women with injuries at or above the T-6 level have an increased risk of experiencing autonomic dysreflexia during labor, and sometimes, during pregnancy. Dysreflexia during pregnancy increases the risk of miscarriage or premature labor.

Systemic Lupus Erythematosus

The most important concern is your state of health at the time you are considering pregnancy. All recent studies indicate that pregnancy does not affect the long-term course of SLE. Also, pregnancy termination does not appear to improve the course of SLE, and is not therapeutic for disease flares. Pregnant women do not seem to experience flares of symptoms any more frequently than nonpregnant women, but about 60% will have some worsening of symptoms; possibly some exacerbations are related to emotional stresses of pregnancy. Disease flares usually, but not always, improve after pregnancy. If conception occurs during a remission, exacerbations are less likely to occur, and those that do occur are less likely to be severe (chances of a flare are as low as 10%–30% during remission, but two or three times greater when disease is active.) There are various recommendations as to how long the remission should have lasted before conception— six months is common.

An important part of the decision-making process is an evaluation of kidney function. If function is very poor, pregnancy is dangerous for both mother and fetus. It is not clear whether pregnancy has a long-term effect on kidney function (studies differ), but it is clear that severely damaged kidneys may fail under the additional stress of pregnancy. A woman with reasonably good kidney function, whose disease is in remission, may be advised to conceive as soon as possible, before ongoing disease causes further damage.

While improved treatments seem to have reduced the incidence of disease flares and fetal death, the risks of pre-term birth, growth retardation, or fetal death remain greater than average. Again, disease status is crucial: the fetal survival rate is as low as 50%–75% when disease is active, as high as 88%–100% during remission. While most miscarriages occur no later than the fourteenth week, they can occur as late as the twenty-eighth week when the mother has SLE. Fetal death in early pregnancy often relates to placental damage; in late pregnancy it is related to high blood pressure and kidney failure. Antibody testing and appropriate treatment may improve pregnancy outcomes.

Systemic lupus erythematosus, and the medications used to treat it, do not increase congenital birth defects. However, there is an association between SLE and a heart problem known as *complete cardiac heart block.* While most women who have SLE have normal babies, studies of infants with heart block found that these babies are more likely to have mothers with connective tissue disease. Antibody testing and prenatal monitoring can help identify a fetus at risk for heart block, and surgery may improve survival rates.

Some newborn babies have temporary SLE symptoms such as skin lesions or blood abnormalities. It is not yet known whether these symptoms predict the risk of developing the disease during adulthood.

Getting Personalized Information About Pregnancy and Disability

The list above is very general. To make your own decision, you will want to gather additional current, specific information. Perhaps in the past you have been advised to expect certain problems if you become pregnant, or advised to avoid pregnancy. The more time that has passed since you were given that information, the more important it is to find out whether recent research confirms or contradicts what you were told. For example, not very long ago women with MS were told that pregnancy might cause their symptoms to flare up, but more recent studies show that MS often stabilizes or improves during pregnancy, and worsens temporarily during the six months after birth, an exhausting time for even the healthiest women. New research might also revise the information given here. Especially if new information would change your decision, we urge you to contact the organization concerned with your disability.

Other chapters in this book provide more information about the kinds of problems women experience during pregnancy and childbirth, ways of adapting to them, and medical treatments. Your own doctor can also advise you in more detail about the interaction between pregnancy and your disability, taking into consideration particular facts such as the severity of scoliosis, the level of spinal cord injury, or the length of time you have had a particular disorder. Make it clear that you are asking for more than a general recommendation.

Your doctor may not offer specific advice on your first visit. He or she may want to review recent research or consult other specialists before making any suggestions. It is usually best to begin by seeing a disability specialist, but if you are seeing an obstetrician or family practitioner, you might like to share written information you have about disability, including the bibliography of this book, which refers to many studies of the interaction between pregnancy and disability. Your doctor may also need to order some diagnostic tests. Such tests might include blood tests to evaluate kidney function; pulmonary function tests to evaluate whether women with respiratory difficulties can withstand the additional stress of pregnancy; hip or spine X-rays to determine whether deformities will interfere with fetal growth, or complicate labor; cervical spine (neck) X-rays to determine whether intubation during anesthesia would injure an arthritic woman; or blood tests or muscle function tests to determine the effectiveness of medication

Below are several questions you may want to discuss with your doctor:

1. *Will my disability affect the health or development of my baby?* For example, "Is my scoliosis severe enough to cause premature labor or labor complications that would endanger the baby?"
2. *What problems or pregnancy complications is my disability likely to cause?*
3. *How severe would these complications (if any) be? Mildly painful, severely painful, life-threatening?.Would they be likely to temporarily or permanently worsen my disability?*
4. *Could complications be prevented?* For example, how much will physical therapy and exercise reduce the risk of clots?
5. *Could complications be treated?* The answer to this question may be crucial to your decision. For example, *autonomic dysreflexia,* an extreme fluctuation in blood pressure which often occurs in spinal-cord-injured people under certain conditions (including labor), can be life-threatening, but it can be watched for, it can be managed with medication, and women who experienced dysreflexia during labor have successfully given birth.
6. *Would treatments for complications have any risks or disadvantages?* For example, would the medicine that would be prescribed for a given problem have unpleasant side effects, or be dangerous for the fetus?
7. *What would be the long-term effects of treatment?*
8. *Is my disability likely to cause problems during labor or delivery?* For example, if you have hip dysplasia, you can discuss whether it is severe enough to necessitate cesarean surgery.
9. *Is there anything we can do before pregnancy to prevent or minimize problems that might occur during pregnancy?* For example, an exercise program to strengthen low back muscles before they are stressed by pregnancy, or a new medication regimen to stabilize symptoms of autoimmune disease.

Many women said that they had received different advice from different doctors. What then? In the next chapter, we examine this question from the viewpoint of women who are already pregnant, or those who are sure they want a child. For them, the question is, "How will I find the right person to help me carry out my decision?" Here, the question is, "Whose advice will help me make the right decision?"

It may be that doctors who disagree are both (or all) correct. Perhaps different research reports have suggested different conclusions, and each doctor is inclined to rely on the research that confirms his or her own experience. Or a doctor may justifiably believe that a research finding or a method of treatment is too new to be relied on until more research confirms its value. To understand these differences of opinion, simply tell your doctor or other adviser that you have heard different advice from different sources, and would like to hear more about his or her thinking. If some of your information is written, such as magazine articles or research reports, bring it to your doctor(s) and include it in the discussion.

If it seems to you that there really is room for legitimate differences of opinion, your options are to

- Rely on the advice that makes most sense to you, and/or the person you trust the most.
- Wait until further research provides more information about the effects of pregnancy on your disability (unless you feel that your age makes it inadvisable to delay a decision).
- Make your decision on another basis. For example, Michelle had no way of knowing whether pregnancy would end her remission of MS. She decided, "Even if I'd have to be permanently disabled, I'd rather take the consequences than not have the baby."

Additional Concerns About Pregnancy and Disability

In thinking about the interaction of pregnancy with your disability, the first questions that come to mind concern safety, but other questions also must be asked. Very possibly, any complications that occur will involve discomfort or inconvenience, rather than real danger. How would you feel about living with these discomforts? Answering this question is not easy—you are thinking about an unknown quantity, like every woman who considers having a child. No one can predict whether she will experience morning sickness, fatigue, or other problems that sometimes occur with pregnancy. Becoming acquainted with other women's experiences may put the possibilities in perspective. Some women compared their pregnancies with those of able-bodied women:

Claudia: "It felt good to be part of the sorority."
Sylvia: "I got jealous of [women who had] easier pregnancies."
Patricia: "It made me feel better because I had a better pregnancy than they did."

Other women compared the pregnancies they had before the onset of disability with those occurring after onset.

• Samantha had two children before her spinal cord injury and one afterward. She said: "I naturally compared. I had a friend who delivered three weeks before me, and we compared a lot. This pregnancy was so much like the other two. My second and third were almost the same...."

• Paula also compared pregnancies before and after polio: "Compared to the first it was different. Physically, I was in totally different shape—I wore two leg braces. But I thoroughly enjoyed being pregnant.... Not worrying about the baby—that part felt intact—felt so nice."

• Renee had experienced the first, painful onset of rheumatoid arthritis while she was pregnant with her first child. Later, she heard that women sometimes have a remission of symptoms during pregnancy. She was not sure at first that she wanted another pregnancy because she feared that, after she gave birth, the return of her arthritic pain would be unbearable. She eventually decided to have another child.

• Sylvia had the worst pregnancy, physically, of anyone interviewed. She experienced severe muscle spasms, bowel problems, and autonomic dysreflexia which caused episodes of premature labor, and several other problems that were milder, but still unpleasant. Not surprisingly, she sometimes wondered, "What the hell am I doing?" Later she said, "I came to the realization that nine months is a long time.... I kept wondering if it was ever going to end."

Even when pregnancy is comfortable and free of problems, it can seem as though it will never end. The mother-to-be grows tired of carrying the extra weight, waking up several times a night to urinate, and lying on her side to sleep. We doubt that there is anyone who does not fantasize that her baby will be born a week or two early.

But some of the other physical changes that take place may heighten your sense of anticipation. The sight of your growing abdomen is visible proof that something really is happening. If you are planning to breastfeed, the changes in your breasts can be very satisfying. Probably most exciting is the sensation of fetal movement. In spite of all her problems, Sylvia recalls the joy she felt when her baby moved, "It was great to notice the difference between her and bowels and gas."

Whatever problems or discomforts occur, your way of coping with them will affect how you feel about your pregnancy. Pam needed bedrest to relieve many discomforts, but it was very hard for her to slow down. As she resisted the need to rest, she wore herself out even more, adding to her stress by putting emotional strain on her marriage. Pam commented, "I had learned to manage by pushing myself and ignoring my limitations. It was hard to adjust to being pregnant. I didn't rest as much as I should have, because it felt like I was pampering myself."

Indeed, a woman with physical disabilities often has to meet life's obstacles with great stubbornness and a powerful refusal to be held back by her physical limitations. Her experience has taught her not to "pamper" herself.

It can be difficult to change deeply felt patterns and confront your problems by "pampering" yourself—resting, taking special care of diet, avoiding stress—as pregnancy often requires.

Making the change is not impossible, however. Arlene, who usually resented having to rest, thought "having a baby was a great reason.... I was able to say to myself, 'I have more time to read'." Some women tell themselves, "I'm not being lazy when I lie down. I'm working hard at growing a baby."

Physical Consequences of Childcare

Portia, who has five children, stressed that the problems of pregnancy are temporary. When asked what advice she would give to women considering pregnancy, she replied, in part, "Pregnancy, labor, and delivery are the first steps to go through to reach the goal of being a parent." It is true that, for the most part, *any physical consequences of having a child will be experienced during pregnancy and birth, or within the first six weeks after giving birth*. But afterward, as any mother will tell you, caring for children can be exhausting. Knowing this, Stephanie, was "pleased and excited to have children... [but] also reluctant, because of the physical care of the children." Marsha's doctor did not worry that pregnancy would worsen her MS, but worried that she would be overly fatigued by caring for a toddler. In fact, Marsha found that toddler care was not too hard for her, but that breastfeeding was exhausting.

Like the difficulties of pregnancy, the physical stresses of childcare are unpredictable. Some women, especially those whose disabilities are worsened by fatigue, may be worried by these possibilities:

- *Loss of sleep:* New-borns have irregular sleeping patterns, and awaken frequently needing food or comfort. Toddlers and small children wake up with wet diapers, wet beds, nightmares, illness. If you are the kind of person who never falls back to sleep after the telephone has rung at 2:00 a.m., you may expect to feel tired often during your child's first years.
- *Physical stress:* Being a playmate in your child's active games, or supervising an especially active and curious toddler, can be very tiring. Even if yours is a quiet, "easy" child, extra housekeeping chores—laundry, cooking, dishwashing—will create new physical demands.
- *Emotional stress:* Sometimes your child will be very difficult to live with. The "terrible twos" and the teenage years are the most notoriously difficult stages of development. Do you respond physically to emotional stress? If you get headaches when you are angry, or lose sleep when you are worried, be prepared for plenty of headaches or sleepless nights.

We are emphatically not saying that the physical demands of parenting are impossible to fulfill. They can be met, and most parents feel the effort is worthwhile. To many women interviewees, such problems were not an important consideration. Sara, who felt "overwhelmed" by both of her pregnancies, said, "I was more concerned about birth defects, not so concerned about the physical aspects of taking care of children." Still, we do wish to emphasize that the physical consequences of your decision extend beyond a possible pregnancy. You might like to consider babysitting for a friend's toddler and finding out just how tired you get. This is not a perfect experiment. If you were to have a child this age, you would have grown used to each other, so your own child might be less tiring. But babysitting is likely to give you a real sense of what having a child is like. If you are tired the next day, imagine what it would be like to feel that tired and still have a small child to care for.

THE POSSIBILITY OF HAVING DISABLED CHILDREN

One set of questions included in the interviews was, "What were your expectations, fears, and fantasies about the baby? Were they related to your disability? If so, how?"

Sara's answer touched on many themes we will discuss:

My first thought was the baby could be disabled. I just hoped it would be okay....I didn't know whether it [Sara's disability] was hereditary, but if the child was disabled, I knew I'd be the best to cope with whatever was there.... I had constant fear that the baby would be disabled, and went to the university hospital to make sure it wasn't hereditary. When I found out it wasn't hereditary, I was able to breathe easier.

Half the women interviewed had been afraid, some intensely, that their children would be disabled. We do not know whether these women felt any more concern than would a group of women without disabilities. One might think that women who had been born disabled would be more likely to fear for their children, but several women with spinal cord injuries also worried that their babies would have problems. Sometimes it seemed that a woman's own difficulties or discomforts during pregnancy made her more pessimistic. Some women, like Dawn, felt that "fear...was not related to my disability. Every mother goes through that." Sasha's fear was certainly related to her disability: Sasha, who was "surprised that [she] could do anything so normal" as getting pregnant, could only imagine that she would have a disabled child.

Some women felt that their concerns about their babies' health were caused by their feelings about their own disabilities. Several women explained, "Since my body didn't work in other ways, I couldn't help feeling that it wouldn't work when I was pregnant." Celeste, who had always felt less competent than her able-bodied mother, couldn't help feeling that, "If my mother had a [disabled] kid like me, I couldn't do any better." Clara's comment was especially illuminating: "I was really excited to have a baby..., [and] I did not want my kid to be disabled. Being disabled myself, and working with disabled people, gave me the sense that physical disabilities are much more common than they really are, and that was scary."

Some people reacted to their fear with denial. Celeste was so afraid her baby would be stillborn that she "protected [her]self against having any expectations." Others suppressed the fear itself: Arlene felt "some fear...[but] didn't let it rule me"; Corinne said of her fear, "I didn't dwell or obsess on it."

Corinne and Arlene's refusal to dwell on their fears was not unreasonable, as they had assured themselves that their disabilities were not hereditary. Hilary also said she consulted a genetic counselor; she did so to reassure her parents-in-law. Leslie, whose pregnancies always involved the risk of miscarriage, pointed out that sometimes the choice to live with some fear is simply an aspect of trying to have a child.

There are really two separate questions to ask about how your disability might affect your child. One is, "Will my disability affect fetal development?" The second is, "Can my disability be inherited?"

Some women with disabilities might have a greater risk of giving birth prematurely, or of having difficult labors which could affect their babies. For example, the blood pressure fluctuations of dysreflexia might precipitate premature labor, and premature birth can cause disability. In the previous section, we suggested questions you could ask your doctor about how your disability might affect your child.

To find out whether a congenital disability can be inherited, it is important to consult a genetic counselor. Counselors have found that parents often over- or underestimate the likelihood that their disabilities can be inherited.

The term "congenital disability" can be confusing. The word *congenital* refers to any problem which is present from the time of birth. However, not all congenital problems are genetically caused, although the two words sound similar. Some congenital disabilities are due to problems in the prenatal environment, such as certain illnesses in the mother. (A well-known example is hearing loss in children whose mothers had cytomegalovirus infection during pregnancy.) Research into the causes of congenital disability continues, and a genetic counselor can give you the most recent information about yours.

Some genetic conditions are inherited. In these conditions, a defective gene is passed from generation to generation, and at least one parent is carrying a similar defective gene in every cell of his or her body, just as all the body cells contain the gene for, say, eye color. Tay Sachs disease and sickle cell anemia are well-known inherited disorders. Other genetic conditions are not inherited. The parents do not carry the defective gene in their bodies; instead, when a sperm or ovum cell was being formed, a "mistake" was made in the formation of the genes. Most instances of Down syndrome are examples of the second kind of disorder, although some cases of Down syndrome are familial. A person who has relatives with an inherited disorder like Tay Sachs disease should certainly look into genetic testing, while someone who has a relative with a disorder like Down syndrome may not have a greater than average risk of having a child with this problem. A genetic counselor can advise you about the appropriateness of testing.

Two disabilities which have caused much confusion are spina bifida and MS. It is now definitely known that spina bifida is caused by a combination of genetic and nongenetic factors. Some families may be more susceptible to this condition, though most cases occur in families with no previous history of the problem. Spina bifida is an example of a multifactorial condition, one that appears to result from a combination of genetic, nongenetic, and environmental factors. Current research indicates that a "familial factor" is among the causes of MS; this factor does not involve a certainty of developing the disorder, but a tendency that may run in families, like the tendencies of some families to be susceptible to ear infections, and others to sore throats. There also may be a viral component that interacts with the genetic background of susceptible individuals.

It is important to remember that new discoveries about the causes of congenital disorders are constantly being made. Hilary received different advice from genetic counselors at different times. Ask your counselor when the research about your disability was conducted, and whether any new studies are in progress.

Not all genetically caused disorders have been identified, and the genes responsible for many of them have not been identified. However, literally hundreds of disorders, most of them extremely rare, can be diagnosed, and this number is growing.

Where prenatal testing is not possible, a counselor may be able to give you statistical information as to how likely it is that your disability can be inherited.

The genetic counselor can use the following information in helping you assess the likelihood of your child's inheriting your disability: your age; your family medical history; and, sometimes, results of tests including blood tests of you and/or the father, sonography, chemical analysis of the *amniotic fluid* (fluid surrounding the fetus), and examination of fetal cells. There are two methods for collecting the cells, *amniocentesis* and *chorionic villus sampling*. In both procedures, the fetal cells which have been obtained from within the uterus are analyzed for the presence of genes causing specific disorders. Amniocentesis and chorionic villus sampling procedures are described in Chapter 6.

In deciding whether to use genetic testing, you need to weigh your desire for information against the possibility the procedure could cause a miscarriage. Your genetic counselor can provide statistics that will help you compare the risks related to testing with the risk that a specific disability will occur. For example, it is known that, for women over 35, the risk of having a child with Down syndrome is greater than the risk that amniocentesis will cause a miscarriage. Some genetic counselors believe that unless a woman is sure she would terminate the pregnancy if test results were positive, she should not have genetic testing. They point out that the same information will be available when the child is born. Other counselors believe the risk is worthwhile because, if the information is available sooner, parents have much more time to adapt emotionally and to plan ways to cope with any problems that are diagnosed. A genetic counselor can provide information about agencies to contact for help in the care and education of disabled children.

A genetic counselor can also help you think about how you would feel about raising a child with a disability. This question was not fully explored in our interviews, partly because none of the women had disabled children, and partly because the interviews focussed on pregnancy and birth. Women's passing comments made it clear that, while some had thought ahead about how they might cope with a disabled child, certainly nobody hoped to do so! Margie, looking back on her pregnancy fears, commented, "I didn't worry as much before my kids were born. Then they were still abstractions. Now that I know them, I worry more about something happening to them."

On the whole, women with disabilities express the same feelings as able-bodied parents do about the idea of having a disabled child. But women with disabilities do have a special slant on the question. When participants in one survey were asked whether a woman should have an abortion if she knows her child would be disabled, their responses strongly reflected their feelings about themselves. Some women favored abortion, emphasizing the loneliness and unhappiness disability had caused in their own lives. Others rejected abortion, explaining that their own lives have been worthwhile, and that they dislike the implication that they should not have been born. Others said that the decision should depend on whether the parents feel able to raise a disabled child.

When a woman with a disability considers what life would be like for a disabled child, she brings special empathy and insight to the question. However, like any other parent, she may have trouble making sure she does not project her own feelings, assuming that her child feels (or would feel) whatever she felt. Therefore, the questions we suggest you ask yourself are closely interrelated.

1. *How will I feel about my child growing up with the possibility of physical or psychological pain?* Remember Margie's observation that these feelings strengthen as your love for your child grows.
2. *How did you feel about yourself while growing up, and how do you feel about yourself now?* Many people feel differently about themselves as adults than they did as children. Often they have conquered frustration

and loneliness and like themselves much better. The same could happen for their children.

3. *What was it like for me, growing up with a disability?* Answering questions 2 and 3 can help you imagine how life would be for your child, but must be balanced by answering question 4.

4. *Will my child's life be like mine?* Are there changed circumstances that might make your child's experiences different from yours? Have there been improvements in therapy for this disability? Will improved educational opportunities and adaptive devices for children with disabilities make a difference?

5. *Have you compared your childhood experiences with those of other disabled persons?* Doing so will help you decide which of your experiences and feelings were typical, and likely to be shared by your child, and which were unique.

6. *How would having a disabled child change my life? How is this different from having an able-bodied child? Would it be possible to provide the extra care a severely disabled child might need?*

There are also a few special issues you might want to consider:

- Your thinking might be colored by memories of growing up with your parents. But it would be different for your child—you would be the parent. You would bring to the situation different strengths, different weaknesses, different knowledge. Sasha felt that her parents' overprotectiveness led to her lack of self-confidence, and she would have tried to avoid being overprotective herself.

- One special advantage you would have—one Sara had in mind when she said, "I knew I'd be the best to cope with whatever was there"—is that, in you, your child would have a role model. Most disabled children never hear about successful disabled people; they see no lists of famous disabled Americans to parallel books about famous minority Americans. Often they do not even see disabled adults in everyday life. Some even fantasize about growing into able-bodied adults. But in you and, possbly, your friends, your child would have a constant example of a disabled person(s) meeting the challenges of adult life.

- Many people with disabilities have felt angry with their parents for bringing them into the world. It is not a surprising reaction in a child, no matter how illogical. They may feel angry even though their parents could not know they would have disabled children. How would you feel about encountering this anger if you had known you would give birth to a disabled child?

- Unavoidably, there would be situations in which you would feel as though you were reliving your own childhood. For example, on a day your child is particularly frustrated by physical therapy exercises, you recall the anger and helplessness you felt as a child. Such a situation has a number of possibilities: Your insight into your child's feelings might lead you to give her understanding and support in dealing with the frustration. You might be able to help the therapist find a more effective way of approaching your child. You might identify with your child's feelings so intensely that you become furious and have an angry argument with the therapist. Working with educators, therapists, doctors and possibly social workers, you would frequently find yourself retracing the path of your childhood. How comfortable are you with the idea of handling these situations?

PARENTING

Physical Aspects of Childcare

If you are wondering whether to have children, you do not need to ask whether it is possible for parents with disabilities to be happy, effective parents. Researchers have already found that the answer to that question is "Yes!" Our interviewees gave the same answer. Though all the interview questions were about pregnancy and childbirth, several women commented on their experiences as mothers. Not one felt that her disability had detracted from her ability to mother her children. Stacy, hinting at the need to be flexible, simply said, "You work it out—the fears about nursing, dressing, carrying, and changing." Sasha, who had always had a very close relationship with her teenage daughter, said, "You make up what you can't do, with love." Arlene wisely observed, "It takes more than the ability to change diapers to be a mother. I knew I could love and sing to my child."

The question we are considering here is, *Just what is parenting like for a person with disabilities?*

Disabled women are not alone in wondering how difficult parenthood will be. Many pregnant women find that their joy is mixed with fears of inadequacy; they even have nightmares about failing as mothers. One of Judi's students told her, "In one of my dreams, I suddenly realized I hadn't fed my baby for days." Another dreamed that she had left her baby someplace and couldn't remember where. A third woman said, "My fear was, what would happen if the baby needed me in the night, and I couldn't go to him?" The third woman was the only one who had a disability.

While physical limitations pose some difficulties, they are not insurmountable. One study of one hundred "handicapped homemakers" included a questionnaire asking, "What do you consider your most difficult problem in caring for your children?" For most of the tasks listed, very few women reported problems. For example, only seven women reported difficulty bathing children, and only two felt inadequate in emergencies.

The most difficult physical tasks were those involving lifting and carrying (13 women). The most frequent problem, reported by only 29 women, was discipline, and since the children involved were young, the problem may have been a function of their age. It would not be surprising if 29% of an able-bodied group also reported difficulties in disciplining their young children!

Many childcare tasks may be simplified by planning and preparation before childbirth. For example, bathing and dressing children could be made easier with adaptive equipment and adapted clothing. Not only is adaptive equipment for the disabled useful, but according to women we interviewed, equipment that has been designed to make infant care easier may be very helpful. For example, some women would dress their babies in a commonly available "safety harness," and use the straps for lifting their babies. Others mentioned that they preferred feeding tables to high chairs because the tables were more stable.

The Occupational Therapist's Role

An occupational therapist can be a valuable resource in planning for childcare. He or she can help you select adaptive equipment and appropriate childcare equipment, modify childcare routines such as bathing and diaper changing, adapt childcare equipment and clothing, and change furniture layouts for greater convenience. The occupational therapist could be most helpful as you plan how to child-proof your home. In a child-proofed home, medicines, sharp objects, electrical outlets, and other sources of danger are blockaded or moved out of reach of the crawling, climbing infant or toddler. The trouble is, child-proofing may make the home parent-proof as well! Tools locked in high cupboards, or medicines in safety containers, may be inaccessible to you, too. Yet, if you lack mobility, you can use help in keeping your child safe. Your best plan is to find and evaluate safety strategies and equipment before you need them.

You may feel uncomfortable with the idea of working with an occupational therapist. Some occupational therapists have found that women who were recently disabled were more willing to listen to their suggestions for work simplification than those who had been disabled for a longer time. Judi, who has been disabled from birth, and is an occupational therapist, knows both sides of the story. She knows from her own experience that a disabled woman is more familiar than anyone with her own strengths, limitations, and adaptations. She also recalls that not all suggestions from occupational therapists have been helpful. Yet her training and work have taught her that an occupational therapist's reading, practical training, and contact with other clients may well have given her some ideas you would not think of yourself. It would be worthwhile to consider suggestions for a few days before deciding whether to try them out. The suggestions of a therapist or an experienced parent may be especially helpful during the first few months after childbirth;

these months are often a time of tension and exhaustion, when the suggestions of a knowledgeable but uninvolved person are really valuable.

Arranging for Help

Another step of your decision-making and planning process should be to find out what help would be available to you in caring for your child. Some women, including some mothers we interviewed, feel that parenting is a way to prove you are self-reliant. In reality, no parent works alone—we all rely on help from day-care centers, baby sitters, friends and schools. For some, the availability of help makes a critical difference. Some questions to consider are:

1. *Who would help—husband, babysitters, paid attendants or household help, roommates, relatives from either side of the family?*
2. *How much help can you realistically expect?* Stephanie said she "got reassurances from both families," but people were not always able to keep their promises.
3. *What kind of help would you prefer?* You might want help with jobs like bathing the baby. Or, you might want help with housekeeping chores, so that you could devote more time and energy to your child. To be of most help, any assistants need to be told clearly just what you expect of them. Sometimes, it is all too easy to slip from "helping" into "taking over." Pam said that at times there were problems because her child was confused about who was really in charge. She had to work with her attendants to clarify that *they* were helping *her* with the job of parenting.
4. *If the help you have arranged becomes unavailable, will you still be able to manage?* For example, if a helpful neighbor is married to someone whose work involves frequent moves, or if you and your husband were divorced, would other help be available? Faith, who had Friedreich's ataxia, knew that she would be able to care for an infant, but might die before her child grew up. Faith's relationship with the father was shaky, so she could not be sure who would be responsible for the child in the long run. Still, on the basis of her strong religious beliefs, Faith decided to put her trust in God and continue her pregnancy.

Emotional Aspects of Parenting

Even as mothers talk about the physical challenges of caring for their children, they often mention emotional aspects of parenting, such as the need to maintain love and respect. Children, for their part, need much more than physical care; if a baby has all of her physical needs met, but isn't given enough emotional contact, s/he will not even thrive physically. Also, a child outgrows the need for physical care, and as the years go by, other factors become more important to your relationship. People are often surprised to learn what the real demands on them will be, like Arlene, who commented, "I never would have guessed that helping with homework and class projects would make me feel like I was going to school all over again."

We will discuss three sets of factors which influence the kind of relationship you would have with your child: your contribution to the relationship, the child's contribution to the relationship, and the influence of other people in your family and community. In discussing these concerns, we will refer frequently to interviews with Jane Carpenter Bittle, who kindly shared the results of research she was conducting on disabled parents' feelings about parenthood and their relationships with their children.

The Parent's Contribution

When thinking about what you would bring to a relationship with a child, it helps to ask two questions: *What personal qualities do I bring to the relationship?* and *What expectations do I bring to the relationship?*

The first question might be rephrased as, *Do I have what it takes to be a parent?* There are two useful approaches to answering this question. The first is to list what you consider the most important traits for a parent to have (five is enough), and ask yourself whether you have these traits or might be able to develop them. If you think you would need to change somehow to be ready for parenting (for example, by becoming more assertive or more patient), but you do not feel ready to change, give yourself room to decide, "For now, at least, parenting isn't for me."

The second approach is to ask yourself what your strong points are. Are these strengths important to child-rearing? Perhaps, for example, you have a wonderful sense of humor. It might not have occurred to you to list humor as important to parenting, but, as you think of how your sense of humor has helped your relationships with friends and family, you begin to see how it could help you as a mother. In fact, many experienced parents would say a sense of humor is vital. For reasons that will become clear as you read further, we'd suggest that you consider assertiveness, and the ability to give and receive emotional support from other adults, as valuable parenting skills, although they are not ordinarily mentioned as such. You might also try listing benefits a child would receive from being raised by you.

Some women feel that their disabilities have been a source of emotional strength. When Sharon described her feelings about starting a family, she said, "I knew I could deal with the challenge both mentally and physically, because I had been able to adjust to becoming disabled. It makes you know you can do it."

When disabled parents speak of the advantages they have to offer, they stress their concern with independence. They know how precious self-reliance is, and make special efforts to teach their children the necessary skills. The women Jane Bittle interviewed backed up their opinion that their children were more self-reliant than their peers, listing specific skills such as shopping, check-writing, laundry and yard work, and helping with family businesses. Parents of teenagers added that their children were using these skills to earn spending money. Mothers taking part in another study also noticed that their children were learning skills such as dressing and using keys, and genuinely helping their parents, earlier than peers whose parents were able-bodied.

Besides identifying your strengths, you would be wise to ask yourself what aspects of your personality might be sources of strain in family life. For example, some parents' concern about dependence and independence is not always an advantage. While parents with disabilities are often concerned to raise independent children, many are equally concerned not to be dependent themselves. Some parents work so hard at being independent that they seem rather distant from their children. Another possibility is that a mother who is unhappy about her own need to depend on others will be uncomfortable having a child depend on her.

Other parents find that their dependence poses a problem. A mother who counsels other mothers with disabilities told us, "Sometimes a woman's dependence makes her need a dependent child." She added that disability-related fatigue can affect parenting: "I have multiple sclerosis, and on the days I'm exhausted, I get angry at my children more easily. My son thinks I'm angrier than other mothers, and he's right."

Feelings of inadequacy are another special concern. In light of Bittle's finding that "The largest contributing factor to feeling competent as parents was a basic sense of self-esteem," it is important to discuss some of the fears and self-doubts parents have expressed. For example, one of our interviewees said, "I wanted to bond with the baby right away—so he wouldn't be afraid of my hands, so he could get used to me." Her remark is doubly significant. First, she had not yet learned what is important to a baby; a newborn infant does not notice people's hands, it concentrates on simple features of human faces. It will be years before the child is aware that her mother is different from others. Second, and more important, a mother who feels that her appearance is frightening may be less spontaneous with her child.

Another story about a hand will illustrate what we mean: Clara recalled a conversation in which she expressed very intense feelings. Her friend reached out to take her hand and comfort her, and Clara responded by reaching across her body with her unaffected hand. One of her hands is affected by spasticity and she will not let anybody hold it. A few days later, her friend asked, "Do you let your kids hold either hand?" and was relieved to hear that the answer was yes. If Clara were to pull away when her children reach for her hand, they might interpret the gesture as a rejection, or they might infer that there is something untouchable about their mother. Either way, the mother's lack of self-acceptance would affect her relationship with her children.

Even people whose self-acceptance is strong may meet new challenges when they adopt a new role by becoming parents. The parents Jane Carpenter Bittle interviewed felt that the physical tasks parents must do are comparatively easy; what bothered them was a lack of social support. Once again they had to win social acceptance, now from pediatricians, teachers, and other people they met through their children.

Conflicts with children can also threaten a parent's sense of self-acceptance. Clara described how she felt when her small son would dart into a busy street and she would have to use all her strength to drag him back, kicking and screaming. Not only was she fearful for her son's safety and angry at his disobedience, but she was frustrated by her physical limitations and angry at her son for "rubbing her nose in them."

A mother Jane Bittle interviewed has arguments with her children because they resent her refusals to take them to a public swimming pool because she, an amputee, feels embarrassed. All the parents said that at times they had similar conflicts with their children. The children were disappointed or resentful; the parents regretted that they could not provide certain experiences. Some parents were so saddened that they cried and wondered aloud, "Have I ruined my child's life?"

It is important to put the last few paragraphs in perspective. They are not meant to imply that having children is primarily a painful experience, but to illustrate some of the strains that can arise in a family's daily life. Parent–child relationships have their ups and downs like other emotional relationships. While some parents expressed sadness about particular problems, the parents we interviewed felt very good about their children, and all the parents Jane Bittle interviewed felt that their communication with their children was better than average. It is not unusual for parents to feel at times that they are somehow failing their children. The supposed failing might not be physical disability, but poverty, lack of education, or a short temper. On a bad day, you can even feel guilty for not baking cookies as often as a neighbor does.

One reason it is important to have supportive relationships with other parents is that they can help you keep your experiences in perspective. Portia told of an incident in which she refused to do something for her teenage daughter, and the girl said angrily, "All my problems are because you're in that wheelchair!" Portia dismissed this silly remark with a matter-of-fact, "That's tough!" Still, the argument bothered her somewhat until she told the story to a friend who commented, "My daughter tried the same line on me. She said that I've caused all her problems by being fat."

To some extent, these children were blaming their parents (as teenagers do) for not meeting some imaginary ideal. Parents, too, find that they enjoy their children more when their expectations are realistic. Sheila commented, "I felt I was trying to be an ideal mother, which takes an incredible amount of work. I knew the fantasies and realities of parenting never matched."

Many parents spend the nine months of pregnancy telling their friends, "I don't care if the baby's a boy or a girl, I just hope it's healthy." Then when the child is born, they realize that they cared very much. If the child is the same sex as they discover they had been hoping for, they feel a burst of joy; if they realize that they had been hoping for a child of the opposite sex, they feel disappointment. Some people feel guilty for having been disappointed, and guilt feelings can bother them for years, even though they have good relationships with their children. We can be hurt by unacknowledged or unrealistic expectations about ourselves or our children.

In our culture, the ideal mother is all-accepting. She is not supposed to care whether her child is practical or intellectual, quiet or outgoing, calm or excitable, but to give the same love, "no matter what." Expecting ourselves to live up to this ideal would be as unrealistic as expecting a shy teenager to try to be a cheerleader. Sometimes our children do things we dislike, and if family members think parents must always act accepting, then somebody— either the parent or the child—is likely to fill the gap between wishes and reality with feelings of guilt.

Another common ideal is the mother who, from the moment of birth, automatically loves her child deeply and ecstatically. Yet many women are like Michelle, who said, "It took a while to have maternal feeling. I wasn't sure I had it." Counselors and pediatricians who have worked with many families have learned that love grows slowly as the mother and baby get to know each other. Like any other relationship, a parent's relationship with a new baby has highs and lows. Some days seem like an endless, boring round of feeding, burping, and changing diapers; others are remembered for special moments like the first time a baby turns towards his mother's voice, or watches her face while nursing. One day, the mother realizes that for some time now, she has not only loved her baby because it is her baby—she has formed a bond with the special, unique person that the baby is.

We are all influenced by the images of motherhood presented in advertising for baby food and paper diapers—serenely joyful models who look as though they could be advertising skin cream and hair conditioners. If you visit a real person who has just had a baby, you will see that no matter how happy she is, she has dark circles under her eyes from staying up all night with a colicky baby, or stringy hair because she has been too busy to pick up a brush. Having a support system that includes friends who are parents or prospective parents can help us form realistic expectations.

If you tried making a list of five traits a parent should have, now is the time to take a second look at the list. Ask yourself exactly how important each trait is. For example, you may have mentioned patience. But is the good parent patient all of the time? 90% of the time? something more than 50% of the time? Next, think of some friends who are good parents and give them scores for how often they act like your ideal parent. Now give yourself a score. Is your score closer to your friends' scores than to your ideal score?

Most likely your friends' scores are not like your ideal. And to be a good parent, like them, you can allow yourself imperfections like theirs.

It is also worthwhile to give some thought to the ways that your feelings towards your parents influence your expectations about motherhood. Several interviewees compared themselves with their mothers: some didn't see how they could compete, others expressed their determination to "do the opposite of what my mother did." Our memories of how we felt about our mothers can help us understand our relationships with our children, but these same memories can give us an unrealistic view of our new relationships. One author tells of a mother who had resented not having any privacy with her dates when she was a teenager, so, on the evenings that her daughter had a date, she often managed to be away from the house. However, the daughter felt insecure coming back to an empty house, and had her dates bring her "home" to a friend's house where some family member was always present.

Finally, you need to examine your expectations about what your children will be like. The hopes and fears women expressed about themselves as mothers were based on specific beliefs about what their children would be like. One mother believed a child would be frightened by deformity; another believed a child would care most about the love she gave; Corinne, who said, "I worried about not being able to participate in activities like roller-skating," believed children expect parents to share in their play. The next section will give you some information about children's changing needs, and how their response to disability changes as they mature.

Children's Contribution to the Relationship

Children's awareness of parental disability changes as they grow, and their feelings about disability change as well. So, we will describe four age groups: infants, pre-schoolers (2.5–5 years old); school-aged children (5–12 years old), and teenagers. Children's own adaptability and growth patterns affect what will happen at each age. Life with each age group offers characteristic challenges and rewards.

Infants Infants are completely unaware of disability, at first because their awareness in general is limited. As they approach toddlerhood, they will continue to be unaware of disability because their experience is limited. An infant's needs are such that the mother's disability is irrelevant to their relationship.

In this earliest stage of life, the child's most important emotional need is simply to establish a strong bond with an adult. Infants need to feel loved and cared for, and they need continuity. Babies as young as 5-6 months old recognize individual adults, and may be upset by change; for example, mothers notice that a baby who has a new babysitter becomes more irritable for a few weeks until s/he is accustomed to the change. Your baby will not be judging you in any way; all s/he needs is for you to be available on a consistent, daily basis.

Most of the stresses and challenges that arise during the first months of parenthood are not related to the mother's mobility. Until the baby's eating and sleeping patterns settle down, you may often be tired. It will sometimes be frustrating to try to understand your baby: is s/he crying because of hunger? a wet diaper? the need to be rocked? But it is not a disaster if you are a little slow in getting to the crib. Even when a woman has limited use of her hands and arms, she is well able to build the foundations of love with her baby. She can feed the baby with the help of a sling or supporting pillow, lean her head forward and tickle the baby with her hair, or play peekaboo by shaking her hair over her face. A mother may feel frustrated by needing other people to warm bottles or to bring the baby to her, but the baby will not care. (Examples of specific infant care methods that disabled mothers have devised are given in *Chapter 9*.)

A growing infant's general adaptability can easily include subtle adaptations to maternal disability. Portia said her infants would crawl to her wheelchair and cling to her arm in a manner that allowed her to lift them. She took this behavior for granted until she babysat for an able-bodied friend whose babies did not know how to help her lift them. Another mother commented, "I change my baby's diaper more slowly than other people do, but she's always more patient with me than she is with other people."

At the end of the first year, when parents and child have become comfortable and familiar with each other, a new challenge arises as children begin to crawl, then walk and climb about the house. Just how challenging the situation is will be depends on a number of factors. First, the child's personality: A child who likes to stay near adults and is often looking over his shoulder for approval, will be easier to supervise than a bold, independent child who "gets into everything." Many parents notice that while some infants are willing to play in a playpen or crib, others are frustrated by any confinement. These individual differences are often more important than anything a parent does, and certainly no one should blame her physical limitations for problems that may have other causes.

Supervising children seems more taxing for people with sensory impairments, however, and Jane Bittle found that sometimes it was difficult to know whether it was a parent's personal style, her disability, or her feelings about her disability that made childcare a challenge. One practical problem is that devices meant to protect the child may create obstacles for the mother; for example, safety gates and playpens may get in the way of maneuvering a wheelchair.

Once children start crawling, discipline becomes an issue. The best ways of dealing with a child will change constantly as s/he develops. Distraction can be a very effective technique for keeping a one-year-old out of mischief, but it will not work with a strong-willed two-year-old. Every child requires some amount of physical discipline—not necessarily punishment, but simply being picked up and removed from dangerous situations. At this age, a child resisting with all her might while being strapped into a car-seat or carried away from a curb, can make a disabled parent painfully aware of her limitations, especially if the disability is of recent onset. Coping with such problems can take all the self-respect and resourcefulness that have been developed during years of coping with disability. For example, a mother may need to ignore the disapproving stares of strangers if she uses a children's harness and lead to protect an impulsive toddler while out-of-doors. She may need to carefully orchestrate the actions of her attendants so it is clear to a child that her mother directs discipline.

The role of helpers, whether attendants, daycare staff, or other parents, must be to assist the mother in teaching her child to be more and more responsive to verbal commands, rather than responding only to physical discipline. While nursery schools can provide physical activities and other experiences a parent cannot provide, they may also be a source of problems if teachers are very physical in disciplining children, or do tasks for children that they must do for themselves at home (for example, dressing).

Fortunately, the difficulties parents experience during this stage are balanced by some wonderful rewards. As children interact more and more with the world around them, they are more and more interesting and fun to be with. For example, children in late infancy begin to engage in make-believe games, and watching a child pretend to be a puppy, or feed a doll with utter seriousness, is delightful.

Up until age two, the goal of discipline is to teach children what is and is not acceptable behavior. Babies get into mischief because they do not yet know what is a "no-no." A baby who is beginning to understand the world around her will try something just to make sure she understands. Her smile of glee as you take her away from the stove for the thousandth time is *not* delight at your frustration, but the delight of discovering, "Yes, I've got it right, the stove is forbidden territory."

Pre-Schoolers Sometime near the second birthday, however, a child becomes deliberately defiant. There is no doubt that a two-year-old who breaks rules is looking for a battle of wills. Much of a toddler's willfulness is just one side of the coin; the other side is her strong desire to take care of herself, and her increasing ability to do so. The two-year-old whose refusal to use the potty makes his mother almost long to return to diapers, will be the three-year-old who feels thrillingly adult when wiping up his own accidents.

Two- and three-year-old children are increasingly aware of mothers' disabilities, but not in the ways one might expect. In certain subtle ways, they continue to adapt to their mothers' limitations. Clara recalls being unable to lift her small daughter Sarah when pregnant with a second child. Once, when Sarah fell on some steps, she picked herself up, walked over to her mother, climbed into her lap—and then began to cry! This is the kind of behavior that gives disabled parents the impression that their children are unusually independent. But very young children cannot be expected to make concessions to parental limitations if they're in a battle of wills. Most children under five or six are simply too young to imagine another's feelings, and a child who hides behind the dresser to avoid a spanking, far from worrying about how her mother feels, will stay there just because her mother cannot reach her. (Each of Sheila's children used this trick. Her solution was to simply wait them out!)

Two- to five-year-olds seem to think of disability as being similar to any other individual characteristic, such as red hair or freckles. If other children ask what's wrong with their mother, they reply, "Nothing." When they do make comparisons, it is from a viewpoint that assumes disability is ordinary. For example, a two-year-old girl who has grown up with a brother whose legs are paralyzed, might have difficulty understanding that her new friend is a boy, because she thinks that "boys can't walk." A friend of Judi's, whose father had lost his hands because of a war injury, remembers expecting her little brother's hands to fall off when he grew up.

Parents naturally want to end their children's confusion. They need to keep explanations simple and clear without triggering needless fear. For example, a mother who explains that she is disabled because she was injured in an auto accident might find that her little one becomes frightened of riding in cars. Parents will need to differentiate between "big" and "little" injuries and illnesses, and may still find that their children have fears that they cannot explain. Such fears may be difficult to distinguish from the kinds of fears two- to five-year-olds normally experience, such as fear of animals, of being left alone by their mothers, or being carried down the drain with the bathwater. Often, however, if parents have been matter-of-fact about disability, it does not occur to small children to worry about it.

School-Aged Children At about the time they start kindergarten (at five years of age) children become much more aware that a disabled parent is different from other adults. Their intellectual development may be partly responsible for this change. Certainly they encounter much more curiosity, and even teasing, from their peers. Here are two examples of the change in children's awareness of disability: When Clara's daughter was four, she simply did not think of her mother as different, even when others commented on her disability. At five, however, she said, "You can't be my mother, because we don't walk the same way"! Clara's son, at four, often imitated the speech of a friend who has speech difficulties; since entering kindergarten, he has begun to claim that he cannot understand what his friend says.

The parents Jane Bittle interviewed said that as their children grew older, they worried more about their parents' difference from other people. They also commented that while a five-year-old was still quite closely identified with parents, a nine-year-old would be more concerned about what peers think. These age-related changes occur in all children.

As children cope with the issues of difference and disability—in their own parents and in other people—there may well be times when they will disappoint their parents. In one study of mothers with disabilities, mothers said that their children were much more sensitive toward children who were different from their peer group, and often made a point of befriending those who were teased by others. The women Jane Bittle interviewed also said that, "Having a disabled mother makes my child more accepting of people who are different." These parents also told of their children's defending classmates who were teased, or refusing to care about another child's different appearance. Still, even children of disabled parents can have trouble learning to accept differences, as an experience of Jane Bittle's demonstrates: Jane is blind, and her eyes make frequent random movements. Since it was not always possible to find childcare for her young daughter when she had interviews scheduled, her daughter would sometimes accompany her on the interviews. On one such occasion, when Jane was interviewing a deaf woman, she brought her daughter along to play with the woman's son. Afterward, her daughter told her that the nine-year-old boy had made fun of Jane's eye movements.

Clara recalls that when her daughter imitated the walk of a disabled child in what seemed to be a mocking manner, "At first I was absolutely furious." When she had had time to think about it, she decided that possibly her daughter's behavior represented a very direct, childish attempt to understand what she was seeing. Small children often use imitative play as a means of learning about others, and they may use the same process in understanding disability.

Innovative programs for teaching children about disabilities include opportunities for children to experience what a disability is like. For example, children may walk blindfolded while led by another person, or try to write, eat, and dress with only one hand. Some parents whose children are being teased might wish to introduce one of these programs to teachers. Another parent might prefer to approach the children more informally, like the mother who told Jane she visited her child's classroom to discuss her deafness.

Between the ages of five and ten years old, a child's ethical development takes a new direction, as s/he begins to think in terms of the general concepts of "good" and "bad," and to judge the goodness or badness of self and others. Disabled parents have an exceptional opportunity to teach their children to be sensitive and accepting of individual differences, but the challenge will be as great for them as it is for other parents.

When children reach this age, it becomes easier to manage without physical discipline. Since physical discipline is difficult for parents with disabilities, it is fortunate that as children are growing larger, they are also growing more responsive to such punishments as the withdrawal of special privileges.

Beyond these special concerns, we must simply say that the joys and challenges parents will encounter are too numerous to describe—children five and older are very complicated individuals! Children's unique personalities, their strengths and weaknesses, become very apparent, and living with them will be as delightful and as exasperating (perhaps a bit more delightful and exasperating!) as living with an adult.

Teenagers What about teenagers? Adults often think of them as a breed apart—not children, not adults, sometimes, even, not quite human. However, the joys and terrors of living with teenagers are only an intensification of what has gone before. It is not surprising that a fourteen-year-old questions rules that were taken for granted when s/he was twelve. A child who is changing physically and preparing for adult rights and responsibilities naturally looks at these rules in a new light, asking, Why do these rules exist? Why are these behaviors considered good or bad? Not only are parents disturbed by these questions, but they may be worried by their teenagers' attempts to practice adult skills and responsibilities before they seem ready. Finally, since the typical teenager's struggle to build a new identity often involves close identification with a small group of friends, s/he may worry her parents by seeming intolerant of individual differences.

Many people have compared the kind of clumsy defiance a teenager displays towards parents with the belligerence of a two-year-old's bid for independence. Teenagers seem to think all is fair in their war for independence, and will attack any apparent weakness, as Portia's daughter did when she blamed Portia's disability for her own problems. Most teenagers, as they try to become as much as possible like their friends, become ashamed of their parents for a few years. Nobody enjoys teenagers' criticisms, but parents with disabilities can take comfort from knowing that able-bodied parents are in the same situation.

Some parents manage by taking a humorous approach to rebellious behavior. A blind mother laughed when she told Jane Bittle that, "My son thinks I don't know it when he kisses and hugs his girl-friend in front of me."

As teenagers renew their childhood struggles to balance independence and cooperation, impulsiveness and responsibility, they will win some new victories. Of the people Jane Bittle interviewed, parents of teenagers felt they had unusually good relationships with their children. While they certainly did not claim to have perfect relationships, they felt that they had had to make a special effort to communicate well with their children, and that now their effort was paying off in better than average communication with their teenagers. They also felt that new responsibilities were less troublesome for their teenagers, who had already shared in household chores for years. Where small children unconsciously adapt to disability, teenagers are capable of a new kind of sharing. One father said his son, who is very athletic, joins him in wheelchair sports; for the boy, it is a way to build upper-body strength—and a sensitive, creative way to share his interests with his father.

One woman Jane Bittle interviewed said, "I had children to create the kind of family I didn't have." She was echoing the hope of many people—disabled and able-bodied alike—to create a climate of love and acceptance they may not have experienced as children. This can be a reasonable hope. Fulfilling the hope demands a lot of work; parents with disabilities share the universal feeling of "giving more than I get." Children cause many disappointments and frustrations as they mature, but they have the potential to give much happiness as they respond to loving guidance. It was the mother of a loving, sensitive teenager who told Judi, "You make up what you can't do with love."

The Parent's Relationship with the Community

Another important aspect of the parenting role is that it changes the parent's relationship with the surrounding community. As they discussed their hopes and fears for motherhood, many interviewees commented that much of their social life had centered on friendships with other disabled people. They wanted to enjoy more friendships with able-bodied people, and looked forward to meeting new friends through their children. Meeting other parents was not seen as a reason for having children, but as a pleasant fringe benefit. Some women felt, too, that having children would make them appear more normal and acceptable in their communities.

Parenthood is very demanding, and all parents benefit from social support for their role. As much as they need the kind of practical support that is found in car-pools and babysitting exchanges, they need encouragement from friends, other parents, and their children's teachers. As Jane Bittle commented about the people she interviewed, "The largest contributing factor to their feeling competent as parents is a basic sense of self-esteem. What they need from society is respect, acknowledgment, and support for their parental roles."

However, our society is still in the process of changing attitudes towards people with disabilities. People who meet a disabled parent often react with surprise. Our mass media rarely portray disabled people as parents, so it is often difficult for people to understand how a person with mobility restrictions can raise a child.

Sometimes the attitude of surprise that a disabled parent encounters is also one of admiration and encouragement. Sometimes it is disapproving, and such negative reactions, besides being unpleasant, can interfere with the parent–child relationship. Several women told Jane Bittle that they were not allowed to care for their babies in the hospital. One woman was told, "Our insurance rates might go up if you dropped the baby and it was injured." A student of Judi's told her, "They would never leave me alone with my baby to nurse. They said I might drop him. What did they think I was going to do when I got home?"

Parents of school-aged children may need to make a special effort to work with their children's schools. Sometimes parents find these efforts rewarding, like the woman who makes a point of visiting her son's classroom to talk to the children about disability. Others are annoyed, like the blind mother who had to call a teacher and tell her, "Please phone me when my son has acted up in class. When you send a note home, he simply doesn't read it to me!" Many parents mention the problems created by lack of physical access to schools; for example, many schools have ramps to building entrances, but no way for parents to visit second-floor classrooms.

While you may not be able to predict how people will react to you as a disabled parent, it is reasonable to suppose that their reactions will be similar to those you already encounter in your community. The important question is, how will you feel about people's reactions? Both Jane Bittle's interviewees and the women interviewed for this book, gave the impression that the parents who felt most isolated were those who were either less self-confident, or generally more sensitive to other people's reactions to disability. Some older parents commented, "People's discomfort was there all the time. Now that I'm older and more self-confident, I feel I could have handled it differently, and reached out more."

Besides wanting social support for your parenting efforts, you will want your child to see you being treated with respect by others. You can accomplish these goals partly by including people with disabilities among your network of friends. You can also educate your community about disability. It can be very effective to help schools teach children about disability, so that children's new attitudes spread to their parents. The attitudes of the community at large will not be as important to you and your child as what happens in your smaller social world. Your own friends and family, and a few good friends in the school community, can give you the support you need for a solid relationship.

THE COST OF HAVING A CHILD

It is difficult to speak of the cost of having a child in simple dollars-and-cents terms. It has often been noted that the average-sized family (containing 2.2 children!) simply does not exist—and the same is true of the average cost of having a child. Estimates of the cost per year of maintaining an eleven-year-old child range widely from $5,000 to $11,000, taking into account variations in optional expenses such as music lessons or summer camp.

However, it is possible for you to give some thought to how you personally would be affected by having a child.

The first step, naturally, is to examine your insurance policy to see whether it includes maternity coverage. Many people who do not have such insurance delay pregnancy while they obtain it. Usually maternity insurance will not pay medical benefits until one year after the policy was started. It may be necessary, too, to find out what costs might not be covered by a standard policy, and start saving to pay such expenses yourself. Your disability specialist might be able to advise you about such special treatments or medications.

If you are employed, it is important to consider opportunity costs—the income lost if you must stop working, or when you miss work to keep medical appointments, care for sick children, and so forth. If you continue working, you may need to explore such arrangements as job-sharing and part-time work, and plan on a reduced income. For many people, the loss of employer-paid health benefits is as great a problem as the loss of wages.

Women who would need help with the physical care of their children must investigate the cost of additional attendant care. If you receive welfare assistance, ask your social worker to explain the regulations to you. Unfortunately, these regulations may be very unrealistic; for example, in some states, no additional attendant care is funded unless the child herself is disabled, regardless of the parent's disability. It may be possible to make adjustments using increases in other benefits, such as rent allowance, but careful planning would be needed.

Many people with disabilities have limited incomes and must manage their budgets carefully. Yet parents often have to meet unexpected expenses, such as costs for extracurricular activities and dental care. Even the cost of clothing can be a problem when your child grows faster than your budget. Will you be able to handle such strains on your income? Do you have a few luxuries, such as an occasional night out, which you would have to give up if you had a child? How would you feel about that?

It is also important to ask whether it is really practical for you to use the money-saving methods other parents often use. For example, some women have difficulty arranging childcare exchanges because their neighbors do not understand that a disabled woman can care for their children as well as her own. Shopping for bargains in used toys and clothing is a task which some women relish, and others find too demanding physically. Generally speaking, people with limited incomes must substitute time and energy for money, and if these resources are already limited, the adjustment can be difficult.

Still, many of the additional expenses associated with having a child are temporary. For example, by the time your child is three years old, dressing and feeding herself independently and spending several hours a day in nursery school, you will not need as much help with her care. When your child starts school, childcare costs will be reduced further, but of course there will be expenses for school supplies. If you start a college fund, your teenager can contribute to it as well. By planning for different expenses at each stage of your child's life, and for possible changes in your earning power, you may be able to plan a long-term budget.

MOTHERHOOD AND MARRIAGE
· ·

The arrival of children appears to have the same impact on a couple in which one partner is disabled as it has on couples in which both partners are able-bodied. The women interviewed for this book repeatedly raised the same issues that appear in the work of family researchers. For example, most commented that their marital relationships began to change not after they had given birth, but as soon as they knew were pregnant, and the same has been found to be true for all new parents. Some women, like Mary, found that the prospect of having a child increased their intimacy: "I felt more fulfilled as a woman, prouder, and that it made it easier for us to come together." Other women, like Dawn, grew more distant from their husbands: "I was more involved in being pregnant than [in] my relationship with my husband." Again, these types of changes are common occurrences. This means that women who want to explore this issue in depth do not need to restrict themselves to literature written specifically for people with disabilities; all the wealth of research on family life is potentially useful. Here we discuss some general issues that interviewees emphasized in their answers to direct questions about how their relationships were affected by children. For information about some of the changes that occur during pregnancy and the first weeks after childbirth, see the sections on "Emotional Concerns" in Chapters 6 and 9.

First, many women emphasized that the quality of the marital relationship before pregnancy offers a good idea of what will happen if children appear on the scene. Arlene said, "Any problems with a relationship are going to be compounded with the birth of a child," and others agreed that areas which were normally sources of tension became more sensitive. For example, couples who have difficulty communicating about their sexual relationship experienced even more difficulty when stress and fatigue were increased by the demands of pregnancy and child care. The most frequently mentioned sources of tension were finances, sexual relationships, fathers' jealousy when mothers seemed absorbed in their new babies, and some women's difficulty in accepting more help than usual. Margie remarked, "I think the difficulty with our relationship is that I react to my MS by feeling and acting dependent. I'm not sure that pregnancy itself was stressful." Positive changes women mentioned most frequently were increased intimacy with their husbands, pleasure in receiving more care and attention than usual, and shared delight in the new baby. It is interesting that no one mentioned disagreements about how children ought to be raised.

For some women, the birth of a child was a motivation to change or end an unsatisfactory relationship. Sybil said, "My husband was drinking all the time, and I thought my child deserved better." For others, the changes associated with pregnancy were an opportunity for re-evaluation and growth, and these women stressed the importance of frequent and honest communication. Sylvia, who said, "A lot of times we were at each other's throats," added, "During this time we became aware of how important it is to be open in a relationship."

Four women reported that their husbands had not wanted children; all of them experienced considerable strain on their relationships, and two of the four eventually divorced. Sasha said, "Communications broke down totally and there was a switch in the relationship. He became unsupportive and negative." However, she valued her relationship with her daughter and felt that she had made the right choice. Carla simply said, "Having children was not healthy for the relationship." These statements contrast strongly with those of women whose husbands also wanted children. Heather recalled, "It was like we were pregnant together. We were ecstatic. He spent time waiting to feel the baby kick." Christina, who had not been married long when she became pregnant, said that during her pregnancy she and her husband learned to work as a team. These women's experiences suggest the importance of involving your husband and other family members in the decision-making process, as Hilary did when she consulted a genetic counselor in order to reassure her in-laws. Try to have them accompany you for some of your visits to counselors and other advisers. Then, even if they do not entirely agree with your decision, they will have some of the same information you were given, and feel that their concerns were taken into account.

Perhaps the most important issue that arises during pregnancy is the mother's need for support. All pregnant women need emotional support, and those who can rely on the help and approval of friends and family tend to be most satisfied with their pregnancies. For women with disabilities, this issue has special significance for two reasons.

First, many women have strong emotional conflicts about their need to depend on others for help, and these emotions may intensify painfully. Others find that their conflicts are reduced when they are pregnant; knowing that all pregnant women need some extra help and attention, they feel they can relax and enjoy the situation. Christina explained, "I was always so independent that when he took charge it lessened the clash. My needing help was good for both of us, and it was nice to see how supportive he was."

Second, the father really does assume new burdens when he must help with infant care or compensate for a temporary increase in the mother's physical limitations. When some women discussed how their relationships were affected by pregnancy, they responded in terms of the stress created by such practical problems. Celeste, for example, remarked that, "My housework was not as effective, and my husband had to take time off work to drive me back and forth to the doctor." Pam, whose husband left her when their child was eighteen months old, felt that her pregnancy had disrupted the delicate balance they had created to cope with her disability, commenting, "I was so sick—much sicker than most pregnant women—and is was so much harder for me to get around, that it just put too much pressure on him."

Arlene and Renee each made a point of scheduling additional attendant care to ease their husbands' burdens, and Pam speculated that her marriage might have survived if she had created a stronger support network. Unfortunately, many public and private agencies will not pay for additional attendant care, assuming that the husband will act as unpaid attendant. It may be necessary to ask for help from others, if only to give your husband an occasional break. For some women, this is not always pleasant, especially if they must turn to very protective parents who are already anxious about the pregnancy. Discussing solutions to these problems before they occur can help considerably. Roberta felt that she and her husband, by making careful plans before her child's birth, minimized the stresses of the postpartum period, a time which is often very difficult because the demands of infant care are great and both parents are fatigued.

Perhaps the most stressful circumstances are those in which people feel helpless. Renee said that even though her husband did not have extra work, "He felt pressured because there was little he could do when I was in pain, and he was worried." Undoubtedly your relationship, like those of most couples with children, will undergo some strains you cannot control or predict. But these women's experience demonstrates that for couples who have developed patterns of cooperation and good communication, such stresses can even provide an opportunity for growth. And, if the decision to have children is a joint one, there is every possibility that your relationship will be enriched. As Stephanie said, "Our relationship got even better because we shared something so important."

COMBINING CAREER AND FAMILY

We often hear this issue discussed in extreme "all or nothing" terms, as if a woman must either avoid all employment outside her home until her youngest child is at least ten years old, or go back to work full time when her baby is six weeks old. In reality, women work out a variety of ways of combining work and career, depending partly on the nature of their jobs. For example, a teacher or professor might time her pregnancy to coincide with her sabbatical year; a nurse or hospital technician might arrange to change shifts, or change to "on call" work, after her maternity leave; a clerical worker who wants to spend several months with her baby might leave her job, then find another full- or part-time job when she feels ready. Some types of employment are inflexible and the mother really must make a decision about changing or interrupting her career.

Any of these arrangements can support a satisfactory family life. Each arrangement has its own satisfactions and stresses. For example, a full-time mother may be pleased that she is able to see her child's early accomplishments, or enrich her child's education by volunteering at school, yet regretful that her family's income is limited by her not working, or lonely for more adult contact. An employed mother may enjoy her work, or value her earning power, yet wish for more time with her children, to help them with their homework or simply enjoy their company. Whether a woman is generally satisfied with her situation usually depends on whether she feels she has chosen it freely.

These issue can be more troublesome for women with disabilities because their choices may be more restricted than other women's. Besides facing barriers to employment in some fields because they are women, they must deal with bias against disability. A woman with disabilities is likely to have more difficulty adapting her work schedule, and if she must give up a good job, she may not find another easily. This is not a problem for a woman who feels that parenting is the most enjoyable job of all. However, many women who have interrupted or given up their careers resent their children at times, especially when they are being difficult or demanding, and some disabled women may find themselves in this situation more often. You may not be able to create the balance you think is ideal, but it is important to your happiness to feel that you have made the best decision you could.

If you want to continue your career, it is important to assess what the demands on your time will be, and how you will meet them. Not everyone is as fortunate as Julie, who said, "I got a tremendous amount of support from my family to make it possible. Plus, I worked for a good firm that was very flexible and supportive. If I needed to take time off for a pediatrician's appointment, it was okay." It might be necessary to make some compromises; for example, while your child is small, you might choose to work for an employer who offers a more flexible schedule, but fewer promotions or less interesting work.

Meanwhile, there will be varying demands on your free time. Julie said that working was actually easier when her child was younger, because "He would be happy to see me and then go to bed. I had more time to relax. When he got older, he started needing help with his homework. Now I have less time for myself."

While it is true that, as a popular bumper sticker says, "Every mother is a working mother," it is also true that an employed mother feels as if she comes home to a second job. The more susceptible she is to fatigue, the more important this issue. It is essential to have help. Couples in which both parents are employed will find that sharing chores can be a major issue in their relationship, and it is valuable to discuss these concerns as part of the decision-making process. Some questions to ask are

- *What are the chores that each of us is willing to do? Can we learn to accept each other's ways of doing tasks, not criticizing different methods of folding laundry or loading the dishwasher?* (Start practicing before you are pregnant.)
- *Should we depart from some traditional ways of sharing tasks?* For example, should the father take the baby to the pediatrician because his schedule is more flexible?
- *Can we agree to change our expectations?* For example, by deciding together that dirty dinner dishes can wait till after the baby is asleep.

Whether to combine parenthood and career, and how best to combine them, are very individual decisions. As with other major decisions, living with your choice can be very satisfying at some times, and stressful at others. What is certain is that with careful forethought you can have something better than the myth of "having it all," and that is the reality of choosing what you want.

CLOSING COMMENTS
. . . .

At the end of Chapter 1, we reported that disabled mothers believe that a pregnant woman with disabilities should be seen primarily as a pregnant woman. In the same way, disability is not necessarily the most important concern for a woman who is deciding whether to have children.

Every question explored in this chapter is one that needs to be considered by *all* potential mothers, whether or not they have disabilities. All women need to decide whether they can afford to have children, to learn the extent of the risk that pregnancy will affect their health, and so forth.

Even the feelings some women expressed that having children proves that their bodies "work right," or that they really are "like other women," are shared by many able-bodied women. Although our society is changing, we still live in a world in which women's worth is frequently measured by the old yardsticks of beauty and fertility. Sometimes these standards are applied more harshly to women with disabilities, but the fact is, these standards can never be fair.

While disproving stereotypes about disability can be a pleasant fringe benefit of the decision to have children, what is important for a woman with disabilities—and all women—is to make the choice that contributes most to her personal health and happiness.

3 TEAMWORK— GETTING THE HEALTH CARE YOU NEED

··

The previous chapter discussed a number of questions that could help you decide whether to have a child. Once the decision is made, new questions arise. The questions that occur to many women at this point are *How do I find a doctor? How do I interview a doctor?* and *How do I learn how knowledgeable a doctor is about disability?* This chapter answers these questions, and also addresses the related concerns of deciding where to give birth, consulting with specialists, and—most importantly—assuring that *all* your health care needs are met.

SELECTING AN OBSTETRICIAN
···

When To Begin the Search

Since early prenatal care is extremely important, we suggest that a woman begin to search for a doctor as soon as possible. In the previous chapter we suggested that a gynecological examination can be a first step in deciding whether to become pregnant, and possibly at that time you found a doctor with whom you could be comfortable. But if this is not the case, or if you have become pregnant unexpectedly, you need to choose an obstetrician as soon as you think you may be pregnant. The importance of finding a doctor as soon as possible cannot be emphasized strongly enough, since babies whose mothers received late prenatal care, or no prenatal care, have an increased risk of dying in infancy.

Beginning your search early for a doctor gives you more choices than if you wait too long. You want to avoid finding out that the doctor of your choice already has several patients with a due date near yours, and cannot manage any more patients.

Time is also needed to find a doctor who will have a positive attitude toward your pregnancy, for you are likely to meet with a wide variety of reactions. Some of the women we interviewed met doctors whose first reaction was to advise an abortion (in one case, the woman was *5 months* pregnant). Other doctors were doubtful or cautious, but still supportive. Still others were enthusiastic and welcomed the challenge, as did Portia's doctor, who, she said "was happy when I came in. It broke up the boredom of his day."

A woman's body changes drastically during pregnancy. A doctor can assess these changes better and provide better care if s/he has come to know you early in your pregnancy, or even before you were pregnant. Such considerations are even more important for a disabled woman. Few obstetricians have had the opportunity to work with many disabled women. You will be glad if you allow time for the doctor to learn what is normal for *you*, and how your disability may affect your pregnancy.

Health problems that are not necessarily related to your disability may need early attention. Weight reduction, correction of anemia, and updating rubella vaccinations, for example, are best taken care of *before* pregnancy. If a woman is taking medications that must be avoided during pregnancy, they can also be changed before pregnancy.

How to Find a Doctor

The best way to find an obstetrician is by recommendations from people whose judgement you trust. Ask for suggestions from the doctor most familiar with you and your disability. This doctor may even call the obstetrician for you, providing an introduction and setting the stage for future cooperation in your care. Also, friends who have had children can give you personal impressions of their doctors. If you are interested in giving birth at a particular hospital, you can ask for a list of obstetricians who work there. If you are interested in using the hospital's alternative birth center, take a tour of the facility, and, if you are satisfied with it, ask for the names of the doctors who use it most often.

Evaluating a Doctor's Practice

It is very difficult to judge a physician's ability if you are not medically trained. Asking for referrals from people you trust can help in evaluating a doctor's ability and practice. The impressions of a doctor's patients and colleagues can be of help in assessing his/her skills and in determining what your priorities are. For example, one doctor might have the best surgical skills, whereas another might have the best ability to help a woman relax during a difficult labor. Friends may even report very different experiences with the same doctor: "I always appreciated the way s/he took time to answer my questions," says one friend, while another reports, "It seems like s/he tried to rush through labor faster than my body could handle it." You may feel more comfortable relying on the experience and intuition of an older doctor, or you may believe a younger doctor will be more up-to-date. The choice of a doctor is a very personal one. As Portia pointed out, there is no single list of requirements for everyone. Instead, you need to "know what *you* like in a doctor."

You will also want to be aware of a doctor's training and experience. If you choose a doctor who has specialized in obstetrics, you know that, after medical school, s/he had to have a minimum of three years of experience in this field in order to be certified. You can ask a family practitioner how many babies s/he has delivered. Hospitals try to ensure that doctors on their staff meet certain standards.

Even before meeting a doctor for the first time, it is a good idea to talk to the receptionist about office policies, such as the following:

- *Fees:* Is there is an inclusive fee for maternity care? What is it? Is the fee different if a cesarean birth is necessary? Which services are covered by the fee? (For example, there may be additional charges for laboratory tests, but your doctor's fee may include special services such as nutritional counseling.)
- *Payments and insurance:* What kind of insurance will this office accept? Will they accept payment by your insurance carrier, or do they prefer to receive payment from you and help you to obtain reimbursement? If you cannot meet their usual payment schedule, can they make other arrangements?
- *Affiliations:* What hospital(s) (or birth center) does the doctor work with?
- *Special requests:* If you are interested in "prepared" or "natural" (unmedicated) childbirth, and/or being accompanied by your spouse or another supportive person, ask whether the doctor(s) in this practice are willing to accommodate such requests.
- *Special accommodations:* If you use a wheelchair, ask whether the office, and the bathrooms, are wheelchair accessible.

The answers to these questions will help you decide whether to spend time and money meeting the doctor(s) in this practice.

If you belong to a prepaid health plan, you will not need to ask questions about finances. However, when choosing from a list of available doctors, or visiting your clinic, you still need to find out what kinds of services are provided.

You may wish to request that you come only for consultation for your first visit, and delay a physical examination until you are sure which doctor you will have. It is a good idea to bring the baby's father or your advocate along for this appointment. Then you will have someone to share impressions with, and to help you make sure that all of your questions are answered. (We will say more about the role of advocates later in this chapter.) Writing a list of all of your questions before your appointment will help you to make sure that you do not forget anything important.

Interviewing a Doctor

When you meet a doctor for the first time, the most important question to ask yourself is, "Am I comfortable with this person?" You are beginning a 9-month relationship, and during the last few weeks of your pregnancy, you will see the doctor at least once a week. Choose someone who is respectful, takes the time to answer your questions, and answers them *willingly*.

You will learn most about the doctor's philosophy by asking open-ended questions. For example, you may feel strongly that you do not want an episiotomy. If you begin by saying something like, "I think you should know I really don't want an episiotomy," you are effectively closing off discussion. It is more useful to ask something like, "What is your policy on episiotomies?" or even, "Do you think I could give birth without an episiotomy?" This way, you will learn how the doctor feels about the subject, while leaving room for further discussion. If s/he tells you, "I usually do episiotomies" (for whatever reason), you have the opening to say, "I'm really hoping not to have an episiotomy. If I practice Kegel exercises and perineal massage, do you think I could avoid having one?"

The following questions are phrased in such a way that the doctor's answers will give you information about his or her knowledge and attitudes, as well as what you might expect during pregnancy:

What are the pros and cons of pregnancy for me?

If the doctor has not raised these issues, be sure to ask whether he/she has any special concerns about working with your disability. Some of our interviewees' doctors were excited and proud to have the opportunity to work with them. One even went out of her way to buy a special birthing chair. You need to hear both positive *and* negative opinions your doctor has about this issue.

If the doctor seems opposed to your pregnancy, *ask why*. The doctor may point out risks that deserve your serious consideration. Then again, his or her concerns may not really apply to you. The first doctor Marsha talked with immediately asked if she wanted an abortion, stating that it would be too exhausting for a woman with MS to care for a toddler. Marsha decided to continue the pregnancy, and later found that caring for an infant was much more wearing than caring for a toddler. In any case, whatever the risks of pregnancy the decision is yours and you need a doctor who will be truly supportive. As you listen to what the obstetrician says about the pros and cons of pregnancy, compare his or her opinions with those of your specialist.

What information do you have about my disability?/How much experience have you had working with disabled women?

Every woman we interviewed stated that it was important to be aware of a doctor's experience. But many women also felt that it is not important for your doctor to have special knowledge about your disability, as long as s/he is willing to work with you, learn about your needs, and adapt to them. Arlene said, "Even though a doctor doesn't have experience, an open mind is most important."

Roberta, however, felt that her treatment had been adversely affected by her doctor's lack of experience. She said she could not talk openly because she felt that her doctor did not know what to expect. This was so even though the doctor was very supportive. She added, "I had a team.... I wasn't comfortable unless my obstetrician consulted my rheumatologist." Roberta had been referred to her obstetrician by her primary care physician. The two doctors conferred frequently, and she felt that these conferences filled any gaps in her obstetrician's knowledge about her disability.

How will you work with my regular doctor?

During your first talk with your obstetrician, make sure that s/he agrees to confer with your regular doctor. A competent doctor should be quite willing to work with the specialist who is most knowledgeable about your disability. Disability specialists writing about pregnancy emphasize the importance of a team approach to prenatal care.

Of the women we interviewed, the ones who were happiest with their prenatal care were those whose obstetricians had conferred with the doctors concerned with their disabilities. The following are examples of three situations in which such teamwork was helpful.

1. Roberta felt that her obstetrician minimized her disability at first. She described his initial attitude toward her arthritis as being limited to "take aspirin and the pain will go away." However, she said that his conference with her rheumatologist made him more aware of how her disability specifically affected her pregnancy.
2. A student of Judi's knew that she might need a cesarean section. She told her doctor she was worried about having spinal anesthesia because she had had lower back surgery. Her doctor then offered to use general anesthesia. She was unhappy about this alternative because she wanted very much to be conscious when her child was born. The solution to the dilemma was a telephone call to her neurosurgeon, who assured her that spinal anesthesia would be no problem for her.
3. Patricia's doctor was very doubtful that a woman with postpolio syndrome

could withstand the physical stresses of pregnancy. Nevertheless, he conferred with her regular doctor and read more about her disability. Then he was able to narrow his concern to specific problem areas, and perform the appropriate diagnostic tests.

After asking your obstetrician to confer with your primary doctor, be sure to follow up. Michelle remarked that her obstetrician agreed to confer with her regular physician, but did not do so. On your second visit, ask whether your obstetrician has met with your regular physician, or spoken with him/her by telephone. Don't worry about nagging—your doctor needs to know that this issue is important to you. Have a deadline in mind. One reason you found a doctor early was to give yourself time to make a change, if necessary. If your deadline has passed and you do not want to change obstetricians, ask your regular doctor to make the first contact.

If I experience unusual symptoms and don't know whether they are pregnancy- or disability-related, who should I call?

It can be difficult to know whether worrisome symptoms are caused by pregnancy or disability. Beth, a student in Judi's birthing class, had kidney stones which eventually caused premature labor. Her response to the earliest symptoms was to assume that they were caused by disability. When she called her disability specialist, she was referred to her obstetrician. Cheryl attributed a normal pregnancy symptom to disability, until her obstetrician reassured her that muscle spasms in her lower abdomen were a reaction to stretching caused by uterine growth. The specific advice your doctor gives you is not as important as the willingness to cooperate in your care with other physicians.

How will labor and delivery be affected by my disability?

Make sure to ask for explanations about anything you do not understand. Your doctor's reply to this question may include positive solutions to special problems. For example, Julie's doctor said they would use a birthing stool, rather than a bed, to give her more hip abduction (so she could move her legs farther apart).

How will we get the hospital's cooperation for treatment which is different from their usual policies?

This question needs to be raised if there is any reason to expect that the birth may be out of the ordinary. The doctor may not be able to answer this question in detail at first, but you need to be assured s/he will cooperate in this matter. You may need to ask this question again at a later visit.

Do you think I will need cesarean delivery? Why? Would you set a date, or wait for labor to begin spontaneously?

Again, your doctor may not be able to answer this question until your pregnancy has progressed further. If you feel that the doctor's opinion reflects incomplete knowledge about your disability, be sure that your disability specialist is consulted. Chapter 9 contains a discussion of the indications for cesarean surgery.

Can you give me a referral for genetic counseling?

If you want genetic counseling, your doctor may be the best person to help you find out where this service is available. If you are asking about genetic counseling because you know you might decide to terminate your pregnancy, you also need to know whether this doctor would help you.

You may have a number of questions about your pregnancy which have nothing to do with your disability. If you have checked with the hospital and learned that certain aspects of your care will be up to the doctor (for example, how many people you could bring to the birth), now is the time to ask. If you have questions about any medical procedures that could be used during labor and delivery, you may want to ask them now.

Most likely, not all of your questions will be answered during your first consultation; certainly more questions are bound to come up in the course of your pregnancy. By the end of your first visit, you should know who in the office or clinic will answer your future questions. A nurse, nutritionist, or health educator may be responsible for providing some information about what to expect and how to care for yourself.

The Physical Examination

The questions you ask are not your only means of evaluating a doctor. Notice how s/he behaves when examining you. Does s/he make an effort to let you know what is happening by making comments such as, "Now I'm going to insert the speculum" or "You'll feel a slight pressure now"? Does s/he give you time to relax? The doctor's behavior during an examination is a good indicator of whether you will be treated with sensitivity and consideration during childbirth. Notice, also, what questions the doctor asks *you*. Does s/he ask specific, relevant questions about your level of sensation, your mobility and flexibility, or physical positions most comfortable for you during the examination?

The Doctor's Partners

It is important to meet your doctor's partners and the physician on call. Schedule one of your regular office visits with the partner(s) as early as possible. Since you cannot predict when labor will start, you cannot predict which doctor will care for you. Childbirth is likely to be a more satisfying experience if there are some familiar faces among the people helping you. Also, you need the chance to make sure that the other doctors who may care for you fully understand and support any plans you have made with your own doctor. You cannot assume that all partners in a practice will take the same approach. Sybil had found a doctor who was highly supportive, but it was her doctor's partner who attended the birth. This partner was horrified that a woman with spina bifida should be having a child, and pressured Sybil and her husband into signing forms permitting him to sterilize her during cesarean delivery. Michelle, on the other hand, found her doctor's partner to be even more helpful than her regular obstetrician, and more careful in taking her disability into account. If you have strong disagreements with one of your doctor's partners, bring up the problem with your own doctor. S/he can help you to resolve the problem, or arrange for another doctor to attend your delivery if s/he is not available.

If you and your doctor make special plans for your care, make sure they are written in your record. When you meet with his/her associates, tell them, "I'm sure you've noticed in my chart that Dr. X and I have discussed (a particular aspect of your care). I'd like to go over these plans with you." These precautions may help you avoid a disappointment like Hilary's: She had planned very carefully for her cesarean delivery. She took a required class, and, hoping she could have regional anesthesia, found a position in which she could receive the spinal injection. She met with an anesthesiologist who was willing to give her husband the required permission to be at the birth. But when Hilary's labor started, both her obstetrician and the anesthesiologist she had visited were out of town. The anesthesiologist who was available would not allow her husband in the operating room, and the obstetrician could not or would not call for a different anesthesiologist. Hilary's disappointment was deepened because her disability prevented her from receiving regional anesthesia. She had planned on trying hypnosis but it did not work for her and she had to have a general anesthetic. When Hilary was asked, "Did you have an unplanned cesarean section?" She answered, "Yes," because nothing had happened according to plan. To the question, "How did you cope?" she answered, "I cried."

SELECTING A HOSPITAL

Hilary's story suggests another strategy for planning your medical care—begin by choosing a hospital or birth center. In some hospitals, she would not need special permission to have her husband with her. It would be enough to take a class on cesarean birth given by the hospital. If you live near more than one hospital with maternity facilities, call each one to learn about their policies. If only one hospital is available to you, it will still be useful to know the answers to most of the questions below. You may ask, with regard to any hospital policy, how much flexibility is possible—whether the hospital will make an exception at your doctor's request or for other reasons. Whenever an exception is to be made for you, *get it in writing!*

Hospitals differ in the services they offer and in some of their rules. The main differences you can expect to encounter are covered in the questions examined below.

What birth-related services do you offer?

Hospitals may offer a number of services in this area including classes about birth in general and the hospital's own procedures in particular (given by nurses and doctors on the staff); classes about cesarean birth; classes about preparing for childbirth; prenatal exercise classes; classes for children who will be present at the birth; referrals to classes given outside the hospital and other information sources; nutrition counseling or referrals.

Do you permit the husband or another support person to be present during the birth?

A support person might be a labor coach, a trusted friend, or a relative. If the answer is yes, be sure to ask how many people may be present. The hospital may have some requirements, such as having your husband accompany you to a childbirth preparation class. You may need more people with you than hospital policy usually allows. When Clara was in labor, her leg went into spasm. Since her husband had to hold her leg, this interfered with his job of coaching her and they needed one more person. If you think you will need extra help, find out if the hospital can change its policy or make an exception.

Do you require any special preparations for delivery?

Such requirements might include taking an enema, shaving the pubic hair, or not eating solid foods after labor begins.

Do your nurses provide ongoing support and coaching during labor?

Some hospitals have regular staff members who provide this service; others will refer you to a coach or allow you to bring someone with you. You might also want to ask whether it is a good idea to bring an additional coach, in case staff members become busy with many patients.

Do you have an alternative birth center?

If the answer is yes, find out who may use these facilities. Also find out what the procedure is if the birth center is in use when you arrive at the hospital. More information about alternative birth centers will be given below.

When do you require fetal monitoring?

Since fetal monitoring equipment can be uncomfortable or interfere with mobility, you may wish to defer its use until it is clearly necessary to evaluate the well-being of the fetus.

Do you require the use of an IV?

This question is not as simple as it seems. An IV is a hollow needle inserted into a vein to deliver fluids and medications. You may need an assurance that an IV would be used only when specific needs arise, and not as a matter of routine. If you have the use of only one hand, and that would be the hand in which the IV would be inserted, you would lose much of your ability to move freely during labor. (The use of IVs and fetal monitors is discussed in more detail in Chapter 7.)

Do you allow rooming-in?

This means that the baby stays with you in your room, rather than in the nursery. Some mothers prefer that the baby be cared for in the nursery; they want some rest. Others want to keep the baby near them. If you are breast-feeding, rooming-in is *much* more convenient. Hospital policies about rooming-in vary: rooming-in may be around the clock, daytime only, or may require your doctor's consent. Find out what your hospital's specific policies are. If the hospital is not set up for rooming-in, you will want to know if the nursery is wheelchair accessible.

In some hospitals, if you are willing to pay for a private room, your husband may be able to spend the night in your room.

If I breast-feed, is the hospital flexible about the feeding schedule?

Find out whether babies are brought to mothers on demand (when they cry from hunger) or according to a schedule. If a schedule is used, you will want to know if it reflects the needs of newborns to nurse approximately every 2 hours.

Do nurses help mothers learn to breast-feed?

You might want to ask friends who have given birth in the hospital what their experiences were like, and/or talk with some of the nurses. Beth recalls that she was never left to breast-feed in privacy. She could not understand why an attendant should be necessary when she knew she would be alone with the baby at home. But some nurses, especially those who have breast-fed their own children, can give wonderful support and advice.

If I have a cesarean section, can the father and/or anybody else be with me?

The hospital may want you to meet certain conditions for the father to be present, such as taking a class or getting the consent of the obstetrician. The same applies to anyone else who might come with you. They will certainly limit the number of people who can be with you.

Does the hospital have facilities for taking care of babies with special problems?/Would the baby be transferred to a children's hospital?

If the baby would be transferred to another hospital, you will want to think about how close it is to your own hospital and to your home.

Does the hospital permit siblings to visit?/Can my child be present during the birth?

Some hospitals allow the brother- or sister-to-be to watch the birth. The usual requirements include the following: the child is above a certain age; an adult is present to care for the child; and the child takes a special class about what s/he will see happen during the birth.

Will I be able to stay with the baby after the birth?

In some hospitals the baby is taken to the nursery immediately after birth to have its health evaluated, and/or to be cared for until the mother is moved to her room. Sometimes, when the baby is born at night, it is kept in the nursery until morning.

Someone in the financial office will tell you what the hospital's basic charges are, and what you might be charged for additional procedures (e.g., forceps delivery). You can take a tour of the delivery rooms, alternative birth center (if any) and nursery. Be sure to find out in advance when these tours are scheduled. On the tour you can see for yourself what the facilities are like—whether the nursery is accessible to wheelchairs, whether any of the delivery rooms have birthing chairs, whether there is a shower in the alternative birth room. Pay special attention to whether the facilities in the labor suite and in the hospital rooms are accessible. You will also have a chance to see what kind of people work there, and to discuss for the first time any special needs they should know about.

It may be difficult to find a hospital that has everything you want. You will have to make decisions such as choosing between a hospital that allows rooming-in and one that is closer to home, or between one that has facilities for premature babies and one that has more flexible policies regarding who may attend the birth. If you strongly prefer a particular hospital, then ask for a list of obstetricians who work there.

ALTERNATIVE BIRTH CENTERS

We suggested that you ask hospitals if they have alternative birth centers (ABCs). (Different hospitals have different names for these facilities, such as "family birth center.") One purpose of these centers is to keep the family together at this very special time when a new member is arriving. It is assumed in the policy of the center that the father or other close friend or relative will stay to give you needed emotional support throughout labor and delivery. The baby will not be taken to the nursery unless s/he is having difficulties. The baby will stay with you for holding, loving, and generally getting acquainted.

Another purpose of ABCs is to help the mother achieve the relaxation and security she needs to give birth comfortably. Rather than the sterile, clinical setting of conventional labor and delivery rooms, the alternative birthing room will be rather homey (many people compare them to nice motel rooms). The room will be comfortably furnished with an ordinary bed and perhaps a couch or comfortable chairs for support people, pleasant wall decorations, and a private bathroom, ideally with a shower. In the regular labor and delivery suite, each nurse may be responsible for more than one patient. But in an ABC, it is likely that one nurse or nurse/midwife will stay with you, monitoring the progress of your labor and helping with breathing and contractions. This nurse will also be trained to care for your baby after s/he is born. In many labor and delivery units, the mother labors in one room, then transfers to a delivery bed or birthing chair. The transfer can be uncomfortable. After birth, mother and baby are moved again. In the ABC, the mother labors, gives birth, and recovers all in the same bed. Some medical procedures that may be routine in the regular facilities are dispensed with in the ABC, which does not use fetal monitors, IVs, and certain medications.

Alternative birth centers are for women who do not have any complications of pregnancy, such as diabetes or high blood pressure. Other health problems and some disabilities will preclude use of the birth center. If there is reason to think the baby may have problems, for example, if it is in breech position or seems to be undersized, then the alternative birth center would not be used. It is important to keep in mind that there is no guarantee you will ultimately give birth in an ABC, even if you meet the standards of the birth center, obtain your doctor's permission, and make all the necessary arrangements. If your health changes at any time during pregnancy, up to and including the moment you go into labor, you may have to change your plans. When a woman is admitted to the hospital, her blood pressure and temperature will be checked before she is sent to the ABC. If labor is not progressing normally, or if there are signs that the baby is in distress, the mother will be transferred out of the ABC.

Some people worry that in hospital-based ABCs (as opposed to home birth or free-standing birth centers), the staff may be biased toward doing medical procedures at the least possible indication. Others have found that in many hospitals, working in an ABC has deepened the staff's appreciation of natural childbirth. In these facilities, there may be little difference between giving birth in the ABC or in a regular labor room. For example, the staff in the labor room may encourage the mother to squat on the table rather than to lie on it, or allow her to give birth without moving to a delivery room.

In addition, there are a number of possible variations. We know a woman who was moved to a delivery room when it seemed that she might need assistance with forceps or suction. However, she was able to give birth without this assistance, and as soon as her episiotomy was repaired, she and her baby were returned to the ABC. At a local hospital which does not have an alternative birthing room, parents may arrange to have an additional nurse so that mother and baby can stay together after the birth. Some hospitals may omit the transfer from a labor bed to a delivery bed. You will learn the most about such possibilities not only by questioning hospital staff but by asking people who have used the hospital to tell you about their experiences.

There may be a free-standing birth center in your city. This type of center is physically separate from any hospital and is exclusively a childbirth facility. It should have the same professional staff as a hospital and the necessary equipment for normal birth and minor emergencies, and be near a regular hospital delivery unit in case the mother needs to be transferred.

Sometimes, a birth center will have an early release program, which allows you to go home within 12 hours after giving birth. Such a program should also provide for a home visit by a nurse on the third day after the birth.

HOME BIRTH

We know a number of women, all of them able-bodied except for a spinal-cord-injured woman interviewed for this book, who have had good experiences with home birth. However, many women have problems such as multiple pregnancy or high blood pressure, which require the facilities a hospital provides. It is clear to us that while home birth can be a good choice, it is a choice that demands very careful consideration.

First, think over your reasons for considering home birth. Some common reasons for choosing home birth are the following:

- A desire to keep the family together—to ensure that father and/or siblings will not be excluded from the birth, and that mother and infant will not be separated afterwards.
- The desire to maintain control of the birth process and avoid some unpleasant hospital routines.
- The conviction that childbirth is a safe, natural process and medical intervention is best avoided.
- The wish to have a midwife as the birth attendant. Many people feel that a midwife is most likely to give sensitive, personalized care.
- The desire to avoid the expense of a hospital birth. A normal uncomplicated home birth, whether attended by a physician or a midwife, is certainly less expensive than a hospital birth. However, you should consider the possibility that if complications do occur, delays will make treatment even more expensive.

Whatever your reason for considering home birth, understanding exactly what you want will help you decide if home birth is really best for you.

The concerns we just mentioned are the same ones motivating consumer demands that have caused changes in many hospitals all over the country. Many procedures which used to be routine are now done less frequently. You can infer from our list of suggested questions for hospitals that it is possible to have a satisfying childbirth experience in a hospital setting. You can ask some of those questions and find out whether a local hospital has features, such as nurse/midwives or permission for sibling visits, which also satisfy the goals you wish to achieve with home birth.

Certainly it is true that pregnancy and childbirth are natural processes, and a woman should not be treated as though her pregnancy is an illness. But it is also important to remember that "natural" does not automatically mean "safe." Another natural process is fever—it is your body's defense against invading germs—but a fever that rises too high is dangerous. Similarly, pregnancy usually poses no threats, and the associated physical changes serve useful purposes, but, occasionally, there are serious complications.

The question is, how safe is childbirth *for you?* For home birth, too, you need to begin by getting a medical opinion about your general health and the risks posed by your disability. You may want to delay discussing home birth with your doctor if you think this information will affect his/her evaluation of your general health. Once your general health has been assessed, you can explain that you are considering home birth and ask what s/he thinks the advantages and disadvantages might be. Remember, the course of a pregnancy can be unpredictable. We have a friend whose doctor was willing at first to attend a birth in her home, but, when her blood pressure became too high, advised her to give birth in the hospital. Since many changes can occur during 9 months, the decision to give birth at home is always somewhat tentative.

The question of where to give birth involves both practical and emotional considerations. We cannot give you the answer, but we want to emphasize again the importance of deciding carefully. Think about your goals. Investigate the potentials of both hospital and home birth, and compare the advantages and disadvantages of each situation. The more information you have, the clearer your answer will be. Some questions you may want to consider are discussed below.

Will home birth be convenient for me, considering my disability?

You may need help to change position during labor. At a hospital, staff should be available. Would there be people available to help you at home? At any hour? Would a birthing chair or other equipment at the hospital make labor significantly easier for you? Weigh any advantages against the advantages you are seeking from home birth.

Who will give prenatal care?/Who will attend the birth?

One possibility is a doctor, or doctor and midwife team. How will they share the task of caring for you? One common pattern is for the midwife to come to the mother's home when labor begins, and call the doctor when labor is well advanced and/or when problems arise.

If you want to work with an independent midwife, choose her as carefully as you would choose a doctor. If your state licenses midwives, find out what the licensing requirements are and decide whether they are the qualifications you want. Whether or not the state licenses midwives, talk to several mothers who have worked with the midwife. Be sure that midwifery is not illegal in your state.

Make sure you are comfortable with the midwife as a person. Meet her and have a long talk. Find out how flexible she is about working with your disability, just as you would with a doctor. Ask how she will care for you, and how the services she provides differ from a doctor's care. Discuss how to differentiate between normal pregnancy symptoms, signs of a problem pregnancy, and warning signs that your disability is causing problems.

Find out whether the independent midwife can refer you to a doctor. Possibly your regular doctor will cooperate in such matters as adjusting your medications or prescribing prenatal vitamins. At the very least, is there a doctor who will admit your midwife's clients to the hospital in emergencies? If not, a trip to the hospital could become a nightmare that involves waiting while emergency staff find a doctor for you.

How can you prepare for emergencies?

Ask the person(s) who will attend your birth what emergency equipment they can bring. Does it include oxygen, IV equipment, and saline solutions? The most dangerous complications of childbirth (again, excluding disability-related complications) are blood loss for the mother and oxygen deprivation for the infant. If you will not have emergency equipment, find out if it is available from paramedic or ambulance services. Find out *exactly* what emergency services are available in your community. A public librarian could help you locate such services or you could contact the fire department, since many paramedic units are attached to the city fire departments.

How far are you from the hospital?

The distance between your home and the hospital is an important factor to consider. We interviewed an emergency physician who found it very difficult to be precise about how close you should be. He did say that severe blood loss should be treated within 30 minutes, and he pointed out that part of this time might be spent getting an ambulance, transferring the person to the ambulance, and driving to the hospital. He stated very definitely that the further you are from the hospital, the greater the risks are from losing a lot of blood. He added that, after arrival at the hospital, saline solutions could be injected, but it would take time for blood typing before transfusions could be given. He suggested the precaution of going to the hospital early in labor for blood testing, then returning home to give birth.

Prolonged labor or difficulty in delivering the placenta are some of the less immediate emergencies that might occur. If you do not use an ambulance, you would need a car in good running condition, with a full gas tank, and somebody besides the doctor or midwife to drive.

MEETING OTHER HEALTH PROFESSIONALS

Your obstetrician may not be the only specialist you need to consult. In some situations, you may want to get a second opinion about a particular aspect of your care. For example, you may want to try vaginal delivery after a previous cesarean section, and you want more than one recommendation. It is always your right to get a second opinion. Your doctor can refer you to another physician. Or, if you are uncomfortable asking for this referral, use any of the methods suggested for selecting your obstetrician. Another source of information would be the National Second Opinion Hotline (see *Resource Directory* in Appendix B).

Anesthesiologists

An anesthesiologist is a physician who specializes in administering pain medications (and related medications) and monitoring the patient's response to these medications, usually during surgery. It is a good idea to visit an anesthesiologist whether or not you are planning to give birth by cesarean. Sometimes pain medications are used during vaginal birth as well, and the anesthesiologist can explain why anesthesia might be used and what the effects are of various medications, and determine which procedures are most appropriate for you. You may feel better prepared for this visit if you read the information about anesthesia in Chapters 7 and 8.

As we mentioned before, some hospitals require the permission of the anesthesiologist for the father to be present during surgery—permission you will want to obtain in case an unplanned cesarean section becomes necessary. Our consultant commented, "I could not agree more with the concept of talking ahead of time to one or more members of the anesthesia department before labor.... The secret to a happy outcome for everyone is communication and understanding between the mother, obstetrician and anesthesiologist."

She went on to say that most hospitals routinely allow the father to be present during cesareans performed under regional anesthesia, adding that most anesthesiologists would not want to be distracted by a father's presence while they are actually administering anesthesia, but would be comfortable allowing him in the delivery room during the baby's birth.

You or your physician(s) may need to give the anesthesiologist information beyond what is usually required. Be sure to ask the anesthesiologist to contact the doctor most knowledgeable about your disability. Heather's experience can give you an idea of the kind of advance planning you could do with your anesthesiologist. After anesthesia was given, Heather was instructed to lie flat on her back. She was very uncomfortable lying on her back without a pillow because she has a congenital hip dysplasia and scoliosis. But the doctor had given firm instructions that Heather should lie flat, and she had to put up an argument to get a pillow. By meeting an anesthesiologist ahead of time, she could have arranged for permission to use a pillow, or to lie on her side, since many hospitals allow patients to do this after receiving spinal anesthesia.

The anesthesiologist may also need time to schedule diagnostic tests that help to determine the choice of anesthetic. For example, women who have myasthenia gravis may need thyroid function tests and an electrocardiogram (a test of heart function).

Even if a cesarean is not planned, the information required for a C-section should be reviewed in case emergency surgery is needed. Faith, who has Friedreich's ataxia, had an unplanned cesarean birth. Since there was no time to determine whether spinal anesthesia would be safe for her, general anesthesia was used, and Faith was very disappointed that she was not conscious when her baby was born. If Faith had consulted with an anesthesiologist ahead of time, the anesthesiologist would have had time to investigate the options. If s/he still found that general anesthesia would be necessary, Faith would at least have known what to expect.

If you have spinal cord dysfunction, the anesthesiologist will need to examine you to learn the muscle tone and reflexes below the level of the lesion. If you need regional anesthesia for control of dysreflexia, or for surgery, this information can be used in monitoring your recovery.

You may have other kinds of questions for which you want answers as well. For example, you might have a friend who had headaches for several days after spinal anesthesia, and want to know if the same thing might happen to you. Some of what you hear and read about other people's experiences will not apply to you. You may hear about practices that are no longer in use, or you may hear about a person who has a rare allergic reaction to medication. The anesthesiologist can tell you how likely it is that you would have any problems that you are concerned about.

We suggest you get some information before you visit the anesthesiologist to help you pinpoint your questions. Besides written sources, you could get information from hospital classes about cesarean births, childbirth educators, or C-SEC, a support group for cesarean parents listed in the "Resource Directory" in Appendix B. Some questions you might want to ask are reviewed below. If it is not possible to consult directly with an anesthesiologist, discuss these questions with your obstetrician.

What are the advantages of each method of anesthesia? What are the risks of each method for myself and for the baby?

See Chapters 7 and 8 for a full discussion of these questions and the related issues of labor and delivery and cesarean section.

What can I expect to experience with each type of anesthesia?/What are the possible side effects?

Your contractions and the sensations you experience will be affected differently by different anesthetics. For example, people who have spinal anesthesia often notice that they cannot feel themselves breathing. The experience can be frightening until someone reassures them that it is normal.

If I need anesthesia, do you recommend a particular type?/What circumstances, if any, would change your recommendation?

You might also want to ask the anesthesiologist to explain the basis for any recommendation s/he makes. Our consultant advised us that most anesthesiologists would feel more comfortable giving regional anesthesia to a patient with a stable neurological condition, such as polio, than to one with a variable condition like MS. If there is any question about which anesthesia would be appropriate for you, the anesthesiologist could refer you to a specialist; you may also want to consult with the doctor who has treated your disability.

Tell the anesthesiologist if you strongly prefer one type of anesthesia.

If s/he recommends against it, ask any questions that help you understand why. If the anesthesiologist's recommendations are based on disability concerns, a consultation with your specialist may be helpful.

What information will you insert in my medical record?/What instructions will the staff will be given when I am admitted to the hospital?

Perhaps s/he would be willing to give you a copy. Then, if this doctor is unavailable at the time you give birth, you will know that you or your advocate can refer hospital staff to important information in your records.

What might be done differently by another doctor if you are not available when I give birth?

For example, Hilary was disappointed because, while the anesthesiologist she interviewed was willing to let her husband attend the birth, the one who attended was not. The anesthesiologist may be willing to insert information in your record that will explain any special arrangements you have discussed, and give you a copy of these remarks.

Perinatologists

A perinatologist's specialty is high-risk pregnancy. After obstetrical training, s/he spends 2 years gaining supervised experience in treating the most common complications of pregnancy, including placenta previa, multiple pregnancy, diabetes (diabetes may be pre-existing or the type that appears in pregnancy), high blood pressure, or a history of miscarriages or premature labor during previous pregnancies. Few of the women we interviewed saw perinatologists. Most who had sought one on their own found that this effort had been unnecessary, for their disabilities did not put them in a high-risk category.

A patient advocate in a high-risk clinic confirmed that physical disability does not in itself necessitate the services of a perinatologist. Not enough disabled people had been referred to the clinic for her to make generalizations about the appropriateness of their referrals. She mentioned congenital pelvic deformity as a disability that may cause a high-risk pregnancy; otherwise, she discussed how specific disabilities might affect or be affected by certain complications.

You have no need to consult a perinatologist unless there is reason to suspect you have a specific complication of pregnancy. If complications develop in the course of your pregnancy, your obstetrician might refer you to a perinatologist or a hospital high-risk center. In some situations, a perinatologist might become your primary doctor, in others, s/he would act as a consultant. Sylvia felt her perinatologist provided technical expertise, but did not offer the kind of empathy and reassurance her obstetrician provided. As a result, Sylvia considered her obstetrician to be her primary doctor.

Genetic Counselors

In Chapter 1 we explained that a genetic counselor can help you determine how likely it is that your child will have a disability, and can help you to explore your feelings about having a disabled child. You can ask your doctor for a referral for genetic counseling, or you can call any March of Dimes agency for information about where to find counseling. If you seek genetic counseling, you will be working with a team composed of doctors and/or ultrasound technicians who perform diagnostic tests, laboratory personnel who grow and analyze the fetal cells, and a genetic counselor.

The genetic counselor is likely to be the person you will work with most directly. The genetic counselor can recommend appropriate tests, possibly in consultation with your obstetrician or your family doctor. Later, the genetic counselor will explain your test results, and provide other information. An important part of the counselor's role is simply to give you emotional support as you absorb the information you're given and reach any necessary decisions. Because it is his or her job to assist you in the decision-making process, s/he should be accepting and non-directive. Arrange to have your counselor send a full report to your doctor, so that your doctor will have all the information necessary for your care. Be sure to discuss the counselor's report with your physician. Discussing this information with two advisers can help you to be sure that you understand your test results correctly.

Many genetic counselors stress the importance of working with an established genetic counseling center. They point out that the procedures for obtaining fetal cells can be done by many doctors, but the crucial step is the culturing and analysis of the cells in a reliable laboratory. Following are some questions you might want to ask when considering a particular genetic counseling center:

- *Are the counselors board-certified genetic counselors, or eligible for board certification?*
- *Does the center offer high-resolution ultrasound and chorionic villus sampling, as well as amniocentesis?* As the term suggests, high-resolution ultrasound provides more detailed images. Chorionic villus sampling is not as widely available as amniocentesis, but it is worth knowing whether the test is available.
- *How long have they been performing these tests? How many have they done?* If you have a choice between centers, you may prefer the one that is more established. However, what is most important is that the *staff* are experienced.
- *What is the miscarriage rate for amniocentesis performed at your center?* The rate at a good center is approximately 1 in 300. In deciding whether this test is appropriate, you will compare this risk with the known risks of your fetus having a particular disorder.
- *If the test results are uncertain or difficult to interpret, will the medical geneticist be available to help explain results?* The geneticist is a physician specializing in this field. Most likely s/he would work with the counselor in explaining test results to you.
- *How much experience does the center have with the particular disorder you are concerned about?* For example, there may be a staff member who is highly experienced in examining ultrasound images for evidence of cleft palate.
- *Who will perform the diagnostic test? How much experience has s/he had with the procedure?* If the center is attached to a school of medicine or a teaching hospital, the procedure may be performed by a resident under the supervision of another physician more experienced in the procedure. Some women might want to request that the procedure be done by a more experienced staff member.

ASSURING THAT YOUR NEEDS ARE MET BY HEALTH CARE PROVIDERS

You may have many unpleasant and even quite painful memories about your medical care, especially if you have had your disability since childhood. Long, anxious waits in crowded waiting rooms; hurried nurses; receptionists who ignored you; painful surgeries and lonely nights in hospital beds; embarrassing examinations by strangers; years of unanswered questions—these may be among your memories. If you add to these memories the vulnerability felt by any pregnant woman, you may feel very unenthusiastic about the idea of facing a new round of doctors, hospitals, tests, and examinations.

Whatever medical attention you need, you need to feel its providers are working *for* you, not *on* you. You need support in coping with your fears, as well as support for your desire to create and care for a new human being. Your tools for getting what you need are threefold:

- Your ability to communicate and plan ahead
- A treatment plan clearly agreed upon by you and your obstetrician
- The assistance of an advocate

When we asked a patient advocate at a university obstetrics clinic what was the most important advice she had to offer, her answer was one word, "Communicate!" Judi recalled an incident related to her by Sharon, who had visited that very clinic. Sharon was assisted in getting ready for an examination, then was left alone for a long wait in the examining room. The wait was not merely annoying but infuriating to Sharon, who is paraplegic and could *not* shift position or get off the examining table. She made a point of telling all concerned that she must not be left alone like that again. The advocate remembered appreciating Sharon's willingness to talk about her needs, and agreed that this incident was a perfect example of the kind of situation in which communication is all-important.

Chances are that you are a pioneer, one of the first disabled patients in your obstetrics clinic or maternity ward. By communicating your problems and needs, you will not only get what you need, but you will smooth the path for other disabled mothers-to-be. There is increasing professional recognition that patients are often the most knowledgeable about their disabilities. Nurses and others can do their jobs best if you make your needs clear. They will welcome the information you give them if you make comments such as, "Please check in with me if the doctor is delayed. Remember I'm stuck up here on this examining table," or, "May I have a pillow? With my scoliosis, I'll need it to lie the way you told me to." Remember, misunderstandings happen *very* easily. When Stacy gave birth, she had not yet made it clear that she had some pain sensation even though she was quadriplegic. When the obstetrician began to stitch Stacy's episiotomy without anesthesia, it *hurt!*

Find out who is the best person to contact for each problem or question. In your doctor's office, a nurse or health educator may answer most of your general questions about pregnancy, while the doctor is the one to ask about decisions relating to you alone. If your doctor refers you to a specialist, ask whether it is the specialist or your own doctor who will explain your test results. Many large clinics have patient advocates, and it is their job to help you make sure that your needs are met.

Advance planning can prevent much confusion and frustration. Obstetricians' schedules can be very erratic—appointments are often delayed while a doctor is detained at the hospital. It is a good idea to call ahead before leaving home and ask whether to come at the appointed time or later. *Do not* schedule other appointments too close together. If you must travel far, plan ahead for delays: Will you need to change your transportation plans or bring along a project to work on while you wait?

If you know you will be covering a lot of information during an appointment, bring along a pencil and paper or even a tape recorder. Keep a written list of your questions to ensure that you cover them all. It can be difficult to search your mind for one last question when your appointment started 20 minutes late.

Whenever you fill out forms, *keep copies*. Bring copies of medical questionnaires with you when you go to the hospital. Information can be misfiled even in the best-run hospital. You will not want to answer questions about your medical history between labor contractions!

Advance planning is a process that you will share with your obstetrician. As the months go by and you discuss a variety of concerns, you and your doctor will develop a more or less detailed plan of action for your childbirth. The important features of this treatment plan should be in written form and signed and dated by your doctor, and you should have a copy to bring with you to the hospital. This plan could include your doctor's instructions to the hospital staff for your care after you are admitted to the hospital. Some aspects of the plan may be specifically related to your disability. For example, you may be using a hospital where enemas are given early in labor (to prevent defecation during birth). If you are at risk for autonomic dysreflexia, your plan should state "no enema." If a nurse starts preparing to give you an enema, you or your advocate can refer the nurse to your doctor's instructions. A common hospital policy is that nothing should be taken by mouth once labor begins; but you may be taking antispasmodics, antibiotics to prevent bladder infections, or other medications that should not be interrupted. Your doctor can give instructions for you to continue your medications, or for you to be given medications by injection.

Other aspects of your treatment plan may deal with issues that concern any pregnant woman. For example, your doctor may agree that your baby can be given to you to hold and nurse right after the birth, rather than being sent straight to the nursery.

Perhaps not all of your treatment plan will be in your signed copy. It depends on what is comfortable for you and your doctor. In addition, some aspects of the plan might change with changing circumstances. For example, if your baby's breathing is irregular or if the pulse is abnormal, you will not be able to hold the baby right away, even if that was the original plan. Some aspects of your treatment plan serve as guidelines for what you may reasonably expect rather than as unalterable procedures.

At times you will want to share the task of assuring that your needs are met. The person you share this with is your advocate. The advocate may be your husband, your friend, or a health professional. The health professional should be someone with whom you are already comfortable and familiar. Your advocate should be someone who is comfortable helping you in the following ways:

- S/he may accompany you on some of your doctor visits. Many of us are uncomfortable asking questions or expressing our concerns. An articulate forthright advocate can help you express yourself. Your advocate may also help you to remember your doctor's explanations and instructions more clearly.
- An advocate may collect written information about your disability for others involved with your care.
- S/he may accompany you on a hospital tour, help you formulate your questions, and work with nursing staff to create special provisions for your care.
- Having an advocate is also very helpful when you are in labor. His or her role would not be the same as in other situations, so you may decide to choose a different person for this role. The advocate's (or coach's) role in labor will be covered in more detail in Chapter 6.

You and your advocate should discuss in advance how you will work together. It should be understood that, while you may want assistance in communicating your needs, *you* are in charge. You and your advocate can help other people see that you are competent and in charge. If, for example, someone asks your advocate a question they could have asked you, answer for yourself.

CLOSING COMMENTS
. . . .

We have discussed a number of issues pertinent to your medical care, and have provided questions you can ask others, and questions you can ask yourself. Answering them should help with all aspects of choosing a doctor: finding someone who is knowledgeable, who is willing to work in a team with you and other physicians, and with whom you feel comfortable. We hope we have simplified and clarified your task in making this choice. We have not tried to give you the "right" answers because, most important of all, we trust you to trust yourself.

4 EATING FOR TWO— NUTRITION IN PREGNANCY

The old saying, "A pregnant woman is eating for two," has a new meaning. It used to mean that a mother-to-be should eat an amount of food that would be enough for two people, but it has been criticized for sounding too much like an excuse for *over*-eating. Yet in one sense, a prospective mother *is* eating for two: She really does not need to eat much more food, but eating the *right* food is very important, and she will need to make good choices for herself and her baby. The difference is clear when you look at the National Research Council's recommendations for nutrition during pregnancy: While the Council recommends an increase of only about 12% in calorie consumption, it recommends a 67% increase in protein consumption, and increases in vitamin and mineral consumption ranging from 15% to 100%. A pregnant woman should not simply increase the *amount* of food she eats; she must make a point of choosing foods that will supply the additional protein, vitamins, and minerals she needs.

Good nutrition is not only vital to the baby's proper development but is important for the mother's health and comfort during pregnancy. So, when we explain the function of each nutrient, we will explain its role in fetal development as well as its value to the mother.

In addition to explaining basic nutritional requirements, we will discuss the special concerns of women with disabilities (including special diets, weight gain and its effects on mobility, and avoiding constipation); the nutrients required for a complete and balanced diet; ways to ensure that a vegetarian diet is adequate for pregnancy; allergies and food cravings; and foods

117

to avoid and limit. Foods that will help you meet the requirements outlined in this chapter are listed in Appendix A.

SPECIAL CONCERNS OF WOMEN WITH DISABILITIES

Women with disabilities have essentially the same nutritional needs as other pregnant women.There are a few minor differences, however, which are related to the effects of special diets and weight gain in women with disabilities.

Some disabled women try special diets in an attempt to alleviate disability symptoms. These diets are based on the idea that eating unusually large or small amounts of some nutrients may alter the body's chemistry. Many of these special diets are controversial, however, and women may hear about the same diet that it is beneficial, useless, or actually harmful. While an examination of these diets is too extensive an undertaking for this chapter, we would like to make one point, and that is that pregnant women should *not try these special diets without consulting a nutritionist.* A pregnant woman and a developing fetus have very specific nutritional needs, and unusual diets could be inadequate or even harmful. Michelle was thinking about trying a special diet she had read about to see if it would improve her MS, but she told us, "My doctor's nutritionist told me I was taking too much vitamin A for the baby." Michelle added that the nutritionist's advice made a significant difference in what she ate: "I would have tried another MS diet I'd heard about, but I found out my baby needs different vitamins."

If a woman has been told by her doctor to modify her diet in some manner related to her disability, she should ask early in her pregnancy whether she needs to change her diet again. It is even better to ask before pregnancy. Also, women who use medications regularly will need to ask their doctors whether to change medications. (For example, a pregnant woman needs more calcium than usual, and, since calcium interferes with the action of some antibiotics, she may need to change antibiotics.) Otherwise, the best plan for a pregnant disabled woman is to follow the nutritional guidelines given below. If she wants to consider modifying this diet, she should consult a nutritionist, or wait until after pregnancy.

Weight Gain

The recommendation that they increase their calorie intake during pregnancy may cause the most concern for women with disabilities. Many women with disabilities worry that weight gain during pregnancy will exacerbate some of their problems. For several women we interviewed, weight gain did, in fact, cause difficulties with mobility. Because the weight gained during pregnancy is not distributed evenly over the body, balance became more difficult for several women. Others found that joints which became painful with weight-bearing were further stressed during pregnancy. The increasing fatigue and clumsiness that all women begin to experience in the second trimester was of greater concern for many disabled women. Several women needed to start using canes or wheelchairs; others found that they simply could not accomplish their normal daily activities because they needed to slow down. If the weight gain is large, the loss of mobility may be even greater. Carla pointed out: "The first time I was pregnant, I gained 50 pounds. It caused a lot of back problems and my range of motion was less. The next time, I was much more nutrition-conscious. I only gained 30 pounds and I had a much easier time." Weight gain is also a factor in the increased risk of pressure sores during pregnancy, although this was not a problem for the women we interviewed, as we will explain below.

Some disabled women try to avoid loss of mobility by keeping their weight down. Pam, for example, was careful to keep her weight gain to 15 pounds. Minimizing weight gain can be a sensible strategy, but should be discussed with a doctor first. While a 15-pound gain may have been adequate for Pam, who is quadriplegic, it is well below the amount recommended for most women. Also, Pam's restricted diet may have contributed to her fatigue. Women who are thinking about restricting their weight gain should consult their doctor or nutritionist.

Because the need to maintain mobility is such a strong motivation to keep weight down, it is important for women with disabilities to understand why they need to gain at least 24 pounds while they are pregnant. Most of the weight increase represents growth of the mother's "products of pregnancy," as shown in Table 4.1.

The weight gain representing fetal growth is very important. It could be tempting to take the same approach as Patricia, who told us, "I actually lost weight at one point, because I was afraid the baby would be too big to go through my pelvis." There was a time when women were often advised to keep their weight down, with the hope that having smaller babies would make childbirth easier. However, more recent studies have shown this approach to be highly inadvisable. Good birth weight is a major indicator of an infant's health. Babies with very low weights (less than 5.5 pounds) are more vulnerable to illness and a number of neurological and learning problems.

Of course, some variation from the recommended weight gain of 24–32 pounds is natural and expected. Women who are underweight at the beginning of pregnancy may be advised to gain from 28 to 36 pounds, while those who are overweight may be advised to gain as little as 16–24 pounds. It may be necessary to modify the usual weight guidelines when considering whether a woman with disabilities is underweight, normal weight, or overweight. For example, a woman who has lost muscle mass from atrophy and

TABLE 4.1
PRODUCTS OF PREGNANCY

Products	Weight Increase (lbs)
Baby[a]	7.5
Placenta	1.0
Amniotic fluid	2.0
Uterine tissue	2.0
Increased blood supply	4.0
Breast growth[b]	3.0
Maternal reserves[c]	4.0–8.0
Total	24.0–28.0

[a]This represents average birth weight of infants.
[b]It should be remembered that, even if a woman does not intend to breast-feed, her breasts will grow, and she needs to eat accordingly.
[c]Reserves are a small amount of fat tissue needed to support the fetal growth spurt in late pregnacy, to provide the mother with energy during labor, and to provide energy during early lactation.

is underweight according to the charts, may be at a normal weight in all other respects. Thus, a woman who *appears* to be underweight might actually not be, and could suffer increased mobility problems, while deriving no benefit, from too great an increase in weight.

Keeping weight gain in the recommended range does not seem to be too difficult for most women. In several studies of maternal weight gain, the average gain was in the recommended range. Weight gain was also appropriate among the disabled women we interviewed. Most were able to remember approximately how much weight they had gained while pregnant. In 33 pregnancies, the average weight gain was 27.5 pounds. Weight gain ranged from 12 to 50 pounds, but for 26 out of 33 pregnancies, the range was between 20 and 40 pounds.

At least as important as the *amount* of weight gain is its *pattern*. A healthy pattern of weight increase is usually 4–6 pounds by the end of the first trimester, and roughly 1 pound a week for the remainder of the pregnancy. A sudden increase in weight can be a symptom of pre-eclampsia. During the first month or two of pregnancy, weight gain may be low as a result of the loss of appetite. However, a pregnant woman does not need to worry if she eats nutritious foods, and if she begins to gain weight normally by the end of the first trimester. (If her appetite is very poor, she may want

TABLE 4.2
DAILY NUTRITIONAL NEEDS DURING PREGNANCY

Nutrient	Nonpregnancy Need	Pregnancy Need
Calories	2,100 (approximate) (may be adjusted for age, height)	2,400 (approximate) (36–40 Cal/2.2 lbs body weight)
Protein	44 g	74–100 g
Vitamins		
Vitamin A	4,000 IU	5,000 IU
Vitamins B		
Folic Acid	400 mcg	800 mcg
Niacin	13 mg	15 mg
Riboflavin	1.2 mg	1.5 mg
Thiamine	1.1 mg	1.5 mg
B6	2.0 mg	2.6 mg
B12	3.0 mcg	4.0 mcg
Vitamin C	60 mg	80 mg
Vitamin D	200–400 IU	400–600 IU
Vitamin E	8 mg	10 mg
Minerals		
Calcium	800 mg	1,200 mg
Phosphorus	800 mg	200 mg
Iron	18 mg	18 mg from food, plus 30–60 mg supplement
Iodine	150 mcg	175 mcg
Magnesium	300 mg	450 mg
Zinc	15 mg	20 mg

to ask her doctor to prescribe a prenatal vitamin.) The slight increase in calories recommended in Table 4.2 will support the slow, steady weight increase that is normal in healthy pregnancies.

Vitamins and Minerals

Some vitamins and minerals that are known to be important to health are not well enough understood to warrant special recommendations for pregnant women. Because very small increases in some of those minerals may actually be toxic, pregnant women are usually advised not to take supplements that would exceed the amounts recommended for all adults. In general, these nutrients are abundant in foods which are rich in nutrients for which there are recommendations. Two important nutrients not mentioned in Table 4.2 are water and sodium (found in table salt). These are discussed in the following section concerning nutritional requirements and their basis.

THE "WHAT" AND "WHY" OF NUTRITIONAL REQUIREMENTS

Calories

Both the mother and the fetus are growing new tissue, and energy is required to support this growth. Many studies have shown that growth of the fetus and the placenta are impaired when a pregnant woman restricts calories in her diet.

Calories are a measure of the energy supplied by foods. In addition to eating enough to meet her energy requirements, the mother also needs to assure "protein sparing." If a woman's diet does not include enough calories, her body will start breaking down proteins to provide the energy she needs. She cannot afford to have this happen, because the protein is needed for building the tissues described in Table 4.1.

It is easy to add the necessary 300 calories by simply eating more foods which are rich in recommended nutrients. For example, if a woman who does not ordinarily drink milk simply adds a quart of fortified skim milk to her daily diet, this will supply all the calcium she needs, significant amounts of vitamins and protein, and 360 calories. A chicken thigh (from a fryer) adds 237 calories, most of the minimum additional protein (29.1 g), and a third of the riboflavin requirement (0.48 mg). A 6-oz serving of cooked red beans, at 236 calories, provides significant amounts of iron and calcium and almost 15 g of protein.

Fluids

All body tissues contain a large amount of water, so a woman needs to drink plenty of water to support her growth and the growth of the fetus. Drinking enough water also helps to prevent the dry, itchy skin that bothers many pregnant women. Pregnant women urinate more frequently, so they need more water for the health of their kidneys and urinary system. Drinking enough water helps prevent urinary infections and heartburn, and may also prevent or relieve constipation by keeping the stools soft.

Women who have disabilities that make them susceptible to bladder infections have even more reason to try to prevent infections by drinking plenty of water. Sylvia recalled, "I drank two or three times as much as usual, and I didn't have any problems with bladder infections." Those women who are unable to exercise may already have problems with constipation, which could become worse during pregnancy. They, too, need to be careful to drink plenty of water.

How much is enough? The equivalent of eight 8-oz glasses of water daily is sufficient for most women. That amount might seem like a lot at first, but it helps to remember that you are not restricted to drinking only plain water. Milk, fruit juice, broth, and coffee substitutes all provide plenty of water.

Protein

Proteins are the essential building blocks of the body. Every living cell contains protein; it is in all tissues—muscles (including heart and digestive tract), skin, blood, organs (kidneys, liver, etc.), even hair and nails. The 75–100 g of protein every pregnant woman needs daily are required for fetal growth, as well as the growth of the maternal tissues described in Table 4.1. Protein is found not only in meat, eggs, and dairy products but in a variety of vegetable foods, as is discussed in the section entitled "Vegetarian Diet." Complete and incomplete proteins are also discussed in that section.

Some research studies indicate a possible relationship between protein deficiency and pregnancy-induced hypertension (high blood pressure), but other studies contradict this finding. Women who follow the daily eating plan at the end of this chapter need not be concerned about their protein intake, for they will be getting all they need.

Many disabled women have an additional reason to make sure they eat enough protein-rich foods—prevention of pressure sores. Disabled women are often warned that they have an increased risk of pressure sores when they are pregnant because of their increased weight. This risk may be reduced by ensuring that they get enough protein to keep their skin in good condition.

Minerals

Sodium

One important function of sodium is maintenance of the body's fluid balance. It was once thought that excess sodium contributed to *edema* (swelling) and *toxemia* (a pregnancy-related illness we will describe in Chapter 6). That is why many of us have heard our mothers mention that they had been on salt-restricted diets while they were pregnant.

More recent studies showed that some increased sodium retention, and moderate edema, are normal responses to both the increase in blood volume and some hormonal changes associated with pregnancy. Also, some researchers have observed *hyponatremia* (low blood sodium) in the infants of mothers who had been on severely salt-restricted diets. Thus, your physician will not necessarily recommend that you restrict salt.

While pregnant women, like other adults, should avoid eating large amounts of salty foods, such as pickles and potato chips, they usually do not need to make a special effort to restrict or supplement their salt. Sodium is abundant in many foods, and using table salt for seasoning will help women get the 1–3 g of salt they need daily. (Reading a few food labels will show how easy it is to find salt in food.) Women who find themselves craving salt (sometimes because they had been avoiding salt before pregnancy) can satisfy the craving by occasionally salting healthy foods, and should consult their doctors if the craving continues. Iodized salt is also a good source of dietary iodine.

Iodine

Iodine is a constituent of a very important hormone, thyroxine, which regulates the rate of chemical reactions that produce energy. A pregnant woman uses more oxygen and nutrients, and the increase of thyroxine and other hormones makes this change possible. Iodine is also needed for the fetus to grow normally.

Not only will lack of iodine in the maternal diet make the mother sick, but iodine deficiency is a factor in *cretinism*, a birth defect characterized by growth retardation, mental retardation, and a number of physical abnormalities. Excess iodine also causes birth defects. When birth defects in humans have been caused by iodine, the culprit was not excess dietary iodine, but iodine-containing medications for bronchitis and asthma.

While many seafoods are rich in this mineral, the most reliable way to get iodine is to use iodized table salt. Women should make sure that they do not purchase rock salt (some types contain iodine and some do not), sea salt, or any salt which is not labeled "iodized."

Calcium and Phosphorus

Calcium plays many important roles in the body's functioning, but the main reason for eating more calcium-rich foods during pregnancy is to provide enough calcium for fetal development of teeth and bones. Early in pregnancy, hormonal changes cause a woman's body to retain more calcium than usual. In this way, her body builds a reserve supply of calcium which can be used when the fetal skeleton mineralizes in the third trimester. So, even though the fetus is not absorbing much calcium until late in the pregnancy, the mother should be eating plenty of calcium from the beginning. For people who cannot have milk products, we will list other calcium-rich foods.

Calcium combines with phosphorus to make the crystal, hydroxy-apatite, which hardens bones and teeth. Phosphorus is so common in so many foods that nutritionists do not make special recommendations concerning phosphorus-rich foods. In fact, it is possible to eat too much phosphorus in proportion to calcium. While vitamin D helps to counteract a calcium/phosphorus imbalance, it is a good idea to avoid such phosphorus-rich foods as processed meats, snack foods, and cola drinks, which are foods that should also be avoided because they contain too much fat, salt, or sugar.

Studies have shown that babies of mothers who did not get enough calcium have lower bone densities than those born to well-nourished mothers. It has been theorized that severe calcium deficiencies, especially over several pregnancies, may also cause loss of calcium from the *mother's* bones, but not all studies support this theory.

Although the research is not conclusive, there is some evidence that the calf-muscle cramps that bother many pregnant women may be relieved by calcium supplements. Women who are bothered by leg cramps might ask their doctors if calcium supplements are advisable. If a woman's disability already makes her susceptible to muscle spasms, as cerebral palsy does, then during pregnancy she may experience much stronger and more painful leg cramps than other women. Clara's cramps were so intense that only a strong person could flex her foot enough to ease the spasm. Clara said, "I was having lots of problems with leg cramps and when I started taking calcium pills the cramps got better." Antacids, which contain calcium, are an inexpensive supplement and are also handy for women who have heartburn. But taking too many antacid tablets can be harmful, so it is a good idea to check with a doctor. It may be important to control the amount of calcium by following a doctor's prescription.

Iron

Iron is part of the hemoglobin that is found in red blood cells. Hemoglobin carries oxygen throughout the body. A pregnant woman needs iron for the red cells in her increased blood supply, and the fetus needs iron for making hemoglobin.

If the mother becomes anemic—lacking in hemoglobin—she is more easily exhausted and more easily stressed. In addition, an anemic woman is less able to tolerate blood loss during delivery.

It is also possible for women who are not anemic to be iron deficient. In this case, they have enough hemoglobin, but the iron stored outside red blood cells is insufficient.

In early pregnancy, the fetus of an anemic mother can usually obtain enough iron for its developing blood supply. However, the fetus may not build up a good iron reserve, so a premature baby of an anemic mother is also likely to be anemic. Unless the mother's iron deficiency is very severe, the hemoglobin levels in full-term infants will probably be unaffected. However, their iron reserves may be low, and they will have a greater tendency to develop anemia during their first year.

Iron is the only nutrient listed in Table 4.2 for which a supplement is recommended. While it is not too difficult for non-pregnant women to get enough iron from foods, pregnant women cannot get enough without consuming a huge amount of calories. One third to one half of those pregnant women who do not use supplements become anemic. For most pregnant women, the iron included in a prenatal vitamin is enough to prevent anemia if the label states that it contains 30–60 mg of elemental iron. Women who are not anemic need to avoid taking more iron, since too much iron can interfere with the absorption of other nutrients, such as zinc.

Unfortunately, iron tablets cause stomach upset and/or constipation in many women. Some doctors recommend that women who are not anemic should wait until they are 20–24 weeks pregnant before starting to take iron tablets. At that time, indigestion is usually not as much of a problem for the mother, and the fetus is just beginning to build up its iron reserves. Taking the iron tablet with meals or at bedtime helps many women to avoid indigestion. Exercise, fluids, and high-fiber foods like vegetables and prune juice can help with constipation. Laxatives should not be used, except products which add bulk, such as Metamucil. Women who continue to have indigestion or constipation should tell their doctors, because different types of iron supplements are available, and the doctor may suggest a change.

Women with rheumatoid arthritis are often anemic. Iron supplements will not improve the anemia associated with arthritis. However, women who develop pregnancy-related anemia in addition to arthritis-associated anemia can minimize their problem by taking their iron tablets faithfully. Women with immobilizing disabilities who become anemic are more susceptible to pressure sores, and to infection from pressure sores.

Many women whose disabilities make it difficult to exercise have problems with constipation. Like Portia, they may find that their usual problems get worse when they are pregnant. They could be tempted to avoid taking iron tablets because they are afraid of making their constipation still worse. We urge them to resist the temptation and work with their doctors to find other solutions (such as injectable forms of iron).

Magnesium and Zinc

While zinc and magnesium are known to have important roles in metabolism, their functions in pregnancy are not fully understood. Zinc deficiency is clearly associated with birth defects in animals, and there is evidence that the same is true for humans. Therefore, pregnant women who are using vitamin and mineral supplements should use a supplement containing zinc.

Vitamins

Vitamins A, C, and E

Each of these vitamins has several functions. One important function of these vitamins is that they contribute to maintaining the integrity of some tissues. Vitamin A helps maintain epithelial tissues—including skin and the linings of the urinary, respiratory, and digestive systems. Vitamin C is involved in maintenance of connective tissues, such as cartilage. Vitamin E protects the membranes of individual cells and helps to maximize the absorption of vitamin A in the intestine.

These vitamins are usually well supplied in food, so it is rare to find people deficient in them. In some studies, women with comparatively low blood levels of vitamin C were found to have a higher incidence of premature births; other studies contradict those findings. On the other hand, when a woman takes large amounts of vitamin C during pregnancy, her fetus may become so dependent on the vitamin that after birth it develops scurvy, a deficiency disease.

There is strong evidence that both too little and too much vitamin A will cause birth defects.

B Vitamins

Thiamine, riboflavin, and niacin are all important in energy production. It is known that severe deficiencies of thiamine can cause babies to be born with deficiency disease. Deficiencies of thiamine and riboflavin have been associated with extreme vomiting in early pregnancy.

Folic acid, vitamin B_6, and vitamin B_{12} are involved in a number of chemical processes. Folic acid and vitamin B_{12} are especially important in cell division. Vitamin B_6, sometimes independently and sometimes in combination with niacin, is involved in building proteins. Folic acid is involved in the synthesis of hemoglobin, and lack of folic acid causes one type of anemia. The levels of these nutrients change during pregnancy, but the processes involved are still not clearly understood, and no definite effects of vitamin deficiency on fetal development are known. Still, it is clearly important to eat enough foods rich in these vitamins, since they are involved in growth processes which accelerate during pregnancy.

Vitamin D

Vitamin D is involved in the absorption of calcium, and it is needed for proper calcification of teeth and bones. Vitamin D deficiency is associated with malformed teeth and bones and other problems in newborns. For the fetus to get enough Vitamin D, the mother must obtain enough from her diet and from exposure to sunlight. While it is not clear how an excess of vitamin D affects the fetus, it is known that too much vitamin D in the diet can lead to bone demineralization.

Finding the Right Balance

Reading a list of nutritional requirements, not to mention hearing people talk about how good vitamins are for us, could easily tempt us to run to the grocery store and buy lots of little bottles of various vitamin and mineral tablets. That is not necessary! While we have described what can happen with *extreme* excess or deficiency of some vitamins, the fact is that such deficiencies are very rare. A well-balanced diet will meet most nutritional requirements, and the prenatal vitamins or iron supplements that many doctors prescribe are all that should be added to a well-balanced diet. In Appendix A, we provide information on the basic food groups and how to use them to obtain a well-balanced diet.

Vitamin and mineral supplements must be used with care, both because excesses of some nutrients are toxic, and because vitamins and minerals which work together (like calcium, phosphorus, and vitamin D, or vitamin B_6 and niacin) must be present in correct proportions. Getting the right combination of vitamins and minerals is a little like getting a treasured cake recipe from a friend. If you tinker with the recipe too much, the cake won't come out right—too much baking soda makes the cake run over the sides of the pan; substituting butter for oil changes the texture. Using the correct recipe—an adequate diet and well-balanced vitamin supplement—is an important step in assuring a healthy pregnancy.

VEGETARIAN DIETS

Vegetarians may need to change their eating habits somewhat when they become pregnant. The main challenge is to get enough protein from a vegetarian diet. Four of the women interviewed for this book are vegetarians, but they all ate meat while they were pregnant. Sharon said that talking to a nutritionist influenced her decision to change her diet. Sylvia said, "I went from vegetarian to eating *everything*. I craved salty meat.... After the baby was born I was a vegetarian again; I didn't even want meat. But I just couldn't do it while I was pregnant."

Women who eat fish and/or milk and eggs can easily get all the protein they need. Those who avoid all animal products will have more difficulty getting enough protein. They should use the protein combinations listed in Table 4.3 to be sure that they are eating complete proteins.

Proteins are chains of different types of amino acids. Humans need eight different amino acids. A protein chain containing each of the eight essential amino acids is a *complete protein*, while a chain containing only some of the eight is an *incomplete protein*. Animal proteins are complete, but vegetable proteins are incomplete. By combining foods from the vegetable protein, bread and cereal, and milk product food groups (see *Appendix A*), vegetarians can improve the quality of the protein in their diet. Some combinations are better than others. For example, beans and cornmeal are a better combination than beans and peanuts. Combining grain and beans, as in a bean burrito or by eating bean soup with bread, provides complete protein. Table 4.3 presents some particularly nutritious protein combinations.

TABLE 4.3
COMPLETE VEGETABLE PROTEIN COMBINATIONS

Beans	+	Milk products
Beans	+	Cornmeal or tortillas
Beans	+	Rice
Milk	+	Rice, wheat, or potato
Wheat	+	Beans
Wheat	+	Peanuts
Wheat	+	Milk
Peanuts	+	Milk
Rice	+	Sesame (including sesame butter, "tahini")
Rice	+	Soy products

These combinations are found in many comfortable, familiar forms, especially if you enjoy some ethnic foods. Many of these ingredients are also among the calcium-rich foods. Sample meals might include the following: a peanut butter sandwich with whole-grain bread and a glass of milk; scalloped potatoes; burritos (made with corn tortillas) and cheese; pita bread with falafel and tahini sauce; rice pudding; red beans and rice; bean soup with whole-grain biscuits or cornbread.

Vegetarian diets also tend to be low-calorie diets, so it is important to eat enough food so that protein in the diet is spared for building new tissue. Sometimes vegetarians need to make a point of eating energy-dense foods. For example, substituting dried fruit for some fresh fruit, or a serving of cheese for a serving of milk, will add calories without making one feel too full.

Iron is also difficult to obtain in a vegetarian diet, so vegetarians will need to use the same iron supplements non-vegetarians use.

Since strict vegetarian diets also tend to be low in calcium and vitamin B_{12}, supplements are often recommended. Nutritional yeasts and some fortified soy products contain vitamin B_{12}, but women who dislike these foods should consider taking supplements.

A woman who is on a strict vegetarian diet needs to consult a nutritionist because it is complicated to get good prenatal nutrition from such a diet.

ALLERGIES AND CRAVINGS
. . . .

Like vegetarians, women with milk allergies can find nondairy sources of calcium in the list of calcium-rich foods in Appendix A. They might also consider using calcium supplements. Generally, allergies should not pose a problem because most nutrients are contained in a variety of foods. For example, a woman with citrus allergies can get plenty of vitamin C from other fruits and vegetables, such as cantaloupe and broccoli. (The lists in Appendix B should make it easy for you to find acceptable sources of recommended nutrients.)

What should be done about food cravings depends on what is craved. It is not true that a food craving is your body telling you what you need. Some women experience *pica*—a strong desire to eat nonfoods like ice, paint chips, or clay. Women with pica should have their doctors check for some underlying problem. But food cravings can be indulged a little bit, as long as eating the desired foods does not diminish an appetite for other nutritious foods. A craving for fresh fruit will not hurt anybody, and neither will an *occasional* scoop of ice cream.

WHAT TO AVOID OR LIMIT

Smoking

Babies born to smokers tend to be smaller, and to have more health problems, than those born to nonsmokers. Smoking harms the fetus both directly and indirectly. When the mother smokes, nicotine and other toxins enter her blood and cross the placenta to the fetus. Each time a mother smokes, her blood vessels constrict, and the change in blood flow probably reduces the amount of oxygen and nutrients available to the fetus. Over time, smoking damages the placenta, probably enough to interfere with nourishment of the fetus. Furthermore, smokers are more likely to suffer a variety of complications of pregnancy, including placenta previa, premature rupture of membranes, and placental abruption—all of them dangerous to both mother and fetus.

It is never too late to stop smoking! Women who stop smoking during pregnancy are less likely to have placental problems than those who continue to smoke.

Women who cannot stop smoking should know that nicotine enters breast milk and that there have been cases of babies getting nicotine poisoning from their mothers' milk. Also, babies with allergies or asthma will be affected by side-stream smoke.

Some women would not dream of smoking tobacco during pregnancy, but think that smoking marijuana is safe. It may not be. Studies suggest that maternal exposure to marijuana leads to behavioral changes in animal and human newborns, as well as physical changes in animals. Smoking marijuana can also interfere with milk production.

Alcohol

Heavy drinking leads, at worst, to fetal alcohol syndrome (FAS) in which the newborn has growth retardation, mental retardation, and certain typical physical deformities. Many infants who do not have full-blown FAS still have severe health problems, including some of the symptoms of FAS, as well as alcohol addiction at birth.

There is evidence that smaller amounts of alcohol may cause more subtle changes, especially behavioral and emotional changes. However, the effects of moderate drinking are difficult to assess for three reasons:

1. Different studies have used different definitions of "moderate" drinking.
2. Mental and behavioral functioning, which are not always easy to assess, have been studied in different ways and at different times. For example, it can be difficult to determine whether a newborn who is not very responsive has been affected by prenatal drinking, or by anesthetics used during childbirth.
3. Studies cannot take into account possible differences in fetal susceptibility to alcohol.

Still, when all studies are taken together, it is clear that even moderate drinking is risky. Health professionals advise pregnant women to stop drinking alcohol altogether.

Coffee, Tea, and Herbal Teas

Studies of the effect of caffeine on the fetus have given variable results. In animal studies, it has taken huge amounts of caffeine—the equivalent of 12–40 cups of coffee a day in humans—to cause birth defects. Some recent studies suggest a relationship between heavy coffee drinking and lowered birth weight. Many people feel that the safest course is to avoid coffee and tea. Drinking decaffeinated beverages could be an acceptable compromise.

Women who have a hard time giving up caffeine can make sure they drink no more than one cup of coffee a day. This amount is unlikely to harm the fetus, and it gives the mother a chance to taper off. To avoid caffeine completely, check the labels of soft drinks and pain medications, because many of them contain caffeine.

It is not necessarily true that herbal teas are more "natural" or safe. After all, coffee is the extract of a plant seed; ordinary tea is brewed from leaves. Digitalis, a powerful heart medication, comes from foxglove root. Warfarin, which comes from a native American plant, is used in low concentrations as anticoagulant medicine, and overdoses are lethal. Even cocaine and heroin come from plants! No doubt many herbal teas are safe, but one also has to consider the possibility that a tea which does not seem to affect the mother can affect the fetus.

There are some hot drinks which may be used as alternatives to coffee and tea: roasted grain coffee substitutes such as Pero and Postum; hot water with honey and lemon; "teas" brewed from spices such as ginger, cinnamon, anise, and orange peel.

Medications

The entire subject of the safety of medications is extremely complicated. A blanket recommendation to avoid all medications is not appropriate, because the side effects of a medicine may not be as dangerous as the symptoms it treats. For example, you might decide not to take medicine for a mild headache, but you *must* take something for a high fever, because prolonged fever endangers the fetus. (We will discuss this problem in more detail in Chapter 6). The best (if not perfect) solution is not to take *any* medicine without a doctor's advice. This includes nonprescription medications which seem harmless—there is even a case on record of a baby born with FAS because the cough syrup the mother had been using contained alcohol (not all brands do)!

Sometimes people wonder whether they can save money by substituting a cheaper medication for one which has been prescribed. When a pharmacist asks if you would prefer a *generic* medicine, s/he is referring to a less expensive medicine which is similar to the one prescribed. However, many patients report to their doctors that some generic substitutes seem less effective. So, if you might want to use a generic medicine, ask your doctor whether that is acceptable at the time s/he gives you a prescription. Possibly you and your doctor will decide to try both forms of the medication, and see if there is a difference in their effects. In some cases, your doctor may have already learned from experience whether it is feasible to use the generic medication.

The same principles that apply to nonprescription medications also apply to herbal teas and/or alternative remedies—*avoid them!* If they work, they may also have harmful side effects.

"Empty Calorie" Foods

These are foods that do not provide significant amounts of nutrients like vitamins, minerals, or protein, but do provide lots of calories from fat or sugar. Examples of empty calorie foods are soft drinks (which may also contain caffeine or excess phosphorus), chips, most crackers (read package ingredients), candy, cookies, and cakes. Even fruit pies have lots of fat in the crust. Ice milk, frozen yogurt, and "light" ice creams are preferable to ice cream, but still have plenty of sugar. Snack meats and soft cheeses have too much fat in comparison to protein, and often contain too much salt as well.

Besides not being nutritious enough in themselves, these foods can make a woman feel too full to eat the foods she really needs. Let empty calorie foods be occasional treats.

CLOSING COMMENTS
. . . .

Eating a balanced diet during pregnancy offers a number of benefits. It is an opprtunity to make an improvement in your eating habits that can last for the rest of your life. It contributes to your health and comfort during pregnancy. For many women, the greatest benefit is the knowedge that they are doing all they can to assure the growth and health of their babies.

5 GETTING IN SHAPE—
EXERCISES FOR PREGNANCY

In this chapter, we present exercises for women who have a variety of disabilities. There really is something for everyone! For each exercise, we describe variations for women with differing functional abilities. We often begin by describing a variation in which a partner or attendant assists with the exercise, and then offer increasingly challenging versions of each exercise.

A great advantage of exercising is its contribution to a general sense of well-being. Studies have shown that, after exercise, a person's blood contains more endorphins (natural chemicals associated with feelings of pleasure and happiness).

Exercise during pregnancy is important for a number of specific reasons:

- By maintaining strength and flexibility, exercise helps maintain the ability to perform such daily activities as transferring.
- Exercise can preserve and even increase muscle strength, as well as help maintain endurance.
- Exercise can help a woman to feel more comfortable walking and standing as her weight increases, and prepare her for the physical exertion of giving birth.
- Blood volume increases significantly during pregnancy, and exercise can help assure that the circulatory system continues to function well.
- Pregnancy hormones loosen the ligaments, so it is important to strengthen the back and abdominal muscles to keep pelvic joints stable.
- Exercise can keep other joints flexible.

135

- Appropriate exercises can prevent or reduce many pregnancy discomforts: muscle spasms in the calves ("charley horses"), back pain, groin pain, shortness of breath, constipation, and, for women with edema, tingling and numbness in the arms.
- Pelvic and abdominal muscles that have been strengthened by exercise during pregnancy are likely to recover more quickly after childbirth.
- Strengthening exercises can be good preparation for the physical demands of childcare.

It is important to do more than one type of exercise. Stretching exercises alone cannot maintain strength, while strengthening exercises alone can actually reduce flexibility of the joints (think of muscle-bound athletes). A balanced exercise program includes four types of exercises:

- General conditioning or endurance exercise
- Strengthening exercise
- Relaxation exercise
- Flexibility exercise

Often, a single flexibility exercise may be described as either a stretching exercise or a range-of-motion exercise: a stretching exercise is a movement that lengthens muscle fibers; a range-of-motion exercise is a movement that enhances the range of motion of a joint. For example, some range-of-motion exercises assure that the elbow bends and straightens as fully as possible. Relaxation exercises ease or prevent muscle pain and improve circulation (blood flow is better in relaxed muscles).

Stretching exercises often feel relaxing, so we have placed those stretching exercises which relieve specific pregnancy discomforts in one section, and included other stretching exercises in the section titled "Relaxation Exercises." The stretching and relaxation exercises in this chapter can help a woman prepare to use the techniques which have been developed for relaxation during childbirth.

It is important that each woman do whatever exercise she can. Women who cannot do strengthening or conditioning exercises will still benefit from relaxation and active or assisted range-of-motion exercises. **Active** exercise refers to exercise a woman performs independently; **assisted** exercise refers to exercise in which another person moves her body. Since no stretching exercise is active in the sense of requiring voluntary contraction of the affected muscles, these exercises are described as **assisted** or **unassisted**.

Exercises for pregnant women should follow certain safety guidelines. Exercise patterns which are safe and appropriate for non-pregnant women may not be equally safe for women who have undergone the physical and physiological changes of pregnancy. Many pregnancy changes continue to affect women for several weeks after birth, so they must continue to modify their exercise during this period. It is also important to remember that the fetus is affected by changes in the mother's body. Both the American College of Obstetricians and Gynecologists (ACOG) and the American Physical Therapy Association have offered recommendations for appropriate exercise during pregnancy. The recommendations are designed to assure the safety of the mother and the fetus.

A number of physiological changes affect the kinds of exercises women should do during and after pregnancy:

- Joints are more vulnerable to injury because of hormonal effects on connective tissue.
- The growth of the uterus and breasts changes the body's center of gravity and increases strain on the lower back and hip joints.
- The increase in blood volume affects heart function, so pregnant women must exercise less vigorously. Sedentary women and women with anemia must be even more careful not to stress their hearts.
- Late in pregnancy, as uterine growth presses upward, the space occupied by the lungs is reduced. Pregnant women are able to breathe in enough oxygen at rest and during mild exercise, but cannot breathe as efficiently during prolonged, intense exercise.
- Pregnant women become dehydrated more easily.
- The basal body temperature is higher during pregnancy. This temperature increase, coupled with the temperature increase occurring during prolonged, heavy exercise, may be cause for concern since fetal development is affected by temperature changes.
- Blood sugar levels are lower among pregnant than non-pregnant women, and overly strenuous exercise could lower blood sugar still more.
- The fetal heart rate is affected by maternal exercise, and it seems wise to avoid prolonged exercise sessions.

Because of these normal changes, all healthy, pregnant women need to follow the exercise guidelines listed in Tables 5.1 and 5.2.

Specific health problems or pregnancy complications may also make it necessary for a woman to avoid exercise. Women who have one or more of the health problems listed in Table 5.3 should *always* avoid strenuous exercise.

Women who have one or more of the health problems listed in Table 5.4 should be evaluated by their physicians and/or physical therapists. They may be advised to limit exercise, or to avoid specific types of exercises.

Women with disabilities may be advised to modify their exercise program for specific reasons. For example, a woman with MS, who must be especially careful to avoid fatigue, may be advised to shorten periods of intense exercise. In some cases, exercises appropriate for those with a disability may have to be avoided because of pregnancy considerations. Leslie was advised to do range-of-motion exercises, but even these mild exercises stimulated uterine contractions. Because she was already at risk for premature labor, Leslie had to discontinue her exercise.

TABLE 5.1
SAFETY GUIDELINES FOR EXERCISE DURING PREGNANCY AND POSTPARTUM PERIOD

Pregnancy and Postpartum

- Women who are not used to exercising should begin slowly, and very gradually increase exercise intensity.
- If a woman experiences any unusual symptoms, including the caution symptoms mentioned below, she should stop exercising and contact her physician.
- Exercise regularly (three times a week), not intermittently. [a]
- To avoid raising body core temperature, do not exercise in hot, humid weather or when sick with fever.
- Exercise on a firm, but not hard surface, such as a carpeted floor, and avoid bouncy, jerky motions, or rapid swinging movements.
- Avoid exercises which strain pelvic floor or abdominal muscles.
- Avoid extreme bending or stretching of joints. If soreness or discomfort lasts more than 60 minutes after exercising, the stretch was too much.
- Warm up before vigorous exercise with activities like slow walking. After exercising, cool down with *gentle* stretching.
- Check heart rate during exercise. Do not exceed recommended limits (see Table 5.2) .
- Always rise from the floor slowly, and exercise legs briefly after rising, to avoid sudden blood pressure changes.
- Avoid dehydration: drink plenty of water before and after exercising, and stop to rest during exercise if necessary.
- Women at risk for, or who have had, cesarean surgery can have appropriate exercises prescribed, and refer to *Chapter 9.*
- Exercises in the knee-to-chest position are inappropriate postpartum.

Pregnancy Only

- Check heart rate during exercise. Heart rate should *not* go higher than 140 beats per minute.
- Strenuous exercise should not last longer than 15 minutes.
- After the fourth month, avoid prolonged exercise while lying on the back. (If a woman lies on her back too long, the weight of the uterus on major blood vessels will interfere with circulation.)
- Avoid the Valsalva maneuver—holding the breath and pushing as if defecating. Instead, breathe rhythmically during exercise.
- Maternal temperature should not rise higher than 38°C (100.4°F).

Caution symptoms: When a woman experiences any of these signs or symptoms, she should stop exercising and contact her physician—pain, bleeding, dizziness, faintness, shortness of breath, rapid heart rate or palpitations, back pain, pubic pain, or increased difficulty walking.

[a]If you must exercise less frequently, don't try to compensate by exercising strenuously and risking muscle strain.

TABLE 5.2
RECOMMENDED MAXIMUM HEART RATES DURING EXERCISE

Age	Beats per Minute
Pregnant (all ages)	140
Postpartum (20 years)	150
25	146
30	142
35	138
40	135
45	131

This table offers general guidelines. Some women may be advised to exercise less strenuously. For example, a woman who is not used to vigorous exercise might be advised to keep her heart rate lower than suggested here.

TABLE 5.3
CONTRAINDICATIONS FOR STRENUOUS EXERCISE

- Diagnosis of multiple gestation (twins)

- Diagnosis of heart disease

- Incompetent cervix

- Dilated cervix

- Vaginal bleeding, or diagnosis of placenta previa

- Ruptured membranes

- Episodes of premature labor, or high risk of premature labor

- Conditions exacerbated by stress or fatigue, such as myasthenia gravis or multiple sclerosis, unless under medical advice.

TABLE 5.4
CONDITIONS REQUIRING RESTRICTIONS ON EXERCISE

- Hypertension (high blood pressure), anemia or other blood disorders
- Thyroid disease
- Diabetes
- Cardiac arrhythmia or palpitations (irregular heartbeats)
- History of precipitate labor
- History of intrauterine growth retardation (fetus too small)
- Extreme underweight or overweight
- History of bleeding during pregnancy
- Breech presentation
- Extremely sedentary lifestyle (women who do not get much exercise should not suddenly start exercising vigorously)
- Toxemia or pre-eclampsia
- Diastasis recti (separation of abdominal muscles)
- Uterine contractions lasting several hours after exercising
- Phlebitis (inflammation of the veins)
- Systemic infection
- Backache, headache, pain radiating to the legs, pubic pain, or other pain after exercising
- Fatigue

Besides having concerns about safety, women with disabilities some-times have other reasons to feel skeptical about the value of exercise. When Athina's doctor suggested that she see a physical therapist, she felt it would be "more of a hassle than it was worth." She never did see a physical thera-pist, and she says that she does not regret her decision, because "I just had too many negative experiences when I was a child.... Trying to exercise just reminds me of all the things I can't do." Judi remembers thinking as a child that exercise would make her able-bodied. When she didn't become able-bodied, she decided that exercise was useless. It took her time to learn that what exercise *can* do is help a person make the most of her abilities. Working as an occupational therapist, Judi has seen that, over time, exercise increases a person's capacity to meet the demands of daily living. It is especially valuable for coping with the increased physical stresses of pregnancy.

Of the women we interviewed, those who had some sort of exercise—active or passive—felt less tired from daily activities and generally more comfortable. Exercising did not have to be a formal routine. Carla said that "running after a toddler" was enough to make her feel stronger and healthier during her second pregnancy. Sheila had passive range-of-motion exercises during her first pregnancy, but not her second; it was during the second pregnancy that she had problems with muscle spasms. When she compared her pregnancies, Sheila wished she had gone to physical therapy for ranging the second time. Michelle had problems with muscle spasms during only one week of her pregnancy. She said, "I was expecting a lot of muscle spasms, but I didn't get any because of my yoga classes." Both Michelle and Priscilla said that the stretching exercises they did in yoga classes helped them feel even better than they usually felt before pregnancy—their mobility and general sense of well-being improved, and they had less muscle pain. Renee found that doing her hand exercises reduced her pain. She said, "It is a good idea to keep active—it usually keeps the pain down. Looking back, I'd exercise more."

The exercises we describe were chosen because they are useful exercises for pregnant women. Most of them are commonly taught to all pregnant women, and some are modifications of ordinary pregnancy exercises which make them easier for women with disabilities. Some of the exercises were originally designed for people with disabilities, and are included here because they are particularly useful for *pregnant* disabled people.

Think of this chapter as a set of flexible guidelines, not as the last word. Women with particular problems such as high blood pressure, blood disorders, or multiple pregnancy may be advised to avoid vigorous exercise. For other women, some exercises will work better than others. It may not be feasible to follow each detail of the instructions for an exercise. Many women will have to modify some exercises according to their abilities. For example, when Judi does curl-ups with her hands at the back of her neck, she cannot keep both elbows back, but she still benefits from the exercise. Do be sure to follow instructions for coordinating breathing with exercise. Otherwise, modify if necessary to give each muscle group the appropriate exercise. Consult with your doctor or physical therapist and create an exercise program that works best for you. Reading this chapter might also be helpful for physical therapists who are designing exercises adapted for particular women.

While the guidelines in Table 5.1 state that women who are more than 4 months pregnant should avoid lying on their backs for long periods of time, we have suggested some exercises which require lying on the back *briefly*. These are valuable exercises, and it would be worthwhile to ask whether your physician approves of your lying down just long enough to do them. If any exercise you learn from this book, in a prenatal exercise class, or in childbirth preparation class feels too difficult or uncomfortable, *stop* and talk it over with your doctor or physical therapist during your next appointment.

Remember to drink plenty of water and empty your bladder before exercising, and never hold your breath while exercising. If you experience any of the warning signs listed at the end of Table 5.1, *stop* and contact a doctor.

CONDITIONING EXERCISES

General Conditioning

Swimming and walking are good general conditioning exercises. They promote good cardiopulmonary function and increase muscle tone. For additional benefits when walking, swing the arms vigorously to exercise the upper body as well as legs and hips. Conditioning exercises can be adapted to many disabilities, and to the changes of pregnancy. If it becomes difficult to move about during late pregnancy, swimming can be substituted for walking. Swimming is also valuable for women who suffer joint pain during weight-bearing exercises.

Women who are paraplegic can also do conditioning exercises. Stacy exercised by doing laps on an indoor track in a manual wheelchair. Women who have to start using a wheelchair during pregnancy could try doing what some women do all the time: use the chair for going long distances, but maintain strength and flexibility by continuing to walk short distances.

Women who are able to exercise vigorously enough to increase their heart rates should talk to their doctors about safety guidelines.

Exercises to Strengthen Abdominal and Lower Back Muscles

The abdominal (stomach) and back muscles work together to support the spine and pelvis. The back muscles alone cannot support the pelvis adequately, so it is always important to keep the abdominal muscles as strong as possible. Abdominal exercise is even more important during pregnancy, for two reasons:

- As the uterus grows, the forward shift of weight stresses the lower back. The lower back tends to become very sore and painful unless abdominal muscles are strong enough to help support the increased weight.
- Even strong abdominal muscles are stretched during late pregnancy. After birth, these muscles are significantly weakened. However, muscles that were well exercised before birth will recover more quickly.

Pelvic Tilts

The pelvic tilt is a commonly prescribed exercise which strengthens the abdominal muscles and, by stretching lower back muscles, reduces the excessive swayback *(lordosis)* so common in pregnancy. Pelvic tilts are one of the pregnancy exercises specifically recommended by ACOG. They can be done on hands and knees, lying down, standing, or seated. Because getting onto the hands and knees is awkward for many disabled women, we also describe pelvic tilts done in other positions.

In an **assisted pelvic tilt** adaptation, a woman lies on her back, on a bed or table at the attendant's waist level, with her knees bent or supported by pillows, and her head supported. Her attendant or partner gently lifts and lowers her hips. If the partner's hands are not properly placed, the tilt will not be at the correct angle. Figure 5.1 shows the best position for this exercise. The back should be as flat as possible for 5 seconds. With each repetition, the woman should exhale as her hips are lowered.

For an **active seated pelvic tilt**, the woman hooks her arms around the sides of a straight-backed chair, as if to join hands behind her lower back. Or, she hooks her arms back over the top of the chair. Then, she presses her lower back against the back of the chair, feeling the abdominal muscles tighten. For some people, it may be easier to grip the back of the chair's seat while doing this exercise.

To do an **active supine pelvic tilt** (lying on one's back), use the floor or a firm bed. Rest the feet flat on the floor about 18 inches from the hips (shins almost vertical). Arms lie relaxed beside the body. Press the lower back flat against the floor. Rock the hips upwards slightly, gradually increasing the lift as the muscles grow stronger. "Squeeze" the buttocks and tighten the abdominal muscles while lifting. As strength increases, increase the amount of lift. One can lie on a couch with knees resting on the armrest. (It may be necessary to use an attendant's help to get in position.) Press down with the knees, squeeze the buttocks, and tighten abdominal muscles to press the back flat. Hold with the back flat for about 5 seconds, then breathe out slowly while releasing (see Figure 5.2). Rest and repeat. (This exercise can be done with the knees supported by pillows rather than an armrest; however, the armrest is stable whereas the pillows may slip.)

For a more challenging exercise closely related to pelvic tilts, called "bridging," the knees are unsupported. The lift is continued until the body is held in a straight line from shoulders to knees. Hold this position as long as it is comfortable. Then, breathe out slowly while gradually rolling back down. At the end, the hips are once again resting on the floor. This variation, too, is most effective when the buttocks are squeezed and tightened during the lift.

At any point, but especially when it is no longer appropriate to lie on the back, a standing pelvic tilt may be substituted. Stand with the feet apart (at

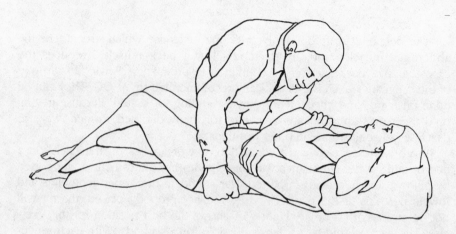

FIGURE 5.1. Assisted pelvic tilt.

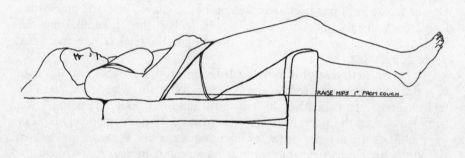

RAISE HIPS 1" FROM COUCH

FIGURE 5.2. Pelvic tilt on couch.

shoulder width), knees slightly bent. The buttocks and abdominal muscles are contracted so that the pelvis is rolled upward. By standing with the back lightly touching the wall at the beginning of this exercise, one can feel the lower back flatten against the wall.

Curl-ups

Curl-ups are especially good for strengthening the upper abdominal muscles (just below the ribs). When the exercise is done properly, more tightening can be felt in those muscles than in the other abdominal muscles.

For an **assisted curl-up**, a woman lies on the floor, knees bent or supported by pillows, feet flat on the floor. An assistant lifts her head until her chin is touching her chest, then raises her shoulders slightly (See Figure 5.3).

For an **active curl-up**, lie in the same position used for the assisted curl-

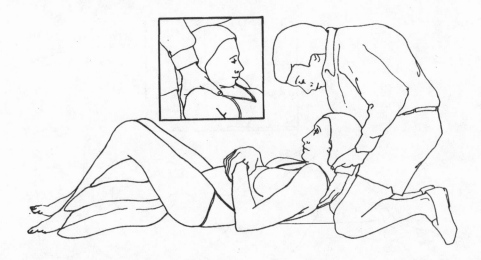

FIGURE 5.3. Assisted curl-up.

up. The hands can be clasped behind the neck, with the elbows held back (upper arms parallel with tops of shoulders), or the forearms can be lightly crossed on the chest. In the easiest curl-up, just the head is lifted from the floor or bed, chin touching the chest. As strength increases, it may be possible to progress to lifting the shoulders away from the floor as well. If this exercise is done with the hands clasped behind the neck, it is important not to use the hands to pull the neck upward. The abdominal muscles should be doing the work. Only curl up until the shoulder blades are off the floor (see Figure 5.4). Lifting to full sitting position could injure the lower back, and it could injure the abdominal muscles in pregnant women. It is helpful to begin by taking a deep breath, then breathing out slowly while curling up.

Women who do not have leg spasticity can make curl-ups more effective by pressing their feet against a vertical surface such as a wall or the footboard of a bed.

Leg Lifts

Leg lifts are especially good for *lower* abdominal muscles (below the navel). When the exercise is done properly, more tightening can be felt in those muscles. When not done properly, leg lifts may cause lower back pain. It is important to hold a pelvic tilt position while doing leg lifts. (One way to accomplish this is to place a rolled towel or firm cushion under the lower back.) After the fifth month, straight leg lifts should be discontinued. As the abdominal muscles are increasingly separated by the growing uterus, they do less and less of the work in this exercise, and the lower back could be strained.

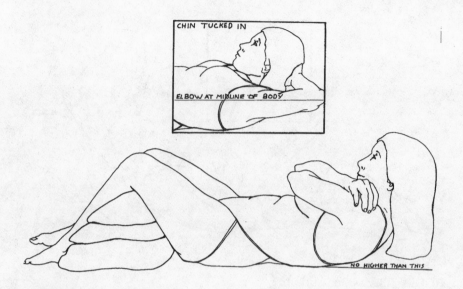

FIGURE 5.4. Correct full curl-up.

For **assisted leg lifts**, a woman can recline in her wheelchair, or lie on her back and have someone else raise and lower her legs.

In another type of **assisted seated leg lift**, the woman acts as her own assistant. She places a loop made of rope, webbing, or a folded towel around her foot, sits on a bed or a firm surface with her back supported, grasps one end of the loop, and swings her legs onto the bed or a nearby piece of furniture. The loop should be long enough to permit her to lean comfortably against the back support as she lifts her leg.

For more challenging **active leg lifts**, sit supported in bed, legs out-stretched, and slowly raise and lower the legs. Or, sitting on a chair, raise the legs onto a footstool, relax, return the feet to the floor, relax, and repeat the exercise. Although this exercise is more effective when the legs are kept straight, doing it with knees bent can still be useful.

There are two more advanced leg lifts. In the easier variation, only one leg is outstretched, and, in the other, the knee is bent, with the foot resting on a footstool or placed flat on the floor. The straight leg is slowly raised and lowered, then the exercise is repeated on the other side. Done this way, the exercise is somewhat less effective than the most advanced variation, but it is safer. More repetitions can make the exercise more beneficial.

For the most advanced leg lifts, lie flat on the floor or a reasonably firm surface, arms resting at the sides. Exercise one leg at a time. The resting leg may be bent or straight. Raise the other leg slowly, keeping it straight, then slowly lower the leg. It helps to breathe out while lowering the leg. During this exercise, the pelvis should be tilted to keep the back from arching upwards; if the lower back arches, it could be strained. For some women, it is helpful to support the lower back by putting the hands under the hips (palms to the floor). This tilts the hips slightly, making the pelvic tilt easier. Others may wish to support the back by placing a small, rolled towel or a foam pad under the small of the back.

Deep Breathing

These exercises will be useful for women who are quadriplegic for any reason. Breathing always involves the abdominal muscles. A number of variations on normal breathing—such as grunting, coughing, laughing, talking in a very deep voice, or special deep breathing—will exercise the abdominal muscles. Any woman can check the effectiveness of these exercises by resting her hand on her stomach and feeling for tightening, or asking someone else to check for tightening.

Doing deep breathing too quickly can make a person *hyperventilate*— she breathes out too much carbon dioxide and begins to feel dizzy. If that happens, just sit down and breathe normally, and the dizziness will go away. Next time, breathe more slowly. Remember, do not push while holding your breath! Also, do not hold your breath longer than 10–15 seconds.

An easy, basic deep breathing exercise consists of taking a deep breath, then slowly blowing out until there is no more air to blow out. Rest before repeating. This exercise can be done in any position, and it is good practice for the slow, deep breathing needed early in labor.

For a slightly more difficult exercise, simply hold the breath for about 10 seconds, breathe out, rest 2–3 minutes, and repeat. To make the exercise easier, rest longer between deep breaths, or hold the breath for a shorter amount of time. To avoid tiring the abdominal muscles, start with as many repetitions as are comfortable, then slowly increase the number.

Laughing is wonderful abdominal exercise—the trick is knowing what will make you laugh. Get silly with friends or children, listen to a favorite comedy tape, or get someone to lightly tickle your ear lobe or neck. Just remember to stop short of getting dizzy or tiring the abdominal muscles.

For another simple exercise, take a deep breath and slowly repeat "ha, ha, ha, ha..." or "oh, oh, oh, oh...." Rest a few minutes and repeat.

"PC" Muscle Strengthening

Like pelvic tilts, these exercises are specifically recommended by ACOG. They are often called Kegel exercises, after a researcher who emphasized the importance of strengthening the muscles of the pelvic floor. The figure-eight-shaped muscle surrounding the vagina and urethra in front, and the anus in back, is named the *pubococcygeal* muscle—"PC" for short. Every woman who can do so, should exercise the PC muscle regularly before, during, and forever after pregnancy—this is exercise for life.

The ability to hold one's urine is not only a matter of bladder control, it is also a matter of PC muscle control. When a woman imagines herself holding in urine, or tries to stop the stream while in the bathroom, she feels the PC muscle working. During pregnancy, bladder volume decreases as the uterus grows and presses on the bladder. A pregnant woman has to go to the bathroom more often, and waiting becomes more difficult. She may have problems with *stress incontinence* ("wetting the pants" when sneezing or coughing). At the same time, hormonal changes contribute to relaxation of the pelvic muscles. Keeping the PC muscle strong helps to prevent urinary problems—during pregnancy, in the postpartum period, and throughout life.

The second reason to do these exercises is to keep the vaginal muscles strong. These muscles will be stretched during child- birth, and they will recover more quickly if they have been exercised beforehand. Some older women may even need surgery for a prolapsed uterus—the uterus actually sags down into the vagina. Exercising the PC muscle may help to prevent this problem. Also, because PC exercises involve contracting and relaxing the muscle, women who have done these exercises know how to relax the vagina during childbirth.

The way to learn the easiest PC exercise may be obvious. Simply stop and start, stop and start, the flow of urine a few times while in the bathroom. By stopping and starting, one is contracting and relaxing the PC muscle. Once the feeling becomes familiar, *it is better not to exercise while urinating*. Too much stopping and starting might prevent you from completely emptying your bladder. Simply contract and relax the PC muscle at other times. The same exercise can be done anywhere, any time, standing or sitting, waiting in line at the bank or waiting for a traffic signal to change. (We have even seen a bumper sticker that said, "Honk if you're kegelling!." But we have never heard anybody honk.) Begin by doing this exercise at least 10 times a day; over a few weeks, work up to 25 times a day. (It is not necessary to do 25 repetitions all at once; 5 at one time and 10 at another is just as beneficial.) Then introduce other exercises, always making sure to do some combination of PC exercises at least 25 times a day.

Next, make the exercise a little more difficult. When urinating, relax slowly, only allowing a few drops to escape, then immediately contract again. Once the feeling is familiar, *do not* do the exercise while urinating, but practice it at other times. For a variation, imagine that the vagina is an elevator: Tighten from the bottom up, stopping at the "first floor," the "second floor," and on up to the "tenth floor." Then relax from the top down, stopping at each "floor"; continue all the way to "the basement," pushing outward a bit.

Some women enjoy tightening the PC muscle during intercourse. Just tighten the muscles against your partner's penis, and hold for a count of five (or longer). Your partner can tell you whether the PC muscle is staying strong, and the exercise will add to the pleasure of lovemaking.

STRETCHING EXERCISES

Stretching exercises should be done immediately after strengthening exercises. Muscle fibers shorten during strengthening exercise, and need to be stretched to prevent cramping. Clara, who swam once or twice a week but didn't take time for stretching exercises, experienced severe leg cramps ("charley horses").

Stretching exercises are easier to do after conditioning and strengthening exercises, because warm muscles stretch more readily. Evening is another good time to do stretching exercises, especially leg stretches. Muscle spasms are most likely to occur while one is asleep, and stretching at bedtime can help to prevent them. Many birthing instructors hear that when their students try doing calf stretches at bedtime, their charley horses disappear. If you do not exercise before stretching, warm and relax your muscles by taking a warm bath or shower, or by applying local heat.

It is very important to do stretching exercises *regularly*. If your daily routine changes, find a new time to stretch. It only takes a few days for muscles to become tight.

It is also important not to bounce while doing stretching exercises. Bouncing alternately shortens and lengthens the muscle, so bouncing makes stretches less effective and can even cause injury. The best way to maximize a stretch is to hold it as long as it is comfortable; usually a slight increase in stretch is felt at the end of the hold. If one exercises regularly, the amount of stretch, and the length of time the stretch can be held, will gradually increase until a given stretch can be held for up to 30 seconds. Remember, the maximum amount of stretch for pregnant women will be less than that for non-pregnant women. Breathing out during a stretch is also helpful. Start breathing out slowly just before beginning the stretch. Repetitions of stretching exercises can be increased gradually. It is better not to push oneself into doing too many repetitions at first. Six repetitions, for a total of 3 minutes' stretching, is a reasonable goal.

Lower Back Stretches

The same pelvic tilt exercises that strengthen the abdominal muscles also stretch the lower back muscles. By helping to maintain good posture, this exercise helps to alleviate the backaches which are so common in late pregnancy.

Seated Trunk Flexion

This is also a useful stretching exercise. Sit with the feet flat on the floor or supported. Grip the back of the chair at the level of the buttocks, then lean forward, resting the upper body on the thighs. Slowly curl upwards, straightening first the lower back, then the middle back, then the upper back.

Calf Stretches

For an **assisted calf stretch**, the person sits with her legs outstretched. The attendant rests the heel of one foot in his/her cupped hand, grasps the ball of the foot in the other hand, and bends the whole foot towards the knee, keeping the leg straight. The exercise is then repeated on the other side (Figure 5.5). Or, a woman could loop a towel around the bottom of her foot and pull the ends to assist in the stretch herself.

Seated Calf Stretch

Unassisted calf stretches can be done standing or seated. One type of seated calf stretch is for people who are able to sit with legs outstretched, another is for those who need to keep their legs bent. To do the first exercise, sit with legs stretched forward, heels supported on the floor, feet at right angles to shins, and toes pointing outward. (The foot is dorsiflexed and everted.) Sitting in this position, bend forward at the hips as if to rest the upper body on the thighs. A stretch should be felt in the calves, and may be felt at the back of the thighs. If the stretch is felt more strongly in the thighs than in the calves, modify the starting position by sitting on a higher chair or placing pillows on the seat of the chair. The idea is to lower the foot with respect to the hip, while keeping the knee straight.

If the seated calf stretch cannot be done with the leg outstretched, it can be done with the foot supported against a large book or block, with the heel resting on the floor.

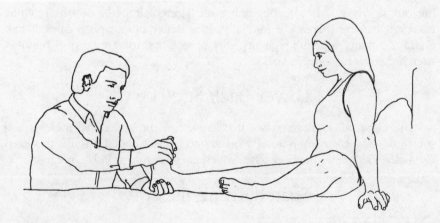

FIGURE 5.5. Assisted calf stretch.

Standing Calf Stretch

For this exercise, start in a modified lunge position. Stand facing the wall, just close enough to lean forward slightly and rest the forearms on the wall. Or, if your balance is good and your wrist joints are not painful, rest palms on the wall with arms stretched straight forward. One leg will be forward, slightly bent at the knee; the other will be straight back, with the whole foot contacting the floor. To do the stretch, lean against the wall, allowing the front leg to bend more, keeping the back leg straight, and feeling the stretch in the calf muscle (Figure 5.6). Repeat the stretch a few times on each side.

Inner Thigh Stretches

The inner sides of the thighs, just where the thighs join the body, also become vulnerable to muscle spasms as the increasing weight of the fetus and uterus put more pressure on the area. Also, many disabled women experience muscle tightness in this area. There are several reasons for doing stretching exercises. First, they may prevent or ease muscle spasms. Inner thigh stretches also help prepare a woman to give birth more comfortably, since she will need to spread her legs as widely as possible, with or without

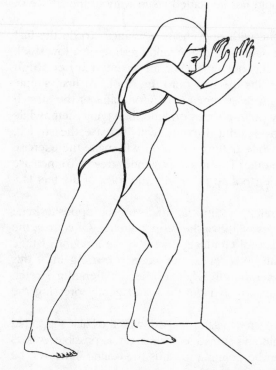

FIGURE 5.6. Standing calf stretch.

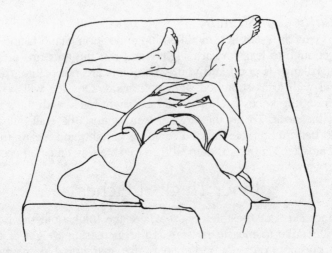

FIGURE 5.7. Inner thigh stretch.

the help of stirrups. Sufficient flexibility may even prevent the need for some C-sections. If any of these exercises cause hip pain, they should be discontinued *immediately*, and they should not be started again without the advice of a doctor or physical therapist.

These exercises can be done with or without assistance. To do the first inner thigh stretch, sit with the outer side of the ankle resting on a low stool, with the knee bent and pointing outward. (For an **assisted inner thigh stretch** variation, an attendant lifts the foot onto the stool.) At first, simply rest in this position for as long as it remains comfortable. As the stretch becomes more comfortable, try putting shoes on, and then tying them, while seated in the stretch position—leaning forward will increase the stretch. Sitting in the stretch position while putting shoes on will make the exercise very easy to work into daily routine. This is a very gentle stretch. To increase the stretch, put both feet on the stool at once, with the soles of the feet facing each other.

For a more challenging stretch, resting the ankle on the opposite knee while putting on and tying shoes will give the proper stretch. Of course, the stretch can be done without shoes! Gradually increase the amount of time the stretch is held, up to about 30 seconds, but *never strain*. Again, if this stretch causes hip pain, stop *immediately*. Another challenging stretch involves taking the position shown in Figure 5.7 and gently pressing the bent knee against the mattress.

For a very practical, effective stretch, sit up in bed, with the back supported if necessary. Sit with legs straight and spread as wide apart as possible. Ankles can be relaxed, or the toes can be pointing towards the ceiling, however, be

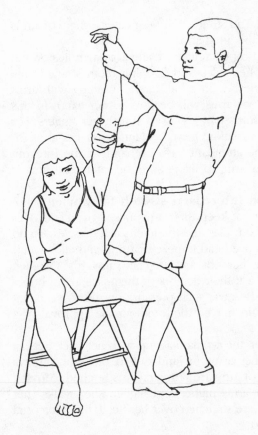

FIGURE 5.8. Intercostal stretch.

sure not to point the toes, because that could cause spasm of the calf muscles. Lean forward (between the legs) for a comfortable stretch. For an **assisted inner thigh stretch**, an attendant could push the legs apart by placing hands on the inner thighs, just above the knees, and/or sit between her legs.

Upper Body Stretches

These exercises stretch the intercostal muscles—the muscles between the ribs. (A "stitch in the side" is usually a spasm of the intercostal muscles.) Stretching these muscles helps to prevent muscle spasms, eases the discomfort of increasing pressure on the ribs during late pregnancy, and sometimes relieves heartburn. These exercises also stretch the arm muscles, and sometimes help with tingling and numbness in the hands.

For an **assisted intercostal stretch**, a woman can sit while an attendant lifts her arm straight up (Figure 5.8), then, with one hand on the wrist and the other hand on the upper arm, gently pulls upward slightly, just enough to stretch the intercostal muscles. The stretch will be greater if the woman is leaning toward the side opposite the lifted arm.

The intercostal muscles can also be stretched while a woman lies on her back. Starting with her arms at her sides and keeping them straight, she slowly sweeps her arms across the bed in a half circle, finishing with arms stretched over her head (her upper arms will be next to her ears). In this position, she can stretch a little further by trying to stretch her fingers. For the **assisted intercostal stretch** variation, her attendant moves her arms for her. For the last bit of stretch, the attendant has one hand on the forearm, and the other hand on the upper arm, to make sure the intercostal area is stretched, not wrists or elbows.

There is a good **unassisted intercostal stretch** for women who, because of spinal cord injury, cannot keep their arms raised overhead. This exercise will stretch both the arm muscles and the intercostal muscles. To do this exercise, a woman grasps an overhead trapeze or strap, and allows herself to sag or hang a bit, so that her ribs are stretched upwards. (Women who cannot grip a trapeze could ask their doctors or therapists about hooking their wrists over the trapeze. Because such pressure on the wrists might be a problem, this variation should not be tried without the approval of a doctor or therapist.)

For a more challenging stretch, the woman sits up with her back against the wall. She begins by lifting her arms up and out to the side, elbows straight, palms facing outward or upward, fingers outstretched. Moving slowly, and gradually raising her arms higher and higher, she "walks" her arms up the wall. When her arms are stretched over her head, her intercostal muscles will also be well stretched.

RELAXATION EXERCISES

Relaxation exercises encourage good circulation and a general sense of well-being. Many of the techniques taught in birthing classes are relaxation techniques, and they will be easier to learn after other relaxation exercises have been practiced. The relaxation exercises we suggest are for areas of the body that were not included in stretching exercises.

Feet

As pregnancy continues, aching feet are more likely to be a problem. The weight increase puts more of a load on the feet, and increased blood volume often leads to swollen feet. Taking time for a good massage not only makes the feet more comfortable, it contributes to a general sense of relaxation.

Some people like to combine a foot massage with an inner thigh stretch by sitting with one ankle resting on the opposite knee or thigh and massaging their own feet. When that is not comfortable, have someone else give the massage. Begin by gently and briskly patting the whole surface of the foot with both hands. Then grasp each toe, one at a time, and gently pull it. Then gently rub the ball and arch of the foot.

Women who cannot bend to reach their own feet can place a tennis ball on the floor and rub one foot at a time over the ball, slightly rolling the ball with the sole of the foot. Women with leg spasticity will need to be careful to rub gently, and, if using a ball about the size of a tennis ball, to press gently to avoid causing muscle spasms *(clonus)*. You may also decide to try this exercise using a larger ball, or avoid it altogether.

Buttocks

Supporting extra weight while seated can cause tension and discomfort in these muscles. Rocking from side to side may release some of this tension. For some women, it will be easier to press their hands on the arms of a chair and bounce up and down slightly. Shifting the weight like this may also help to prevent pressure sores.

Because there is an increased risk of pressure sores during pregnancy, people who cannot exercise may need to change position more frequently, either by transferring between wheelchair and bed more often, or by getting help to change position.

Neck

For many people, it is the neck muscles that are most likely to become tense in response to stress, so relaxing these muscles contributes most to a general sense of relaxation. Relaxation exercises will not only help to prevent neck pain, they can also help to prevent headaches.

Chin Tucks
One of the best exercises for relaxing the neck is chin tucks (dorsal glides). Look straight ahead, and tuck the chin in slightly to make a double chin. Hold about 2 seconds, relax, and repeat about 10 times. During this exercise, the back of the neck will seem to tighten like a rubber band. This exercise should be discontinued if it causes pain or tingling in the arms, or pain in the shoulder blades or shoulders.

Head Rolls
Head rolls are also relaxing. First drop the chin to the chest, breathe deeply, and relax. Slowly roll the head to the right, then reverse direction, rolling toward the center and all the way to the left. Return to center,

breathe deeply once or twice, then repeat the head roll in the reverse direction. Repeat three or four times in each direction. Breathing out slowly while rolling the head makes this exercise even more relaxing. If this exercise makes you dizzy, try pausing before changing the direction of the roll. (Do not bend the neck backwards without the advice of a doctor or physical therapist.)

Neck and Shoulder Massages

Neck and shoulder massages are also very helpful. Begin the massage gently, kneading more firmly only at the woman's request.

EXERCISE TO RELIEVE CONSTIPATION

While conditioning exercises such as walking and swimming help to prevent constipation, there is also an exercise specifically for relieving constipation.

Sit on the toilet with legs stretched out in front. Imagine a line coming down from the ceiling through the center of the toilet, and slowly circle the body around the imaginary line. If it is difficult to hold the legs out, rest them on a chair or footstool. If balance is a problem, hold onto grab bars or the sides of the toilet seat and, if necessary, modify the circling motion— rock slightly from side to side, or back and forth. (Do not use this exercise if you have hemorrhoids.)

CLOSING COMMENTS

We want to emphasize again that disabled women who try the exercises we have described have much to gain. These exercises do not have to be strenuous or painful, and they are effective when a woman exercises to the extent that is comfortable for her. It takes time to see the benefits of exercise. Many women must wait as long as 6–8 weeks to see noticeable results. But the results are very worthwhile: prevention or reduction of discomforts like back pain and muscle spasms, increased endurance, and better general health. The women we interviewed made the strongest recommendation for exercise during pregnancy when they said, "I should have done more."

6 NINE MONTHS OF CHANGE—PREGNANCY

The changes of pregnancy occur in phases called trimesters, each lasting approximately three months. For each trimester, we will discuss the following topics: normal physical changes; common pregnancy symptoms; typical discomforts and ways of coping with them; medical care, including office visits and diagnostic tests; fetal development; possible complications; emotional concerns; special concerns for each trimester (for example, how to choose a birthing class during the second trimester); and the special concerns of women with disabilities.

Table 6.1 lists a number of common discomforts and some disability problems that can be associated with pregnancy, and shows how many of our interviewees experienced these problems during each trimester. This list communicates a sense of what pregnancy can be like—each trimester differing as symptoms appear, intensify, or disappear.

While this table provides a general sense of the experience of pregnancy, it does not include all possible symptoms, and should not be taken as a guide to what every woman might expect. Some common pregnancy symptoms were under-reported, possibly because the interviews often focused on disability. It is surprising, for example, that no one recalled having had headaches, and few women recalled having such common problems as anemia and sleeplessness. In some cases, a symptom may have been misunderstood. For example, some women who mentioned feeling tired or faint may have been anemic without knowing it. Others may have simply forgotten some of their symptoms, like Clara, who remarked during a casual conversa-

Table 6.1
DISCOMFORTS REPORTED FOR 62 PREGNANCIES OF 36 WOMEN

Symptom	Trimester 1	2	3	Comments
Emotional extremes	3	0	1	
Anemia	6	7	9	Including five pregnancies of one woman
Faintness/fatigue	14	8	6	
Nausea	21	0	4	Including one hyperemesis
Sleeplessness		2?		Trimester unknown
Heartburn	0	5	8	
Hemorrhoids	0	0	3	
Constipation	7	5	11	Including five pregnancies of one woman, only two with spinal cord injury
Numb/painful hands	0	2	0	
Felt warmer	2	2	3	
Stuffy nose	0	0	1	
Urinary frequency/ infection	8	6	16	One kidney infection in the second trimester, and an infection associated with dehydration from hyperemesis
Abdominal muscle spasm/stretching	4	0	0	
Leg spasms	3	8	9	
Edema	0	3	11	
Vaginal discharge	0	0	3	
Back or joint pain	3	8	10	
Sore breasts	1	0	0	
Shortness of breath	0	2	10	
Threatened miscarriage	1	2		One clearly unrelated to disability— caused by placenta previa
Miscarriage	6	8		Including one during polio infection; one associated with spinal cord injury; two associated with lupus; two associated with arthrogryposis
Episode of premature labor	2	1		Two women with spinal cord injury
Premature birth	1	4		Two mothers with spinal injury; two such births to one mother with lupus
Dysreflexia	1	1	1	
MS exacerbation	2	0	3	Four interviewees had MS
Pressure sores	0	0	2	
Impaired mobility or balance	0	16	19	

tion that took place after her interview, "I forgot to mention that with one of my kids my nose was stuffy most of the time." Probably several women forgot comparatively minor symptoms because others were more important or memorable. When Celeste was asked what symptoms she experienced during the third trimester, she replied, "I was so afraid I'd have a disabled child, I blocked everything else."

Also, being disabled appears to affect the perception of pregnancy symptoms. For example, most woman who have spinal cord injuries might not be aware of vaginal infection because they cannot feel genital irritation. Sometimes a woman cannot be sure whether she is experiencing a symptom of pregnancy or of disability. Jennifer described the swelling of her feet as a pregnancy symptom, but commented that the sensation resembled arthritic pain. Any woman who is experiencing an unpleasant or confusing symptom should not hesitate to discuss her concerns with her doctor.

FIRST TRIMESTER

. . . .

Initial Signs and Symptoms of Pregnancy

Many of the women we interviewed did not recognize the initial signs of pregnancy until their husbands or friends suggested the possibility. This was not limited to women who did not believe they could become pregnant. While the common symptoms of early pregnancy may have other causes, a woman who experiences one or more of the following should consider the possibility that she is pregnant:

Amenorrhea (absence of menstruation): This symptom is not always noticed. Jennifer, who had been taking fertility medications, said, "I was paying attention to every sign so I was particularly aware of my periods." But Patricia was caught by surprise. She explained, "I wasn't using any birth control, and I was telling a friend of mine about some of my sexual relationships when she said, 'If you go on like that you could get pregnant.' When she said that, I suddenly realized I *was* pregnant—I had already missed one period."

Reduced menstruation: This may also be a sign of pregnancy. Women who experience a light flow at the time they are expecting to menstruate, and even some women who have stopped menstruating, do not realize they are pregnant until other symptoms occur.

Nausea: Morning sickness is the second most common symptom of pregnancy. Sheila commented, "It wasn't till I got sick to my stomach that I started looking for my period, and I realized I was late and I was pregnant." Many women think at first that they really are sick. Julie said, "It didn't occur to me that I was pregnant. I told a friend of mine that I got sick at the same time every day, then felt fine for the rest of the day. I couldn't believe it when she said I might be pregnant, but she badgered me into getting a pregnancy test." While some women feel nauseated at the same time every day (not necessarily the morning!), others become sensitive to particular sights or smells. They may even dislike the smells of foods they normally enjoy. Celeste recalled, "I was watching the movie 'Vertigo,' and when I saw one particular scene, I started feeling sick and the feeling just wouldn't go away. Then I knew I was pregnant again!"

Breast changes: Some women notice changes in the appearance of their breasts. During pregnancy the nipples and areolas darken and take on a bumpy appearance, and the veins become more prominent. Others notice swelling, tingling, or soreness. Fay remarked, "I was sure I was pregnant even before I took the test, because my breasts hurt."

Increase in basal temperature: Body temperature rises during activity; the basal temperature is the resting temperature of the body. It is measured with a special thermometer before getting out of bed in the morning. Basal temperature varies during the menstrual cycle, but it rises in a different pattern when a woman becomes pregnant. Clara said, "We wanted to have a baby, so we were keeping track of my temperature. My husband knew I was pregnant when he took my temperature and it went up and didn't go down again."

All the above pregnancy symptoms, as well as other symptoms such as urinary frequency or fatigue, are easily confused with other conditions. Many women who become nauseated think they have the flu. Stacy said, "I thought I was sick until my husband commented, 'Your breasts are looking bigger. Maybe you're pregnant.'" Or, of course, a woman may believe she is pregnant when she is not.

Even a physical examination can be misleading. The most reliable sign that a woman is pregnant is a positive pregnancy test.

Pregnancy Tests

Pregnancy tests involve detecting the presence of a pregnancy hormone, human chorionic gonadotropin (HCG), in the urine or blood. Many women consider using home pregnancy tests. Common reasons are that they want to be sure they are pregnant before calling the doctor, they want privacy, or they want to avoid the inconvenience of going to a laboratory or clinic. However, doing a home pregnancy test might not be worth the extra expense. Your doctor will include a pregnancy test in your physical examination, and while the doctor's test is covered by medical insurance, a home test is not.

Home tests require only a small amount of urine, and some are 99% accurate. Women who have indwelling catheters can use the home test with a sample of urine taken from the leg bag. Women whose hand control is poor may not be able to use home tests without the help of an assistant, since a sample of urine must be poured up to a measuring line in a small vial, and some test ingredients must be measured with a dropper.

Laboratory and office pregnancy tests also measure the presence or absence of HCG in urine. Blood tests are only used when there is a need to measure the quantity of HCG.

Office Visits

Medical History

The first office visit is usually the longest, since your doctor must ask a number of questions about your medical history, and perform a very thorough examination. The medical history will cover four areas—personal medical history, family medical history, gynecological history, and social history. In a very busy office, you may be asked to complete a questionnaire, or you may be interviewed by a nurse or medical assistant. The doctor will review this information and ask about any unusual answers, and you can ask any questions that concern you.

Personal medical history: Discussion of your personal medical history is most important. Although it can be helpful for you to have copies of your medical records sent to your doctor, there is no substitute for a discussion of your past experiences. S/he may need to ask some questions to gain a clearer understanding of what has happened in the past. This part of your appointment also presents an opportunity for you to ask questions. For example, if you are often bothered by urinary problems, you can ask your doctor what to do about them during pregnancy.

Family medical history: A discussion of your family medical history can alert the doctor to the possibility that you may have certain medical problems. For example, if your mother has diabetes, or had diabetes of pregnancy, you might be more susceptible to the problem, and your doctor might want to make sure you know the warning signs.

Gynecological history: The gynecological history includes a discussion of your menstrual experiences, past pregnancies, and past pelvic or genital infections.

Social history: Social history refers to your current life circumstances, including your emotional and economic situation. Your doctor can care for you better if s/he knows whether you have the help you need for pregnancy and child-care, whether you have other children to care for, and so forth. Because many disabilities (for example, myasthenia gravis and systemic lupus erythematosus) are exacerbated by stress, it is important to discuss these issues thoroughly and honestly.

Medical Issues for Disabled Women

Disabled women will need to discuss a number of special issues with their doctors. As you discuss these questions, you and your obstetrician can decide which questions should be answered by her, and which by your disability specialist.

Current status of your disability: At this first visit, and during all later visits, you will want to discuss the current status of your disability. The problems you discuss will depend on your particular disability. Most women will need to discuss how pregnancy is affecting their mobility and daily functioning. It may be necessary for their doctors to change medications, alter medication dosages, prescribe additional attendant care, or prescribe occupational or physical therapy. Women who have back or joint pain, or morning stiffness, could tell their doctor the extent of their problems so s/he can monitor changes. Women who experience autonomic dysreflexia need to discuss this problem thoroughly with their doctors, including a description of the circumstances that stimulate dysreflexia, so that their care can be planned accordingly.

Bladder and kidney problems: Women who have bladder or kidney problems should discuss their usual symptoms with their doctors. Because pregnancy increases susceptibility to urinary infection, it is important to ask what symptoms merit a call to your doctor's office. Preventing infections is not merely a matter of convenience or comfort; severe infections increase the risk of pre-term labor, and both myasthenia gravis and systemic lupus erythematosus can be exacerbated by such infections. Preventing infection depends on appropriate use of medication, good hygiene, and good bladder drainage. It is important to discuss all these issues with your doctor.

Breathing problems: A number of disabling conditions, including myasthenia gravis, post polio syndrome, high spinal cord injuries, and kyphoscoliosis (scoliosis of the upper spine), involve respiratory difficulties which may grow worse during pregnancy. Upward pressure of the growing uterus is an obvious cause of this exacerbation. For some women, particularly those with high spinal cord injuries, another cause can be pressure from the large intestine if it becomes impacted with fecal matter. Such problems may first become noticeable just at the end of the first trimester, as the uterus begins to rise into the abdominal cavity. Women with these problems must be careful to avoid respiratory infections; they need to call their doctors as soon as they have symptoms, so that a slight infection cannot become dangerous. Breathing difficulties can become hazardous not only for the mother, but also for the fetus, which depends on the mother for oxygen. You and your doctor need to discuss whether respiratory testing is necessary, and what treatment would be required if problems arise.

Pressure sores: Women who have occasional problems with pressure sores should discuss the problem with their doctors. The increased weight of pregnancy, and pregnancy-associated anemia, sometimes worsen pressure sores, and plans can be developed to prevent this problem. For example, your doctor may decide to test for anemia more frequently.

Pregnancy complications: Some disabilities are linked with increased susceptibility to certain complications of pregnancy. You and your doctor need to discuss the signs and symptoms of such complications, so that you are aware of what they might be and will be prepared to contact him or her if they occur. You might want to briefly discuss treatment options, planning to discuss treatment in more detail if and when complications occur.

Exacerbation of disability: Discuss plans for preventing or treating possible disability exacerbation, particularly the possibility that you might be hospitalized for such problems as respiratory difficulty or pre-term labor, so that you can plan ahead.

Medications

A review of your medications is a crucial part of your examination. Your doctor needs complete, accurate information about your medication schedule. To be sure you give him the correct information, you should (a) provide the name of each medication, dosage, time of day it is taken, and any side effects you have noticed; (b) have your medical records sent to your obstetrician before your appointment; (c) arrange for your primary physician and your obstetrician to discuss your medications; or (d) bring all your medications, in their original containers with the prescription labels attached, to your appointment.

When discussing medications with your doctor, be sure to mention any non-prescription medications you use. Perhaps you have never thought of it that way, but if you ever take aspirin for a headache, or a glass of wine to relax after dinner, or sometimes use recreational drugs to cope with disability symptoms, you are medicating yourself. Smoking, drinking, and drug use are not unusual problems among people with disabilities, and it is easy to start using a drug to relieve occasional pain or tension, and then use it more and more often without realizing what has happened. Even if you are not addicted, any medications you take can affect your baby. Stopping as early as possible is the best protection for your baby. Your doctor can help you to stop.

Women are usually advised to avoid even prescription medications during pregnancy, but there are important exceptions to this rule. For some women, reducing or discontinuing medication can be life-threatening. Women with disabilities need to discuss any changes with their doctors, as it is important to carefully weigh the possible risks and benefits of each medication.

Not all medications have the same effects. Some are chemically changed by the placenta before they reach the fetus, others are not. Sometimes only small amounts of a medication the mother is taking will reach the fetus, while others others reach the same concentration in the fetal blood as in the maternal blood. Many medications have been studied in this way, so that it is often possible to treat the mother with a medication that is known to be unlikely to affect the fetus, or to treat a fetus by administering medication to the mother. In certain situations, the risks of medication side effects are smaller than the risks of leaving a condition untreated; for example, the possible side-effects of a particular antibiotic may be less worrisome than the risk that a severe urinary infection will lead to premature labor. Medications used to treat some symptoms may exacerbate others; for example, drugs for treating pre-eclampsia or premature labor can increase the muscle weakness of myasthenia gravis, and medications used to suppress systemic lupus erythematosus symptoms and avert miscarriage increase susceptibility to infection. All these considerations can be discussed by the mother, her obstetrician, and her disability specialist. Since information about the safety and effectiveness of various medicines and their combinations continuously improves, your doctor may recommend medications different from those you or your acquaintances received in earlier pregnancies.

Your obstetrician and disability specialists may need to confer about your medications. Roberta told us, "My obstetrician would order my lab tests, and my rheumatologist would tell him how to adjust my medication. It worked out fine." If your physicians need to confer about a particular medication, or if your dosage will be adjusted according to laboratory test results, make sure you ask whether to continue your medications in the meantime, whether the doctor will call you or you should plan on calling her office, which doctor you should call, and when.

One possibility is that your doctor will ask you to substitute a medication that is known to be safer during pregnancy. For example, Stephanie regularly took an antibiotic to prevent bladder infection, and her doctor prescribed a different antibiotic that was safer for the fetus. If your prescription is changed, be sure to ask about possible side effects. If the dosage may need to be adjusted, ask your doctor to explain signs and symptoms that the dose is too high (for example, ringing in the ears is a symptom of aspirin overdose). Ask about special instructions for taking medication; for example, taking medication with meals can lessen indigestion.

Many doctors prescribe a prenatal vitamin at the first visit. Some women are troubled by constipation caused by iron in this vitamin. If constipation has been a problem for you, your doctor can prescribe stool softeners, which are often prescribed for pregnant women. (Also see Chapter 4 for suggestions for preventing constipation.)

Some of the women we interviewed commented on what happened to them when their medications were altered. Sheila said, "In my first pregnancy, my doctor and I agreed to try stopping my antibiotics, but I had to start them again when I got a bladder infection. With my second, I just kept on taking antibiotics, and it went better." Sharon and Sybil also developed bladder infections when they tried discontinuing antibiotics. When Cheryl discontinued her tranquilizer, she actually felt better. She said, "I noticed I didn't need it. I found I had an inner sense of peace." Michelle, however, had difficulty sleeping when she discontinued her tranquilizer. Sara said, "I did okay when I lowered my dose, but when I stopped altogether I felt very tense and I got more muscle spasms. Staying on a small dose worked best." Roberta did not notice any change after discontinuing some of her medications before pregnancy; she did not say how long before pregnancy she stopped taking these medications, and it is possible that she did not feel any change because pregnancy caused a remission of her symptoms. It is also possible that, at least during pregnancy, the medications which were continued gave adequate relief of her symptoms. Laura said, "I had to start my cortisone again because my lupus flared when I was 5 1/2 months pregnant," and Leslie pointed out, "I didn't get prednisone till my third pregnancy, and that went much better than the first two."

Physical Examination

After describing what happens during a routine office visit, we will discuss some special concerns of women with disabilities. The first examination includes a general evaluation (heart, lungs, etc.), and some tests that will not be repeated at later visits. The pelvic examination usually will not be repeated until the final weeks of pregnancy. Other aspects of the examination—measurement of temperature, blood pressure, pulse, weight, and urinalysis, are repeated at every visit.

Routine Examination Temperature is taken because elevated temperature is often the first sign of infection. High blood pressure is a health problem that requires careful attention. Increases in blood pressure may be a sign of pregnancy complication and/or disability exacerbation. A sudden increase or decrease of weight is also significant. Urine is tested for the presence of infectious bacteria, sugar (a sign of diabetes of pregnancy), and protein (a sign of pregnancy complication and/or disability exacerbation).

Blood Tests Several blood tests are done at the first visit. The blood type is determined, so that the doctor knows whether maternal and fetal blood might be incompatible, and has a record of the mother's blood type in case she needs a transfusion. It is important to determine the Rh type (positive or negative), because untreated Rh incompatibilities can lead to fetal illness, miscarriage, and premature labor. The level of antibodies to rubella (German measles) is determined; if the antibody level is low, the mother will not be vaccinated until she has had her baby, as rubella vaccination during pregnancy is risky. It is important to know whether she is immune to rubella in case she is exposed during her pregnancy. A VDRL test diagnoses syphilis, a venereal disease (women who have systemic lupus erythematosus may react with a false positive). A CBC (complete blood count) can reveal the presence of systemic infection or anemia. The CBC may be repeated at later visits.

If you or any of your sex partners has ever used illegal injectable drugs, consider including an HIV-antibody test among your blood tests. This test can tell you whether you have a risk of developing AIDS, or transmitting the HIV virus to your fetus. Your doctor can advise you about confidentiality (keeping test results secret), understanding test results, and AIDS prevention.

Pelvic Examination The pelvic examination serves a number of purposes. The appearance of the vagina and cervix can show signs of infection. At the first visit, the examination includes a PAP smear and cultures for gonorrhea and chlamydia. (Gonorrhea and chlamydia are sexually transmitted diseases. A baby who is exposed to gonorrhea in the vagina during birth may contract the infection and be blinded as a result.) Examining the appearance of the cervix and the size of the uterus help to confirm pregnancy, and determine how advanced the pregnancy is. The size of the uterus will help the doctor estimate the size of the fetus and the probable date of conception. During the manual examination, the doctor can assess whether the size and shape of the pelvic opening, and the mobility of the coccyx (tailbone) are adequate for birth, and s/he may detect the presence of any unusual masses. The pelvic examination is usually not repeated until the last 4 weeks of pregnancy.

The pelvic examination alone may not give enough information to determine how advanced the pregnancy is. When Pam's doctor examined her, the height of the fundus (top of the uterus) suggested that she had been pregnant longer than the time indicated by the date of her last menstruation (LMP); this discrepancy occurred because Pam's lordosis affected the angle of her uterus. The due date can also be estimated on the basis of the date of the last menstrual period. The due date is not an exact prediction but an estimate, which can be incorrect if the woman does not have a 28 day menstrual cycle, or if she had a light flow after becoming pregnant and does not know her true LMP. Also, there are individual variations in the length of gestation; first pregnancies in particular may last somewhat longer than expected. Sometimes the estimated due date seems almost magical; as women near the end of pregnancy, they can hardly wait for the due date, and they worry after it passes. It is better to mentally add a week to your doctor's estimate.

Sometimes it is important to determine the length of gestation more precisely. Early in pregnancy, if there are signs or symptoms of ectopic pregnancy, a measurement of the quantity of pregnancy hormone in the mother's blood may be done. Later in pregnancy, the doctor's decision as to how to treat complications may depend on using ultrasound to determine the maturity (gestational age) of the fetus.

Special Diagnostic Tests At the first office visit, samples of blood and urine are taken for routine testing. These same samples may be used for special diagnostic tests needed by women with disabilities. You need to ask the doctor what tests you will need, how test results will influence your care, and when test results will be available. These are some of the tests that may be needed:

Kidney malfunction tests: Women who have kidney malfunction for any reason may be tested for levels of chemicals which the kidneys should clear from the blood.

Antibody tests: Women who have systemic lupus erythematosus need to have blood tests for the presence SS-A and SS-B antibodies. The presence of these antibodies indicates an increased risk that the fetus will be born with heart damage. If these antibodies are present, other diagnostic tests will be needed later in pregnancy. The presence of lupus anticoagulant and antiocardiolipin antibodies is associated with increased risk of miscarriage caused by blood clots in the placenta. If these antibodies are present, appropriate medication will be prescribed; these medications have greatly improved the outcome of systemic lupus erythematosus pregnancies.

Muscle strength and lung function tests: These tests may be ordered for women who have myasthenia gravis. Since medication dosage needs continuing adjustment as weight and blood volume change during pregnancy, these tests may be repeated.

Special Issues for Women with Disabilities

Some aspects of the physical examination can pose problems for women with disabilities, but there are possible solutions for each problem.

Blood Samples Having a blood sample taken in the doctor's office or at the laboratory can be a nuisance for women who have spasticity, involuntary movement, or muscle wasting. If you have one "good" arm, decide in advance whether you would prefer to have blood drawn from that arm or the opposite arm. Some women prefer to have blood drawn from the good arm, because it is more difficult to draw blood from the affected arm, and the technician may need to try more than once. Some prefer to have blood drawn from the affected arm, because they do not want a sore spot in the opposite one. Tell the technician if you have a preference, or remember any methods that have been helpful in the past, and tell the technician. For example, "It's usually easier to get a sample if I've had a warm compress on my arm for a few minutes."

Urine Samples Giving a urine sample in the office can be a problem. While some women are comfortable using a catheter in the restroom at the doctor's office, many prefer to bring a sample to the office in a clean jar.

Weighing In Being weighed is difficult for many women with disabilities. Several women solved the problem by weighing themselves on special scales and reporting their weight to their doctors. Sylvia and Sara used a freight scale at a nearby hospital, Stephanie used a laundry scale, and Samantha used a special scale at the nursing home where she worked. One woman laughed when she said, "I even thought about trying a veterinary scale." Most women were assisted by their husbands; the husband stepped on the scale first, had his weight measured, then took his wife in his arms. This may not have been the best procedure for Pam, who tried to avoid gaining weight so her husband would not injure his back while lifting her.

Pelvic Examination Several problems can occur in connection with the pelvic examination. A woman may have trouble getting on the examining table or finding a comfortable position; muscle spasms, incontinence, or dysreflexia may occur during the examination.

If the doctor has an adjustable examining table, it can be adjusted to a height that makes it easier for you to get on and off, and easier for others to assist you. Hilary recalled, "After my doctor lifted me onto the examining table, he decided to order one that had a hydraulic lift." If the table's height is not adjustable, using the widest table available may help. Removing the paper covering makes it less likely that you will slip or slide as you get on. If you get on and off the table yourself, make sure someone is there to put your crutches or sliding board out of the way, and to put them within reach when you are ready to leave.

Women who need help often prefer to bring their own assistants. Sylvia explained, "It's easier to go with your attendant because they know the routine and you don't have to go through a long explanation." Portia, Pam and Stephanie had their husbands help them.

If the office is not too busy at the first office visit, your attendant or companion might show the office staff how to help you. Then the office staff will be able to work with you at later visits.

If you must tell your doctor or a member of the office staff how to assist you, clarify the following points for them:

- Make sure you are not transferred to the examining table until someone is able to remain in the examining room with you. It is often routine to have a patient wait in the examining room for a few minutes while the doctor finishes with another patient. Explain in advance that you can wait in an office chair or your wheelchair, but must not be left alone on the examining table.
- The examining room and other equipment must be ready for you. Somebody may need to move furniture aside so your wheelchair can be brought closer to the table. Explain how to set the brake on your wheelchair, turn off the motor on an electric wheelchair, and move armrests and footrests out of the way. If adaptive devices such as leg braces

must be removed, explain how they must be removed and set aside. Make sure jewelry, loose clothing, and tubing are not in the way.

- Have the examining table adjusted to the appropriate height.
- Any of the common transferring methods described below can be used, depending on individual preference. If you have developed a special method, reading these descriptions can help you decide how to explain your own method. Describe the entire transferring procedure in advance. It is better to have more than one assistant available, but if you have only one, discuss what to do if s/he feels s/he might drop you (it may be safest simply to lower you to the floor, then get help). Possibly have your assistant(s) practice once by lifting you over your wheelchair, and lowering you into the chair. Remind your assistants to protect themselves by keeping their backs straight, bending their knees, and lifting with their legs.

Pivot Transfer: For a pivot transfer, the table should be low enough for you to sit on it. Your assistant stands in front of you, takes your knees between his or her knees, grasps you around the back and under the armpits, then raises you to standing position. Then s/he pivots you onto the table. Once you are seated on the examining table, the assistant can help you lie down. When returning to your wheelchair, have the table readjusted to a position that allows you to place your feet firmly on the floor before you are brought to a standing position.

Cradle Transfer: The cradle transfer is done with one or two assistants. The examining table should be at about the waist height of the assistants. If there is one assistant, s/he squats beside you, puts one arm behind your knees and the other arm around your back and under your armpits. Then she stands and carries you to the table. Or, two assistants can grasp each other's arms behind your back and under your knees, and carry you to the table. They must be careful to coordinate their movements.

Other Two-Person Transfers: Two other types of two-person transfer can be used to lift a woman in a sitting position over the arms of her wheelchair and onto the table. With these methods, the taller, stronger assistant should lift your upper body, and the assistants must be careful to work together. In the first method, you cross your arms across your chest. One assistant starts by kneeling behind you and reaching around you, putting her/his elbows under your armpits and grasping your opposite wrists (right hand on your left wrist). The other assistant supports you under the knees, and they lift together. If you cannot cross your arms, the assistant standing behind you puts his/her hands together, or grasps her own wrists, so that s/he will not lose hold of you.

During the Examination Once you are on the table, you may need some help finding a comfortably balanced position. If you have a catheter in place, it does not need to be removed for the examination, but someone should make sure that the tubing is not caught or kinked. You may wish to put the leg bag on the table beside you, or on your abdomen, for proper drainage.

Many women with disabilities are unable to assume the usual position for a pelvic examination. A number of modifications are possible. Some women are more comfortable with "OB" stirrups which support their knees rather than their feet. Jennifer was able to stay in position for a short time by resting her heel (rather than the sole of her foot) in the stirrup. Celeste had her husband hold up her legs.

If a woman must catheterize herself to urinate, or manually stimulate her bowel movements, the pelvic examination can cause her bowels or bladder to empty. This is less likely to happen if she can empty her bladder and bowels before her appointment. It is also helpful to empty one's leg bag before an examination.

Sometimes the touch of the speculum, or a slightly awkward position, will stimulate muscle spasms in the limbs or abdomen. An assistant should gently support the spasming area; the examination can continue after the spasm resolves.

The internal pressure of a pelvic examination can occasionally cause dysreflexia. Your doctor will perform the examination during the first visit, but at later visits assistants may examine you. They should do so only when a physician is available, and should know that you must not be left alone if symptoms occur. Many physicians have found that applying an anesthetic jelly to the vagina and rectum before they begin will prevent this reaction. Since cold objects touching the legs or feet can also cause dysreflexia, it can be helpful for you to wear thick, warm stockings, or have towels placed on the table and stirrups. If you experience symptoms of dysreflexia, the stimulus must be found and removed (for example, the speculum must be removed, or a kinked catheter straightened). Bringing you to a sitting position may reduce your blood pressure. If symptoms stop, you can try continuing the examination, but if they persist, another examination can be scheduled. If your blood pressure does not drop, or symptoms grow severe (throbbing headache or stuffy nose), the doctor should be called to decide whether you need medication.

Concluding the Office Visit

After the examination, you and your doctor can discuss any remaining questions about your pregnancy. Your doctor will advise you about nutrition and other aspects of your care. If appropriate, s/he can advise you about signs or symptoms of infections or other problems. Many women begin discussing their concerns about what will happen during labor, and continue the discussion during later visits. In the first trimester, office visits normally take place once a month, but your doctor may ask you to return sooner if s/he wants to follow up on a particular problem such as a vaginal infection.

Other Diagnostic Tests

Two other tests that may be done outside your doctor's office are sonography (often called ultrasound) and chorionic villus sampling (CVS).

Sonography

Sonography, or ultrasound, may be done at any time during pregnancy for a variety of reasons. In the first trimester, it may be used to determine the gestational age of the fetus, to verify that the pregnancy is in the uterus (if symptoms of extrauterine pregnancy occur), or to locate the fetus for chorionic villus sampling.

Women who have systemic lupus erythematosus are likely to be scheduled for sonography at the time of the first prenatal visit. Since their babies are at increased risk for both pre-term birth and growth retardation, it is important to determine gestational age accurately, so that a baby who is simply small will not be considered premature.

Sonography resembles sonar, the method submarines use to navigate and locate objects under water. High-frequency sound waves bounce off the fetus, and a transducer sends the resulting image to a screen.

During sonography, the woman lies on her back. A special gel that improves the transmission of the sonogram is applied to her abdomen; the gel feels cool and slippery, and seems to help the transducer glide more easily. In early pregnancy, she will be instructed to drink several glasses of water just before the examination in order to fill the bladder. The filled bladder is more easily distinguished from other organs, and lifts the uterus so that it can be examined more easily. Filling the bladder in this way obviously poses a problem for women who use indwelling catheters, and those who experience dysreflexia when their bladders are full. They will need special instructions from their doctors. Other women should be aware that the examination may become uncomfortable; if they must hold their urine for long, even the light pressure of the transducer can be unpleasant. If they have good control but become very uncomfortable, they can ask whether they can get up and partially empty their bladders.

Chorionic Villus Sampling

This is a method of genetic testing which was developed more recently than amniocentesis. While it is no longer considered experimental, it still is not as widely available as amniocentesis. (Amniocentesis is described among diagnostic tests performed during the second trimester.) Some people prefer CVS because the procedure can be done earlier in pregnancy and test results are available much sooner after the procedure is done. If the mother decides to terminate her pregnancy, she can do so earlier, when it may be safer, and less stressful emotionally. When a woman is deciding whether to use CVS, her doctor or genetic counselor will discuss the advantages and disadvantages, including the risks of infection or miscarriage.

Early in pregnancy, the embryo is surrounded by a sac, the chorionic membrane, which will develop into the placenta. This membrane is covered with small projections called villi. During CVS, some of these villi are removed through a thin tube which is introduced into the uterus through the cervix (transcervical CVS), or sometimes, through an abdominal puncture (transabdominal CVS—this procedure is more complex than transcervical CVS). During the procedure, sonography is used to locate the embryo. If the transabdominal procedure is used, a small amount of local anesthetic will be injected to prevent discomfort. Genetic material in the villi is analyzed for abnormalities.

Physical Changes

The most commonly noticed changes are described below. Other changes that occur during the first trimester are less likely to be noticed by all women. For example, all women's intestines become somewhat less active, but not all women experience constipation as a result. Many additional physical changes are listed in Table 6.1, and are discussed in the sections on pregnancy discomforts for each trimester.

During pregnancy, a number of complex hormonal changes take place, and the amount of each hormone rises and falls in a characteristic pattern. Some changes in levels of hormone in the blood or urine may be measured for diagnostic purposes.

Changes in hormones and other physical changes are not always perceptible. For example, a woman is not aware that there is a change in the way her body uses insulin, she simply knows she feels hungrier.

Blood Volume

The blood volume begins to increase during the first trimester, in order to support the growing fetus, placenta, and uterus, and to create a reserve in case the mother loses blood during delivery. Sometimes the volume increases so quickly that the amount of hemoglobin (iron-containing protein) seems relatively lower; this mild anemia is not unusual.

Uterus, Cervix, and Vagina

The uterus and vagina begin to change even in the first trimester. The non-pregnant uterus is a pear-shaped organ, with the "neck" of the pear, the cervix, extending into the vagina. The uterus does not simply stretch during pregnancy; the muscle tissue in the walls grows. By the fifth week, some enlargement can be found during pelvic examination. By the twelfth week, the uterus is spherical in shape.

The cervix, the area where the cervix joins the uterus, and the muscles in the vaginal walls become softer and looser. These are the beginnings of changes which will allow these tissues to stretch enough for the birth of the baby. Some couples may notice the change in the vagina during intercourse.

The uterine muscles begin to contract slowly and irregularly, like an athlete getting in shape for the uterine "Olympics" (childbirth). The contractions are too slight to be noticeable to the mother, although her doctor may be able to feel them during a pelvic examination.

The lining of the vagina thickens, and the woman may notice a thick white discharge. This discharge is normal, and differs in texture, color, and odor from discharges caused by infection (vaginitis is described among pregnancy discomforts of the third trimester.)

Body Temperature

The increase in temperature that follows conception stabilizes for the remainder of pregnancy. Some women enjoy feeling warmer, while others may be uncomfortable.

Breasts

Several changes in the breasts occur in the first trimester. Many women notice soreness, tenderness, or a tingling sensation in the first few weeks. During the second month, breast size increases noticeably, and the veins become more visible as a network of blue and pink lines. The nipple and surrounding area (areola) darken, and the nipple begins to enlarge. The little bumps on the areola (Montgomery's glands) also enlarge.

Pregnancy Discomforts

Pregnancy affects all body systems—including the digestive, urinary, and muscular systems. The discomforts of early pregnancy often seem most dramatic. Laura spoke for many women when she said, "The first trimester was worst of all."

Nausea and Loss of Appetite

Perhaps the most common pregnancy discomfort is morning sickness. From about the sixth week of pregnancy, approximately one third of all pregnant women experience only a slight loss of appetite, while others become very nauseated or even suffer from vomiting. Symptoms usually improve or disappear by about the fourth month. It is not possible to predict who will be troubled by morning sickness; some women are bothered in every pregnancy, like Paula and Portia, others in only some of their pregnancies, like Samantha and Hilary.

Nausea does not necessarily occur only in the morning, though for many women it occurs at the same time of day. Julie said, "It was like clock-work. It happened between 10:00 and 11:00 every morning." Pam said, "The awful feeling happened around 3:00 or 4:00 in the afternoon." Some women do not become nauseated at a particular time of day, but in response to tastes, sights, or smells. Corrine said, "The smell of coffee made me sick."

The causes of morning sickness are not completely understood. Some suggest that it is somehow caused by HCG, since it is most likely to occur when levels of this hormone are high. Others cite evidence that negative or ambivalent feelings about pregnancy contribute to nausea. While negative feelings may play a role, it is unlikely that they are the sole cause of nausea. Sasha, whose family's anxiety made it difficult for her to enjoy her pregnancy, had no problems with morning sickness. Sheila had morning sickness during both pregnancies, but only felt ambivalence during the second one, when her husband was unsure he wanted another child. A number of remedies have been tried for reducing nausea. No single solution works for all women. Experiment with these suggestions and do what works best for you:

- Eat a few crackers at times you are likely to feel sick. These must be dry, low-fat crackers such as soda crackers or matzoh. Some women, like Christine and Clara, kept the crackers by their bed and ate a few before rising. Dawn was helped by beginning her meals with a few crackers.
- Try sipping carbonated water or hot mint tea.
- Some women like a combination of remedies. Michelle's afternoon nausea was relieved by dry toast and mint tea. Laura, who said her nausea was "horrible," ate popcorn and sipped ginger ale.
- Never allow yourself to become too hungry or too full. Eat small, frequent meals. Make sure each meal includes a high-protein food, which satisfies hunger longer than sugar or starch. Before you get up in the morning, and when you get up at night, eat some crackers or a small amount of yogurt, cottage cheese, or milk.
- Avoid drinking a lot of soup or other liquids with meals. Drink between meals instead, so you get adequate fluids without feeling too full.
- Notice which foods make you feel worse, and avoid them. Leslie said, "I stayed away from greasy food, otherwise I would get sick."
- Take a nap or become involved in some absorbing activity at the time of day you expect to feel nausea. Pam said, "I tried to occupy myself, but sometimes needed the medication."
- Talk to your doctor about anti-nausea medication.

Ordinary morning sickness is not dangerous. However, some women develop a condition called *hyperemesis gravidarum,* which means literally "too much vomiting during pregnancy." If excessive vomiting continues, you may become malnourished and/or dehydrated, and need hospitalization. If you notice that you are urinating much less than usual, or not at all, that may be a sign of dehydration; other signs can be found by examination. It is unwise to allow such severe problems to develop. If you experience frequent vomiting, consult your doctor about the advisability of medication. For some women, it is very helpful; Sylvia commented, "When I started the medication it helped me gain weight."

Nausea creates special problems for women with disabilities. It can be dangerous for women who have myasthenia gravis, who may become seriously weakened if vomiting interferes with absorption of their medications. If these women experience nausea, they should contact their doctors and discuss using injectable medicines. Other women, too, may have trouble absorbing oral medications, or need medication dosages adjusted after weight loss.

Some women have difficulty reaching the bathroom quickly when they feel nauseated, or bending to clean after they vomit. Some interviewees thought it was fortunate that they were nauseated at the same time each day, because they were able to schedule attendant care accordingly. Others made sure to keep a bowl within easy reach.

The fetus is not harmed by mild morning sickness, since it does not require much nutrition in early pregnancy. Taking prenatal vitamins helps assure that mother and fetus are well-nourished, and women who were well-nourished before pregnancy are likely to have adequate reserves.

Some women, far from becoming nauseated, have increased appetites in early pregnancy. Jennifer remarked, "I ate constantly. I was impressed at how much I ate." Clara said, "I usually don't eat breakfast, but when I was pregnant it felt as if somebody else inside me made me eat." Both women said they felt as though they would become nauseated if they did not eat.

Others start craving unusual foods (the "pickles and ice cream syndrome" of folklore). Food cravings are harmless so long as they do not interfere with a sensible diet; cravings for non-foods such as ice or chalk may be a sign of illness, and should be reported to your doctor.

Fatigue and Faintness

Feeling flushed, faint, or dizzy is common in early pregnancy. Many people believe that fatigue occurs because extra energy is required for growth of the fetus and placenta and maternal tissues. That cannot be the only reason, because even more growth occurs in the second trimester, when many women feel more energetic. Many women do not feel equally tired in every pregnancy. Carla commented, "It was easier the second time. I was in better shape from running after my first child, and I had a better idea how my body works."

Anxiety or ambivalence can contribute to fatigue. Sheila remarked, "I think I was more tired the second time because I was having relationship problems and I was depressed."

Sometimes fatigue is a symptom of health problems such as anemia or infection. Such problems are likely to be diagnosed during regular office visits, and treated if necessary. However, if you feel extreme fatigue between office visits, it is reasonable to call your doctor. Most women are given prenatal vitamins containing iron to prevent or alleviate anemia. When iron supplements cause constipation or indigestion, many women are tempted to stop taking them; instead, they should discuss the problem with their doctors, and use the suggestions for avoiding constipation given in Chapter 4.

Even when fatigue is not associated with other problems, many women are simply upset at being unable to accomplish as much as usual. Disabled women may be particularly upset, since they already have difficulties with some daily activities. When Pam needed to rest, "It felt like I was pampering myself." Priscilla said, "It was upsetting. I was used to having so much energy. I read an article about the effects of pregnancy hormones, and that helped me get over my frustration about not keeping up with the demands on my time."

Some women experience faintness in addition to or instead of fatigue. Faintness is somewhat more common during the second trimester, but Stephanie became faint during the first. She noticed that she was especially likely to feel faint after meals, and after her bowel movement (every third day). She found that when she became faint after bowel movements, it was best to remain seated and put her feet up on the bathtub bench. She added, "Often I made sure I carried smelling salts with me. One time when I was out with my husband and I got dizzy, I had him lay me down right there on the ground." It is wise to stop and rest whenever one is dizzy, since ignoring the dizziness may cause you to fall and be injured. Raising your feet may help you recover more quickly. If you become faint at predictable times, like Stephanie, alter your schedule accordingly.

The best solution to fatigue and faintness is to rest as much as possible. Elevating your feet to improve circulation may be helpful.

It is important to arrange times for resting or napping. Paula said, "I would collapse on the couch whenever my children were napping or busy playing." Corrine said, "I felt more tired with my second, so I would nap whenever my first was sleeping." Heather "kept to a regime. I just stopped what I was doing and watched TV. I made sure I kept my legs up."

Some women have difficulty getting into bed or arranging cushions to support their feet. If they cannot arrange additional attendant care, it is hard for them to rest. Some women adapt by using reclining chairs, or reclining wheelchairs. Athina managed at first by carrying a pillow with her; several times a day she would place the pillow in front of her and lean up against a piece of furniture to rest. Eventually, she said, "I realized I would just have to spend more time in bed. I found things I could do in bed and stayed there twelve hours a day."

Several women emphasized that finding ways to reduce housework and other responsibilities is as important as finding time to rest. Margie said, "I worked only part-time," and Patricia said, "I didn't go to work and I cut down on my social life for the first two months." Paula "cut back on everything [she] had to do."

Women who cannot afford extra help must find other solutions. Sometimes one's husband can take over some tasks, but that approach may cause more problems than it solves. Stephanie and Cheryl's husbands did not mind doing more work, but Pam's husband felt so burdened that he left her when their child was 18 months old. Portia rented a spare room in exchange for housework. Some women simply eliminate some chores; Heather said matter-of-factly, "My house wasn't as clean as it had been before I was pregnant."

Some women described their fatigue as multiple sclerosis exacerbation. Michelle said she had experienced an exacerbation in the first trimester, then elaborated, "I was really tired in the first and third trimesters. I felt so tired I stayed in bed." Mary said, "Increased tiredness was my main problem." It is difficult to distinguish pregnancy-associated fatigue from exacerbation of multiple sclerosis or myasthenia gravis, and these conditions may be worsened by fatigue and stress. Women with these disabilities must be very careful to get adequate rest, and to report their symptoms to their doctors in case they need medication adjustment or other treatment.

Urinary Problems

Some increase in urinary frequency is normal throughout pregnancy. The increased volume of body fluids, and pressure of the growing uterus on the bladder, both contribute to frequency. Some women find that pressure is relieved later in pregnancy, as the uterus grows upward out of the pelvis. Others, especially those who have had reconstructive surgery on the urinary tract, may experience obstruction from uterine pressure.

Some women we interviewed were not very troubled by frequency or incontinence. Paula said, "It wasn't any worse than my other pregnancies," which occurred before she became disabled. She added, "I just stayed closer to home."

Other women had more severe problems. Mary and Marsha both stopped wearing underwear so they "wouldn't waste any time." Other women suggested staying close to a bathroom, or wearing absorbent underwear.

Some women, like Sharon, find that it is more difficult to catheterize themselves. Women who are bothered by this problem, or by incontinence, may want to try using a Foley catheter (a catheter that remains in the urethra). This decision should not be made too quickly, because a permanent catheter increases the risk of urinary infection, and because some researchers have found that spinal-cord-injured women who use an indwelling catheter during pregnancy often cannot discontinue its use after they give birth.

A more serious problem is urinary infection. Women whose disabilities increase their susceptibility to bladder or kidney infections are even more susceptible during pregnancy. They must be alert for early symptoms of infection, since severe infection can exacerbate disability or cause pre-term labor. Increased frequency is one symptom of bladder infection; your doctor can advise you as to how much frequency can be attributed to pregnancy, and how much to infection. Other symptoms are pain or burning during urination, and feeling the urge to urinate but only passing a few drops. Symptoms of kidney infection are chills and fever and blood in the urine; sometimes blood in the urine may be caused by local irritation, but this symptom should always be reported to your doctor.

Several women tried drinking large quantities of water to prevent or combat infections. Sylvia said, "I was getting quad sweats a lot, and I drank lots of water to replace the fluids I lost. I must have been drinking two or three times as much as normal. Maybe that's why I never got a bladder infection, even though it's usual to get one." However, Sheila and Samantha reported that increasing fluids was not as effective as taking antibiotics. Adequate fluids can help prevent infection, and increase comfort during infection, but as soon as symptoms develop you should contact your doctor and take medications as prescribed. Treating infections early is important because during pregnancy, the ureters (tubes leading from kidneys to bladder) are dilated, making it easier for bladder infection to spread to the kidneys.

Abdominal Muscle Stretching or Cramping

As the abdominal muscles are stretched by the growing uterus, some women feel a stretching sensation or even have muscle cramps. This can happen at any time during pregnancy. Sometimes it is possible to stretch in such a way as to relieve a muscle cramp. Massage or firm pressure on the cramping muscles might also help. These sensations are not long-lasting, and Carla said, "I just lived with it." Cheryl remarked, "I know it was the uterus expanding, but I still felt maybe my cerebral palsy added to it."

Leg Muscle Cramps and Back Pain

These problems are more likely to occur during the second and third trimesters, and will be discussed in these sections below. Some women whose disability involves back pain or muscle spasms experience exacerbations as early as the first trimester.

Constipation

Some people refer to infrequent bowel movements as constipation. However, the term correctly refers to hard, dry stools and difficult bowel movements involving strain or discomfort.

Some women experience constipation as early as the first trimester, but the problem is much more common in the third trimester, and is discussed among discomforts occurring then.

Headaches

Headaches are most likely to occur during the first trimester. If you have headaches, it may be worthwhile to visit an optometrist and find out whether you need glasses or a change in your prescription. Headaches may also be caused by sinus congestion. Most often, however, there is no obvious cause, and the problem disappears spontaneously by mid-pregnancy.

Do not use non-prescription medications for headaches. Instead, try one of the following remedies: Getting more rest will often prevent headaches. Use neck relaxation exercises to prevent muscle tension which may cause headaches. When a headache occurs, try to rest or at least get into a more relaxing situation. Avoid noise and bright lights. Try covering your eyes with a cold compress. Use heat or massage to relax tense neck muscles; some women prefer scalp massages. If your sinuses are congested, try alternating hot and cold compresses. Call your doctor if your headaches are persistent or severe, or if they are accompanied by swelling of your face or hands, blurred vision, or double vision.

Skin and Hair

Sharon commented, "My hair and skin were never healthier." Women's hair seems healthier because it grows faster and stops falling out during pregnancy, so it becomes thicker.

There is much individual variation in skin changes. Some women's skin becomes dry and itchy, even painfully so. They will be more comfortable if they wash with mild soaps or no soap, and moisten their skin with unscented lotion. Others find their skin is oilier; Dawn recalled, "I started breaking out. I was like a teenager. My skin was oilier and my hair grew more."

Women's abdominal skin is marked with a very faint vertical line from the navel to the pubic hair. Among white women, this line grows darker. Some women experience *chloasma,* in which patches of skin on the face and neck grow darker, especially on the forehead, nose, and cheeks. Some women develop red, spidery markings on their skin, especially the limbs. Many of these color changes are reversed after pregnancy. Since chloasma is enhanced by sunlight, using a sunscreen lotion outdoors keeps it from becoming more noticeable.

Weight increases and anemia associated with pregnancy can worsen pressure sores. If pressure sores become infected, the infection can become systemic. However, only two woman interviewed for this book had problems with pressure sores. Several women noted that their skin had never been healthier than when they were pregnant, and Sasha said, "It was the first time in my life that the sore on my foot healed." Good care and nutrition can prevent worsening of sores. Sylvia said, "When my skin got red over the pressure points, I started using a special pillow, and that kept it from getting worse."

Interaction Between Pregnancy and Disability

Some disability changes are not so obviously related to pregnancy changes as, for example, increased incontinence. It is thought that some remissions and exacerbations of disability are related to hormonal changes, but the nature of these relationships is still being studied.

Although rheumatoid arthritis often improves during pregnancy, sometimes it grows worse. In some cases, arthritic symptoms first appear during pregnancy. It cannot be predicted whether a particular woman will experience remission or exacerbation. Jennifer's joint pain improved starting in the first trimester, but her skin sensitivity worsened in late pregnancy. Roberta's arthritic pain did not improve until the second trimester. Renee's arthritic pain first appeared early in her first pregnancy, and gradually grew worse as her pregnancy continued.

The kind and degree of exacerbation also vary among women who have systemic lupus erythematosus. For example, Laura had increased joint pain; she said, "Each morning when I woke up, different joints were aching." Leslie had no joint pain, and her psoriasis improved when she was pregnant. However, Leslie's temperature fluctuated between 96° and 101°F throughout her first two pregnancies, and until she was given medication in her third pregnancy.

Sometimes women who have multiple sclerosis suffer exacerbations which do not appear related to such pregnancy discomforts as fatigue or urinary infection. Marsha, for example, had difficulty gripping small objects; she could not write, hold cans, or use a can-opener.

Some women with high spinal cord injuries may have more episodes of dysreflexia. It is not clear why this is so, but one possibility is that the bladder and bowel are more easily over-filled as the uterus enlarges.

Complications

Chorea Gravidarum

The Latin name for this very rare complication means "dance of pregnancy." Women who have systemic lupus erythematosus are more susceptible to this disorder, which is characterized by repetitive involuntary movements. There are medications for this condition. There have been few opportunities to study the fetal effects of these drugs, but they seem to be harmless.

Ectopic Pregnancy

This unusual complication occurs when the fertilized ovum implants anywhere other than the lining of the uterine cavity, usually but not always in the fallopian tube (tube leading from the ovary to the uterus). ("Tubal pregnancy" is not the correct term, because some ectopic pregnancies occur elsewhere.)

An ectopic pregnancy occurs when an obstruction such as a tumor or adhesions caused by past pelvic infections interferes with the passage of the ovum into the uterus. This is a dangerous complication because of the risk that the pregnancy will rupture, causing potentially fatal bleeding. The usual treatment is surgical removal of the fetus.

Signs and symptoms of ectopic pregnancy may also be caused by other conditions. For example, abdominal pain and tenderness might also be caused by local infection. However, any of the following signs or symptoms might indicate ectopic pregnancy, and justify an immediate call to your doctor: bleeding or spotting following a missed period or confirmation of pregnancy; severe cramping pain and tenderness in the lower abdomen, sometimes one-sided; in some women, nausea and vomiting; in some women, sharp shoulder pain; sudden dizziness, weakness, or fainting, accompanied by clammy skin and a fast, weak pulse.

The procedure used to diagnose an ectopic pregnancy depends on the nature of the symptoms. If the only symptom is spotting, sonography or testing of blood hormone levels may be necessary. When symptoms are more severe, a diagnosis can usually be made by physical examination.

Miscarriage and Threatened Miscarriage

"Miscarriage" is a common term for spontaneous abortion of a fetus that is too immature to survive after birth. After about the twenty-second week of pregnancy, the fetus has some chance of surviving. Birth after the twenty-second week and before the thirty-seventh week is considered pre-term or premature birth.

"Threatened miscarriage" refers to the presence of signs or symptoms of impending miscarriage.

Miscarriages occur for a variety of reasons, including fetal death (often because the fetus has genetic defects), Rh incompatibility, placental abnormalities, and infection. Women who have systemic lupus erythematosus are at increased risk for miscarriage, because they may have antibodies which cause formation of blood clots in the placenta, and eventual placental rejection. We want to emphasize that *it is extremely rare for falls or accidents to cause a miscarriage.* Many disabled women worry that falling will cause a miscarriage, but the uterine wall and amniotic fluid cushion most blows. Some of the women we interviewed fell during pregnancy, but only Carla had a miscarriage after an incident she correctly described as "a freak accident"; her abdomen was struck by the handle of a baby carriage in just such a manner that the fetus was injured. She realized the circumstances were very unusual and commented, "I didn't feel guilty. Somehow I didn't feel like I wanted to punish myself."

During the first trimester, often the only possible treatment for threatened miscarriage is for the mother to begin total bed rest. Many women feel frustrated and discouraged when they need to neglect their responsibilities and rest. It may be heartening to know that rest was effective for Sara, who said,

"I had some spotting during my second pregnancy. I was told to rest for several days, and I didn't have any problems after that." Resting does not guarantee a good outcome, but offers the best chance. Laura explained, "I knew that I only had a 50% chance of a successful pregnancy, so I took one day at a time. I listened to my body and didn't push myself."

If threatened miscarriage is related to systemic lupus erythematosus complications, appropriate medications will be prescribed. Studies suggest that medical treatment of systemic lupus erythematosus has improved the rate of successful pregnancies. Leslie's experience is an example. Her longest lasting pregnancy was the third, during which she received medication. Her miscarriage of one twin in the first trimester was due to cervical incompetence (cervix too weak to retain pregnancy), and the second twin was born prematurely, then died.

Often sonography is necessary in evaluating a threatened miscarriage. When Cheryl experienced spotting after pregnancy was confirmed, a sonogram showed that her fetus was of normal size and activity, and it was determined that the problem was local bleeding in the cervix. Christina's experience was different. She said, "I wasn't even sure I was pregnant. I thought I might be having either a period or a miscarriage. I went to the doctor who confirmed that I was pregnant. When I kept on bleeding heavily an ultrasound was done. It showed I had placenta previa. They said there was a chance it would improve as the baby grew." (Christina was able to give birth vaginally.)

Symptoms which may indicate threatened miscarriage, or a miscarriage in progress, are the same: bleeding with lower abdominal cramps or pain; pain which is severe or lasts more than a day, even without bleeding; heavy bleeding, or light staining lasting more than three days. Women who experience these symptoms should call their doctors immediately, before blood loss reaches a dangerous level.

Other symptoms represent an emergency. If a woman experiences these symptoms and her doctor is unavailable, she should leave a message and go to a hospital emergency room: bleeding and or cramping in a woman who has had previous miscarriages; unbearable pain; bleeding heavy enough to soak several pads in an hour; passage of clots or grayish material. (Your doctor may instruct you to bring such material to the hospital in a clean container).

If a miscarriage does occur, a "D and C" (dilatation and curettage) may be necessary. In this procedure, the cervix is dilated and instruments inserted to remove pregnancy tissues from the uterus. The D and C prevents infection or bleeding caused by tissues retained in an incomplete miscarriage.

Thrombophlebitis

Thrombophlebitis is inflammation of a vein. When inflammation occurs, blood clots (*thrombi*) may form. Deep vein phlebitis is potentially dangerous because of the risk that clots will break loose and be carried to the lungs (*thromboembolism*). Superficial (near the surface) vein phlebitis is less likely to be dangerous.

During pregnancy the risk of thrombophlebitis in the leg or pelvic veins increases. Women who have post polio syndrome or spinal cord injuries are already at increased risk, and must be especially watchful for symptoms during pregnancy. Symptoms are local pain, tenderness, and swelling. Sometimes the whole limb swells. (Women with reduced sensation need to watch for visible swelling.)

If the problem appears to be in superficial veins, rest, elevation and elastic support of the limb, and mild pain relievers may be sufficient treatment. Deep vein thrombosis is difficult to diagnose; special diagnostic procedures and treatment with anticoagulants (medication to prevent further clotting) may be necessary.

While adequate exercise is important for preventing thrombosis, one should not exercise if symptoms occur. Contact your doctor immediately and rest until you receive further instructions.

Only one of the women we interviewed encountered this problem. Sharon had had phlebitis in one leg prior to pregnancy, and it became more swollen in the third trimester. Sharon did not feel very concerned. She said, "I was conscious of the problem. I made sure I kept the leg elevated both at work and at home." Sharon chose not to use anticoagulants. Sharon's decision worked out for her, but cannot be a guideline for other women. In each case, the relative risks of treating or not treating are different, and should be carefully discussed by the woman and her physician.

Fetal and Placental Development

The fetus remains very small in the first trimester. By the end of the first month, it is no larger than a grain of rice, and by the end of the third month, it is about 3 inches long, weighing half an ounce. Most organ systems (skeleton, heart, liver, etc.) begin to develop in this trimester; the limbs are "buds" in which fingers and toes have not separated, and while reproductive organs have started to form, it is still difficult to distinguish boys from girls at the end of the third month. The fetus can kick and clench its fists, but the mother cannot feel these movements.

The placenta begins to develop as part of a membrane surrounding the fetus, and eventually becomes a large, specialized organ. It attaches firmly to the uterine wall by means of many villi (finger-like projections) which penetrate the wall. Nutrients and oxygen pass from maternal vessels in the uterine wall into fetal vessels in the placental villi. (The umbilical cord contains blood vessels connecting the placental vessels to the fetal heart. Normally, the umbilical vessels close at birth).

Besides being the organ which provides nutrients to the fetus, the placenta is an important source of pregnancy hormones.

Emotional Concerns

Women who have just learned that they are pregnant react with a variety of emotions, including shock, delight, amazement, and fear. One woman may experience any of these feelings, and more, at different times.

For some women with disabilities, the first reaction is surprise that pregnancy is even possible. Stacy, who had thought she was sick, said, "Immediately I was shocked and skeptical. I thought all the X-rays had made me sterile."

Even women who have been trying to get pregnant can have a dreamlike feeling of unreality. Samantha said, "I was absolutely thrilled. I wanted it so long. *I couldn't believe it!*" Emotions are strong, and women who want to be pregnant speak in glowing terms. Sheila and Priscilla both said they were "ecstatic," and Sheila went on to say, "I didn't have any fears for myself or about the baby." Paula said, "It was pure joy."

Most of the women we interviewed had mixed feelings. Faith described her reaction to her first pregnancy as "a combination of emotion between panic and exhilaration." Some women's ambivalence had nothing to do with disability; one woman recalled, "I was ecstatic when I found out I was pregnant with my second child, but I felt some apprehension, too, because my husband and I were having some problems with our relationship." Other women worried about the effect of pregnancy or child care on their disabilities. Stephanie said, "I was excited, but at the same time I was reluctant, because of all the physical work required in taking care of a child." Celeste said, "I was frightened of giving birth and afraid I might not get a C-section." (Celeste gave birth vaginally without any difficulty.) Other women, including Carla, Cheryl, and Sara, worried that their children would be born with disabilities. In Chapter 2, we discuss many aspects of the interaction between pregnancy and disability, and women who have unplanned pregnancies will find many of their questions answered there.

Most women's emotions change over time. A woman who feels pure joy at first may begin to have a few practical worries, or a woman who is shocked at first begins to enjoy being pregnant. Celeste recalled, "I was ambivalent at first because my husband wasn't sure he wanted children. But then we went out and shared a milkshake and we began to giggle and he said that it was wonderful."

Like Celeste, many women find that their feelings are affected by the reactions of others. In the first trimester, a woman has some control of the situation; the only people who can know that she is pregnant are the ones she chooses to tell. However, their reactions can be very influential. Sasha said, "I was horrified when I found I was pregnant, and it's because my family was always so fearful for my health. Because they worried, I never felt able to enjoy my pregnancy."

Julie's story was different from Sasha's. She was very upset by her unplanned pregnancy. She worried that she could not afford to have a child. She feared that her family would reject her for being a single mother, and that pregnancy would worsen her disability. She was at work when she found out that her pregnancy test was positive, and she went to the ladies' room to be alone. However, a co-worker found Julie crying, and when Julie poured out her feelings, she said, "This is such a beautiful miracle for anyone to experience. Forget about anyone thinking badly about you. All that matters is you and the baby." Julie said, "When she was so sympathetic, I began to feel hopeful."

Julie's experience confirms many research findings that women feel better about their pregnancies when friends and family are supportive. Women who want to enjoy being pregnant should make a point of sharing their news with supportive people. If they must tell people who can be expected to be fearful or disapproving, they can prepare by first talking with a supportive friend or counsellor.

As the first trimester continues, many women begin to wonder whether their emotions will ever return to normal. The physical and hormonal changes of pregnancy often cause women to over-react to ordinary situations, or change moods suddenly. A woman may be laughing uncontrollably at a joke that is not very funny, when she suddenly bursts into tears. Some of her emotions are responses to her physical sensations, for example, frustration at feeling tired all the time. Sylvia said, "My mood would depend on how I was feeling physically. When I got sweats or a lot of spasms, it was depressing."

While few of the women we interviewed specifically mentioned being troubled by emotional extremes, many women described strong reactions to particular problems. Undoubtedly the emotional fragility of pregnancy contributed to the fears and concerns they expressed.

Women find a variety of ways to cope with their emotions. They may distract themselves by getting involved in shopping for the new baby, or calm themselves with special relaxation techniques. Many women feel it is helpful to compare notes with other pregnant women. Pam did not like having to spend more time resting but, she said, "I have an able-bodied cousin who was pregnant at the same time I was. I told myself, 'If she can lie down, I can lie down.'" Several women made similar comments. A few enjoyed the unusual experience of feeling better than other people; Priscilla, whose only problem in the first trimester was fatigue, said it helped to compare notes with women who had many more discomforts.

Perhaps the most difficult problem a woman can face in the first trimester is a miscarriage. Some women with disabilities are at increased risk for miscarriage, which can cause tremendous emotional pain. Among the women we interviewed, some who had had miscarriages could not bring themselves to talk about their memories.

It is important that a woman who has had a miscarriage not try to minimize her feelings. She needs to know that it is common for women in her position to feel just as much grief as women who suffer late pregnancy losses. Rather than telling herself (or letting other people tell her) that, "It was only a miscarriage," and that she can "try again soon," she needs to allow herself time to grieve normally. If her emotions seem unbearable, it is appropriate to join a support group for parents who have had similar experiences, or to seek counselling. It is also important for her to take care of herself physically. The blood loss and other changes associated with a miscarriage are stressful, and adequate rest, nutrition, and medical care are important to a full recovery. Physical recovery can contribute to a good emotional recovery. Remember that sleeplessness and loss of appetite can be manifestations of depression; these feelings must be resolved, with professional help, if necessary, so that complete recovery is possible.

Arlene's comments reflect many of the feelings women express after some time has passed. "When I had those miscarriages, I knew it wasn't meant to be. I think now that my daughter has been born, I pushed the other two aside. I have learned to be philosophical, with my background of being disabled and a research example."

If a woman feels emotionally ready to try again, she should first discuss with her doctor whether she is physically ready. At the same time, she can discuss any questions she has about the possibility of preventing another miscarriage.

SECOND TRIMESTER

. . . .

Office Visits

During the second trimester, you will visit your doctor once a month. These visits are usually much briefer than the initial visit, since the full physical examination is not repeated. The visit includes routine measurements of your weight and blood pressure and a urine test. The level of alpha fetoprotein in your blood is measured some time between the fifteenth and twentieth weeks (see "Diagnostic Tests" below). Your doctor may order a blood sugar test if you are at risk for developing diabetes of pregnancy. Your risk of developing diabetes is higher if you are obese, if you previously gave birth to a large baby, or if you have a family history of diabetes or diabetes of pregnancy. If an earlier blood test showed you were anemic, your doctor may repeat this test. Some women with disabilities may need repeat blood tests (for example, tests of medication levels or kidney function).

The uterus has grown enough by now to make it possible to measure the height of the fundus (top of the uterus) at each visit. These measurements help determine the length of gestation and fetal growth rate.

It may not be possible to hear the fetal heartbeat until about the twentieth week, using an ordinary stethoscope. However, when a Doppler instrument (hand-held ultrasound device) is used, it is often possible to detect the heartbeat as early as the twelfth week. Often when the doctor or nurse hears the heartbeat, s/he lets the mother and other family members listen. This is an exciting moment for many parents, and the idea that they are going to have a baby seems much more real. Do not worry if the heartbeat cannot be heard at the twelfth week, because it is possible that your baby's position may make detection difficult, or the length of gestation may have been miscalculated. You will probably hear your baby's heartbeat at the next office visit. By that time, you may have already felt the baby move, since movement is first felt some time between the sixteenth and twentieth weeks.

As usual, the office visit will include an opportunity for you and your doctor to discuss any physical or emotional changes you are experiencing. If you have many questions for your doctor, you may wish to write them down before the visit. No symptom is too unimportant to mention to your doctor, who can then reassure you, give practical advice or, if necessary, do diagnostic tests. For example, do tell your doctor if you have been feeling tired, even though it is common for pregnant women to have fatigue. S/he can ask questions to determine whether to test for anemia or disability exacerbation, or help you plan ways to rest or reduce stress. Try to notice as many details as possible about any symptoms you are experiencing. For example, if you have been experiencing headaches, are they located at the front or back of your head? Is there a constant ache or throbbing? Does the headache occur at a certain time of day, and is it accompanied by other symptoms?

Be sure to discuss any disability symptoms. If your doctor recommends a change of medication (or if you are interested in changing medications), be sure to discuss advantages, disadvantages, and possible side effects. Your doctor can also advise you on how to cope with some side effects. For example, s/he may suggest an antacid if medications for systemic lupus erythematosus are causing indigestion, or prescribe medication for vaginitis, which sometimes occurs as a side effect of taking antibiotics.

Your doctor will also ask whether you have felt the fetus kicking. At first this sensation is difficult to recognize, so we will share some women's descriptions below in the section on "Physical Changes."

If you had genetic testing or other special tests, your doctor will explain the results to you during your office visit.

Diagnostic Tests

Maternal Alpha Fetoprotein (AFP)

This is a screening test for fetal abnormalities. Other tests will be done if results indicate possible problems. Alphafetoprotein is a chemical that is secreted by the fetus and some of it enters the maternal blood stream. The AFP level in the mother's blood may be tested any time between the fifteenth and twentieth weeks. However, it is recommended that the test be done before the eighteenth week because, if the mother needs to consider terminating an abnormal pregnancy, an earlier screening test would allow time for further testing before she must make a decision. Before the screening test is done, the length of pregnancy must be determined so that test results can be interpreted correctly.

Further testing is required if the serum AFP level is not normal. A low level may indicate Down syndrome, while a high level indicates a possible neural tube defect.

Sonography

This procedure may be used for a variety of reasons during the second trimester. Sonography may be used to determine the causes of pain or bleeding, or to make a more accurate assessment of fetal size and age than is possible from external examination. If the fetus seems to have stopped moving, or its heartbeat is difficult to detect, sonography can help determine whether there is a problem. It can also be used as an adjunct to amniocentesis. Sonography produces a "sonogram," an image like a still photograph. "Real-time" ultrasound produces a screen image which shows the fetus in motion.

Sonography can also reveal whether there is a normal amount of amnionic fluid, locate the placenta, and determine whether the fetus is of normal size and activity (both breathing activity and movement of the limbs). Some deformities (including neural tube defects) may be detected during this procedure. Depending on when the sonogram is done, and the position of the fetus, it may be possible to see the fetus' heartbeat, and determine its sex. Many twin pregnancies are also discovered during sonography.

Women who have systemic lupus erythematosus need sonography monthly, starting at the twentieth week, because of the increased risks of growth retardation and stillbirth. They will need this procedure every 1-2 weeks if there is evidence that the fetus has congenital heart block.

During the second trimester, the uterus is large enough that the mother will not need to fill her bladder before the examination. Sonography is often a rather routine procedure during this stage of pregnancy, and many parents feel it is an exciting opportunity to see their baby for the first time. Seeing the ultrasound image on the screen, like hearing the heartbeat, helps them to feel that they really are going to have a baby. In some families' scrapbooks, "baby's first picture" is a sonogram!

Fetal Echocardiography

This procedure uses ultrasound to study the fetal heart. If the fetal heartbeat shows signs of congenital heart block (an infrequent complication of SLE), echocardiography can determine whether there are also structural defects of the heart. This procedure is done at 20 to 22 weeks gestation.

Amniocentesis

In this procedure, a very small amount of amniotic fluid is withdrawn from the uterus for diagnostic testing. A physician uses a syringe to withdraw the sample, after determining the positions of the fetus and placenta by using real-time ultrasound. Since a local anesthetic is used, having an amniocentesis is no more uncomfortable than having a blood sample drawn.

There is a small risk (as low as 1 in 300) that the procedure will cause infection or miscarriage, so the procedure is only used for specific indications. Before you have an amniocentesis, discuss the risks and benefits thoroughly with your doctor and/or a genetic counselor. This discussion could include safety and accuracy statistics at the facility you would use.

For some indications, the amniotic fluid is chemically analyzed and results should be available within 24 hours. If the maternal AFP test or family history suggest that the fetus may have a neural tube defect, measuring the amount of AFP in the amniotic fluid can determine whether there is a problem. Sometimes, amniotic fluid may be examined for the presence of infectious organisms.

For genetic testing, cells which the fetus has shed into the amniotic fluid are collected from the amniocentesis sample and cultured until there is enough genetic material for analysis. Results are available approximately 3 weeks after the amniocentesis. Women who are over 35, or have a family history of genetic disorders, or whose maternal AFP test indicates the fetus might have Down syndrome, should consider genetic testing. Women who would not wish to terminate their pregnancies may also choose genetic testing, like Amy, who remarked, "I had an amniocentesis because of my age, although I wouldn't abort. I just wanted to know." Weighing the value of this knowledge against the risk of genetic testing is a very individual decision. Faith agreed to have an amniocentesis to assist research on her disability. (For more information about genetic testing, see Chapter 2.)

Some women want to know the sex of the fetus after genetic testing, since knowing the sex helps with preparations like shopping for clothing and choosing a name. Others enjoy being surprised, and wait until their baby is born to find out whether it is a boy or a girl.

Stress and Non-stress Tests

These tests are more commonly used during the third trimester, but may be performed in the second trimester if there are signs of fetal distress or threatened miscarriage. Since women who have myasthenia gravis, systemic lupus erythematosus, or spinal cord injuries are at increased risk for pre-term labor, they may need these tests, which are described among other third trimester medical procedures.

Additional Blood Tests

Women who have kidney problems will need frequent tests of kidney function. As of this writing, medical researchers are investigating the possibility that levels of specific serum complements (proteins that work in conjunction with antibodies) can help predict exacerbation of systemic lupus erythematosus, and differentiate it from pre-eclampsia. If your doctor uses this diagnostic procedure, a series of tests will be performed, because the procedure measures the rate at which complement levels rise.

Medical Procedures

Pre-term Delivery

Some women will need pre-term delivery near the end of the second trimester. Since babies born so early cannot survive without intensive care, delivery will only be considered if there is a severe threat to fetal or maternal health, such as placental abruption, impaired placental function, or kidney failure.

Before delivery, if amniocentesis shows that the fetal lungs are immature, the mother can be given an injection of hormones that will cross the placenta into the fetal bloodstream and may speed maturation.

Pre-term delivery in the second trimester is rare but, if it is necessary, labor may be induced, or cesarean surgery may be performed. A stress test can determine whether the fetus can tolerate labor. Since the fetus is small, labor will probably not be as uncomfortable as it is with a full-term baby.

Plasmapheresis

If myasthenia gravis symptoms are severe and resistant to medication, plasmapheresis may be considered. In this procedure, the mother's blood plasma is replaced by donor plasma. The exchange is made very slowly, so that normal blood pressure can be maintained. During the procedure, the mother must lie on her left side (unless a disability problem forces her to lie on her right side). If she lies on her back, pressure from the uterus might interfere with blood circulation. The procedure is not uncomfortable. You simply have to anticipate spending 1 1/2 to 2 hours lying on your side with an IV needle in your arm.

Physical Changes

As the uterus and fetus continue to grow, and the amount of amniotic fluid increases, the abdomen looks more rounded. Earlier in pregnancy, many women like to wear T-shirts proclaiming, "I'm not fat...I'm pregnant!" However, they do not need them by the fourteenth week. Most women need to start wearing maternity clothes early in the second trimester.

Because the uterus has enlarged, you must not lie on your back when you sleep (and the left side is preferable to the right), because the weight of the uterus resting on major blood vessels can interfere with circulation. It is also difficult to lie "on your stomach."

Many changes experienced in the first trimester, such as breast growth, increased vaginal discharge, and changes in skin color, continue during the second trimester. Increased blood flow makes the genitals appear darker and more swollen. Most women notice that their hair and fingernails grow faster, an interesting coincidence since the fetal hair also starts growing in the second trimester.

Fetal Movement

The change that is most delightful is really a result of fetal development. Feeling the baby move is even more exciting than hearing its heartbeat. Christina recalled, "When I first felt him kick, I was in church, but I yelled anyway. I couldn't help myself." Cheryl said, "The joy of feeling life inside me made me glad to be a woman." By the end of the second trimester, most women can share their excitement by inviting other people to "come feel the baby kick."

The fetus starts moving during the second month, but movement cannot be felt until some time between the fourteenth and twenty-sixth weeks, usually about the nineteenth week. A woman who has already experienced pregnancy is likely to recognize fetal movement earlier, since the sensation can be difficult to recognize at first. Sharon explained, "It was muted. It felt more like pressure. Then I would put my hand on my belly and feel the movement." Stacy and Samantha said they saw the movement before they could feel it. Many women describe it as a fluttering movement, and others compare it to gas pains. Both Patricia and Laura said, "It felt like the baby had hiccups," and Laura added, "Sometimes it felt like a fish wriggling."

Several women remarked that fetal movement felt the same as it had in pregnancies occurring before they had become disabled. Most of the women with spinal cord dysfunctions, including those who could not feel labor contractions, were able to feel fetal movement.

Pregnancy Discomforts

Most women find that the second trimester is the most comfortable, since they are no longer bothered by such unpleasant symptoms of early pregnancy as nausea and vomiting. Corrine commented, "The second trimester was the only one when I had no problems at all." Many women feel more energetic, and are not troubled by fatigue until weight gain begins to interfere with their mobility. Christina said, "I felt so good I went out in my wheelchair and did all kinds of things." Also, looking pregnant and feeling the baby kick can be so satisfying that many women are less annoyed by those discomforts that they do experience.

Muscle Spasms

The women we interviewed did not always differentiate between two kinds of muscle spasms—cramping and clonus. Muscle cramps also bother able-bodied women during pregnancy. However, women with disabilities may have more frequent or severe cramps, and if they experience clonus when they are not pregnant, it may become more frequent during pregnancy. These problems usually begin during the second trimester.

Cramps Cramps are strong, painful, involuntary muscle contractions; if you touch the cramped muscle, it feels like a hard knot. Calf muscle cramps ("Charley horses"), which are most common, usually occur at night. The cramp can be relieved by firmly bending the foot upward. Some women sit on the edge of the bed and press the foot against the floor or wall. Others find the cramp so painful that they awaken their husbands, who must grasp the ball of the foot and bend it at a right angle (see Figure 5.5).

Some cramps can be avoided by using preventive measures. Pointing the toe can cause a cramp; tight bed clothes may cause a woman to point her toe as she sleeps, and some women have fewer problems when they stop tucking in the top sheet. Many disabled women prefer satin sheets even when they are not pregnant, because they can move more easily between these slippery sheets and have fewer problems with muscle cramps or tension.

Heat relieves soreness after cramps, and seems to prevent further cramping by relaxing the affected muscle. Many women take hot baths, but for some women with disabilities it is difficult to get in and out of the bath. Sara pointed out that it can even be difficult to check the water temperature so, although she thought a bath might have been more effective, she used a heating pad instead. Sybil used massage, liniment, and a hot water bottle. Twenty minutes of heat should be sufficient to promote relaxation and good circulation. Women who have reduced sensation should check frequently for reddening of the skin when using a heating pad or hot water bottle.

Faith found that ice packs relieved her muscle cramps. Ice may have worked for her because of her particular disability, but other women may find that the cold makes the cramping worse.

Several women discovered that sleeping position affected muscle cramping. Samantha, who only had cramps at night when she was very tired, found it helped to sleep with pillows between her knees, with her legs slightly bent. Sleeping with pillows between the knees also helped Cheryl to prevent groin cramps, and helped several other women to prevent thigh cramps.

Some of the stretching exercises in Chapter 5 can be very effective in preventing muscle cramps. Michelle remarked that she never had cramps until the last week of her pregnancy, when she was too tired to exercise. Calcium supplements may also prevent cramping. Clara remarked, "I never drink milk, and when I took calcium tablets the cramping got better." (For more information about calcium supplements, see Chapter 4.) And, of course, do not use calcium supplements without consulting your doctor.)

Clonus Clonus refers to involuntary movements caused by muscle spasms. Clara remarked that for her, ordinary calf cramps seemed to stimulate clonus. Clonus often ends more quickly when another person holds and supports the affected limb (see Figures 7.1 and 7.2). Women who use anti-spasmodic medications when they are not pregnant should not resume or increase these medications during pregnancy without consulting their doctor about possible risks.

Back Pain

Several physical changes interact to cause back pain in pregnancy. First, pregnancy hormones cause ligaments to relax, and pelvic joints become less stable (this is an advantage during childbirth). Hilary could feel the difference and she commented, "My back wasn't as rigid." Second, because the abdominal muscles are stretched and weakened as the uterus grows, the back muscles must work harder. Third, the weight of the uterus puts additional strain on the lower back muscles.

Women who are disabled are often more vulnerable to back pain, and may experience it earlier in pregnancy, while able-bodied women usually have no problems until the third trimester. Paula commented that she had no back problems during her first pregnancy (before she was disabled), but did experience back pain in later pregnancies after her abdominal muscles were weakened. Faith, too, thought that she felt more back pain in her third pregnancy because her abdominal muscles had become weaker. Several women with spinal cord injuries noticed back pain during pregnancy. It is not surprising that their backs were strained, since their abdominal muscles were weakened, but it is surprising that they were able to feel the pain. Possibly the pain was caused by additional strain on functioning muscles.

Exercises to stretch the lower back muscles and to strengthen abdominal muscles may reduce back pain. Rest, heat, and massage can also alleviate pain. Sitting in a straight-backed chair may also help. When a woman is not pregnant, sitting upright can make back problems worse by straightening the normal curve of the lower back. However, sitting upright can be helpful during pregnancy when the curve is exaggerated.

Women who have difficulty exercising, or who have persistent back pain, should talk to their doctors about getting physical therapy. Besides helping with active or passive exercise, the therapist can suggest ways to avoid back strain when doing daily activities—for example, by reviewing the best ways to bend and lift.

Mobility Difficulties

Able-bodied women usually find that their mobility is unaffected until the third trimester, when the size of the uterus may affect their sense of balance and make them feel clumsier in general. However, women who already have impaired mobility often experience difficulties as early as the second trimester.

An important exception is those women whose rheumatoid arthritis goes into remission during pregnancy, like Jennifer and Roberta, who found that walking was easier than usual. Jennifer commented, "Before I was pregnant, I complained about walking from the bedroom to the kitchen; during pregnancy, I took long walks and enjoyed them." Some women whose disability symptoms are mild also experience less difficulty, like Margie, who said, "I walked the same as before, dragging one leg."

Besides difficulty with walking, some women start having trouble when bending to lift objects. Others begin to have more difficulty transferring or being lifted.

Some women whose mobility is reduced still feel that they have time to adapt. Celeste explained, "Looking back, I see it didn't affect me as badly as I thought, because the body accommodates." Portia remarked, "If I had to go immediately from not being pregnant to being 8 months pregnant it would have been impossible, but I managed because it is a gradual process." Other women cannot adapt quickly enough, like Cheryl, who had difficulty walking for 6 weeks after she fell and strained some muscles in the groin area.

It is important to think about ways to adapt before mobility difficulties become serious. The women we interviewed used creativity and common sense in finding solutions. Paula said, "During my last pregnancy I felt off balance in the second trimester, so a lot of the time I used a baby buggy like a walker." Sharon used a "reacher" that was designed for taking objects from high shelves. She also pointed out that when a woman is pregnant, it is not as easy for her to carry things in her lap, so attaching a lap tray or backpack to one's wheelchair may help. Possibly using a bath chair and a hospital bed can make transferring easier for you or your attendant.

Some women may need to start using an assistive device or a wheelchair, but the decision is not always easy. Psychological factors can weigh as heavily as physical problems. Many women cannot help feeling that crutches and wheelchairs are unpleasant symbols of disability and dependence. However, the risk that a woman really will become more disabled or dependent is greater if she has been injured in a fall, or fatigued by too much exercise. Several women we interviewed wished that they had used a wheelchair, or started using one earlier. Hilary explained, "When I was a child, I was given a lot of positive feedback whenever I used my prosthesis, so using a wheelchair was hard on my self-image. When I consulted an orthopedist about pregnancy, he said I would need to use a wheelchair. I thought, 'Not me,' and I waited until I really didn't have any option, because it was safer and I was falling a lot. It was astronomically easier, and in my second pregnancy I started using the chair earlier."

Faintness and Dizziness

These symptoms are commonly caused by lowered blood pressure. Blood returns to the heart more slowly because pregnancy hormones relax the walls of the veins and the uterus presses on several veins.

Some women notice that they feel faint in specific situations. For example, Amy felt faint after warm baths, and solved the problem by using cooler water. Others feel faint when they stand up after sitting or lying down. They can adapt by getting up more slowly, possibly using a support. Many women find that they can relieve dizziness by lying down, leaning back in a reclining chair, or bending forward with their heads lowered. Stephanie noticed that she felt faint after eating a large meal, and solved the problem by eating small, frequent meals (also a good strategy for preventing heartburn).

There are ways to help prevent dizzy spells from occurring. Stacy remarked that even when she is not pregnant, a maternity girdle improves her circulation, and wearing it when she was pregnant reduced her dizziness. Wearing elastic support stockings is a good alternative. Resting with the legs elevated several times a day can also help.

Sometimes anemia contributes to dizziness or faintness. Renee's dizziness improved after she started taking iron pills. Some women's dizziness is caused by sudden drops in blood sugar levels. Many women, like Pam, Stacy and Sylvia, found it helped to eat small, frequent meals and prevent such extreme variations.

Urinary Difficulties

Ordinarily, the increased frequency of urination that bothers many women in the first trimester is not as much of a problem during the second. However, this is not uniformly true for women with disabilities, some of whom will have more trouble with incontinence, stress incontinence, or urinary tract infection.

Hilary, Sharon, and Sasha all became more incontinent as their bladders were compressed by uterine growth. Sharon said, "I was dripping all the time, and it was getting harder to reach around my belly to put the catheter in." Sharon's incontinence was so annoying that she decided to use a Foley catheter, but after her pregnancy she regretted the decision, because she was not able to stop using it. Sasha saw her problem as "the same old, boring bladder." She tried to reduce her incontinence by restricting fluids. This was not a good solution because it did not affect her incontinence, and may have increased her risk of bladder infection.

Stress incontinence is a condition in which urine leaks when pressure is put on the bladder from ordinary actions such as laughing, coughing, sneezing, or straining. Heather recalled, "Whenever I coughed or sneezed, I leaked. Sometimes I had to go home from work to change clothes. It was wonderful to have an understanding boss." Using the bathroom more often does not seem to help most women. Sometimes "Kegel" exercises (see Chapter 5) help to improve bladder control by strengthening the muscles that hold it in place. For many women, the best solution may be the use of absorbent pads or underwear. If you want to try waterproof underwear, watch for symptoms of vaginitis or skin irritation, which develop more easily when the genitals are warm and wet. Do not use waterproof underwear if you develop these problems.

Few of the women we interviewed developed bladder infections during the second trimester. However, women who are particularly susceptible to bladder infections, such as those with spinal cord injuries, should watch for symptoms because pregnancy increases their risk. Use preventive measures: drink plenty of fluids (at least twice your usual intake), keep the genital area clean, and be especially careful to wash your hands and use proper technique when using your catheter. If you develop fever, frequency, pain or burning with urination, or urgency, start drinking plenty of fluids and call your doctor. Besides prescribing an antibiotic, your doctor may ask you to bring a urine sample to the office or a clinical laboratory. Laboratory testing can determine which antibiotic would be most effective against your infection. Depending on laboratory results, your doctor may then ask you to change from one antibiotic to another.

Nasal Congestion

Hormonal changes and increased blood volume can cause the lining of the nostrils and sinuses to swell during pregnancy. The resulting sensation of a "stuffy nose" is usually a minor nuisance, although some women have trouble distinguishing this condition from a cold or allergies.

The one interviewee who recalled having this problem, Jennifer, said, "I managed to find nose drops that didn't have any harmful ingredients, but they were expensive." Since many medications that relieve nasal congestion contain ingredients which may be harmful to the fetus, none should be used without a doctor's advice.

Many women find that using a cool mist vaporizer, or inhaling steam from a hot shower or a cup of hot water, relieves their symptoms. Others feel more comfortable when they gently massage their sinuses.

Edema

Julie recalled, "I had feet like an elephant." Some swelling as early as the second trimester is not unusual. It results from the normal increase in blood volume. Even when you are not pregnant, some fluid escapes from your circulatory system into the spaces between cells (interstitial space). When the amount of blood increases during pregnancy, even more fluid may enter the interstitial space. There is no need to worry about the mild, gradual swelling that makes your wedding ring a little tight, or your shoes too tight at the end of the day. However, sudden or severe swelling may be a symptom of pre-eclampsia.

Heartburn

Heartburn is most commonly experienced during the third trimester. However, some women with disabilities may have indigestion late in the second trimester. Heather remarked, "I think I got heartburn early because my pelvis is small and I carried high" (putting more pressure on her stomach).

Fetal Development

The placenta, which produces many pregnancy hormones, supplies nutrition and oxygen to the fetus and eliminates fetal wastes, continues to grow during the second trimester. The fetus also grows much larger. Its weight increases from about 1/2 ounce to 1 3/4 pounds, and its length increases from about 3 to 13 inches.

All the organ systems mature considerably. The skeleton begins to harden, and hair begins to grow in the fifth month. It is the increase in muscle mass and strength that makes it possible for the mother to feel fetal movement, and by the end of this trimester the heart beats so strongly it can sometimes be heard by pressing an ear against the mother's abdomen. In the sixth month, the eyelids open and close, eyes move, and tooth buds begin to form.

Some babies born at the end of the second trimester are able to survive with intensive care, although they are far more vulnerable to health problems, especially respiratory problems, than full-term babies are.

Complications

Like the complications that can occur in the first trimester, these complications of pregnancy do not affect most women. They are common only in the sense that they occur more frequently than other complications. They are serious, even though infrequent, and it is important to recognize their signs and symptoms.

Pre-eclampsia

Pre-eclampsia is increased blood pressure accompanied by proteinuria (protein in the urine) and/or swelling (edema), after the twentieth week of pregnancy. While the incidence of pre-eclampsia among all women is only about 5%, it most often affects women who are pregnant for the first time, especially the oldest and youngest members of this group. So, for example, a teenager who is pregnant for the first time has a higher-than-average risk of developing pre-eclampsia. Multiple pregnancy, pre-existing vascular disease, and a family history of pre-eclampsia/eclampsia also indicate an increased risk.

The condition is described as mild when proteinuria and some increase in blood pressure are the only symptoms. However, severe pre-eclampsia or eclampsia, which endanger both mother and fetus, can develop suddenly. Since these more extreme forms are more likely to develop in the third trimester, they are described with third trimester complications. If you had edema or proteinuria from vascular or kidney disease before pregnancy, and these conditions worsen during the sixth month, pre-eclampsia is said to be superimposed on the pre-existing problem.

A woman cannot tell that she has high blood pressure or protein in her urine; these problems are discovered during an office visit. However, she can watch for swelling, which is often the first sign of pre-eclampsia. This is not the mild swelling many pregnant women experience, but swelling accompanied by a sudden weight gain of more than 2 pounds in a single week, or more than 6 pounds in a month. Another sign to watch for is sudden swelling of your hands and face—even your eyelids can look puffy, and your fingers may be so swollen that suddenly your wedding ring is painfully tight. Check for "pitting edema"—a "pit" or dent remaining in the skin after pressing with your fingertip. Call your doctor if you experience severe swelling.

Women who have pre-eclampsia *must* rest in bed for most of the day. If you are not hospitalized, you will need to see your doctor twice a week so s/he can monitor your condition closely.

If the problem does not improve, hospitalization will be necessary. If pre-eclampsia becomes severe, you may need medications to lower blood pressure. Unfortunately, the most reliable medication for this purpose cannot be used for women with myasthenia gravis, since it causes a dangerous exacerbation of muscle weakness.

If you have systemic lupus erythematosus, your doctor may order tests to determine whether your hypertension and proteinuria are caused by lupus exacerbation, pre-eclampsia, or both. If you have lupus exacerbation, your doctor may need to change your medications. If so, you will need to discuss possible side effects with your doctor. Make sure s/he helps you understand as clearly as possible how to differentiate symptoms of pre-eclampsia, systemic lupus erythematosus, and medication side effects.

While pre-eclampsia symptoms can be treated, the only "cure" is the birth of the baby. Your doctor must continually evaluate whether it is best to deliver the baby or allow the pregnancy to continue, especially if symptoms become severe.

Cervical Incompetence

Cervical incompetence is painless dilation of the cervix in the second or early third trimester. The opened cervix is unable ("incompetent") to retain the fetus in the uterus.

Among the women we interviewed, cervical incompetence contributed to one pre-term birth. Bed rest had been prescribed for Leslie, whose placenta was partially abrupted. It was not known that her cervix was incompetent. When she was allowed to try sitting up, she went into labor. Leslie explained that she did not know the signs of labor and, "I was in labor for 16 hours, thinking I had the flu. The contractions were one-sided, and I didn't realize I was in labor until the bag of water broke." Leslie gave birth to her son in the sixth month of pregnancy.

Because dilation may be painless, and pelvic examinations are not routinely included in second trimester office visits, cervical incompetence may not be diagnosed until a woman has had more than one miscarriage. The treatment is rest and, sometimes, "cerclage," in which the uterus is sutured shut. A woman who has had cerclage must watch carefully for signs and symptoms of labor, since her uterus might rupture if active labor begins before the sutures are removed.

Miscarriage and Threatened Miscarriage

Miscarriage and threatened miscarriage are rare in the second trimester, but may occur for a number of reasons, including fetal illness or death. Because

Arlene's blood circulation was poor, her fetus did not receive enough oxygen, and died early in the second trimester. Arlene said, "The first sign that something was wrong was when the doctor couldn't find the heartbeat. Then I had an amniocentesis to find out what was wrong. After the baby died, it was a month before I had a miscarriage. I had a mini-labor and delivery. Physically it was not bad."

Placenta Previa and Placental Abruption

Placenta previa and placental abruption are dangerous to both fetus and mother. Placental abruption is partial or complete separation of the placenta from the uterine wall. In placenta previa, the placenta is placed lower than the fetus, possibly covering the cervix, so that the placenta may separate from the uterine wall during cervical dilation or during labor. (Both conditions are described in detail in Chapter 7.) These conditions can cause threatened miscarriage, miscarriage, or fetal death.

Signs of placenta previa are painless bleeding and, sometimes, passing of clots. With placental abruption, bleeding is accompanied by severe pain. Leslie, who had a partial abruption in the second trimester of her first pregnancy, recalled, "I never have experienced such pain in my life. When I got to the hospital I ended up lying in an uncomfortable position and staying that way because it just hurt too much to move. Because the placenta was large and the abruption was only partial, I was able to stay pregnant." (Leslie's child was born in the seventh month.) When either of these conditions is suspected, sonography can confirm the diagnosis.

Bed rest may prevent a miscarriage but, especially in cases of placental abruption, immediate delivery may be necessary to prevent further blood loss. The mother may need blood transfusions if much blood has already been lost.

Intrauterine Growth Retardation

Intrauterine growth retardation (IUGR) is inadequate growth of the fetus. IUGR is associated with a number of maternal conditions, including small stature, poor weight gain, anemia, vascular disease, and kidney disease. Placental abnormalities, multiple fetuses, and hypoxia (perhaps including lack of oxygen caused by maternal breathing difficulties) also contribute to IUGR. In addition, IUGR can be caused by the mother's use of alcohol, tobacco, or "hard" drugs.

IUGR is diagnosed by sonography. Little can be done to treat it in the second trimester. If the mother is smoking, drinking or using drugs, it may help to stop. If she is undernourished or anemic, improvements in her diet can help. Bed rest may be advised.

When the mother has SLE, IUGR may be caused by placental damage related to the mother's condition. If she is not already taking medication to control SLE, it will probably be prescribed if her fetus is not growing normally.

Choosing A Childbirth Class

In many communities, childbirth classes are so popular that it is important to enroll in one as early as the fourth month—certainly by the end of the second trimester.

Women with spinal cord injuries may wonder why they should take a childbirth class. Sharon remarked that she did not take a class because she did not think she needed one, and Sheila was advised that she did not need one. Yet many women with spinal cord injuries give birth vaginally, and many of them feel the discomfort of labor. Women who have lesions below the T11–L1 level feel labor pain; those who have lesions between T5 and T10 generally do not, but they do experience increased clonus and spasticity during labor. In addition, women with higher complete or incomplete lesions have been known to feel labor pain. Also, childbirth classes have much to offer besides information about coping with labor. They present an opportunity to meet other pregnant women, and to obtain information about medical procedures and medications, pregnancy discomforts, preparation for breast feeding, and normal fetal development. Roberta commented, "I was glad I took a birthing class because I found out my baby was doing fine."

There are a number of ways to find a good childbirth class. Faith checked the bulletin board at the hospital. Sara called the local school for adult education. You could also call a community recreation center, ask a friend or your physician for suggestions, take a class offered by a local hospital or clinic, or check the index of your telephone directory for listings under "Childbirth Preparation." If a variety of classes are available, the next step is to interview instructors by telephone or in person.

It is important to talk to more than one instructor, even in areas where only one type of childbirth class is taught. Michelle interviewed two teachers, and chose the one she thought she could work with more easily. Stephanie said, "I looked until I found one I thought had a positive attitude towards disability." Women's attitude toward childbirth instructors paralleled their feelings toward their obstetricians; they did not mind when instructors were unfamiliar with disability, as long as the instructors were willing to find ways to adapt. For example, Sara found a class in which she could exercise in her wheelchair.

The teacher's personality or class organization is sometimes more important than the method she teaches. Many teachers change their philosophies as they gain experience and continue their education, and different teachers individualize their classes in different ways. For example, one teacher might be interested in helping students experiment with different positions for giving birth, while another might think it is important to have the students discuss the advantages and disadvantages of circumcising newborn boys.

Interviewing instructors is easier after learning something about childbirth methods. Most childbirth educators teach either the Bradley method or the LaMaze method. Bradley teachers are trained and certified by the American

Academy of Husband-Coached Childbirth; LaMaze Teachers by ASPO (American Society for Psychoprophylaxis in Obstetrics).

Both methods emphasize teaching women about the labor process so that it seems normal and familiar, rather than mysterious and frightening. Because women who are not frightened can relax their muscles more easily, they may feel less pain during childbirth, or at least be more likely to find the pain bearable.

The LaMaze method also emphasizes intensive practice of a variety of specific methods for breathing and relaxation. The mother is attempting to learn a new way of responding to pain and tension, so that she will react appropriately during childbirth. The method uses concentration on external objects as a way of distracting oneself from discomfort. Some women find one of the breathing techniques (panting) difficult. During childbirth, the mother may be coached by a LaMaze instructor, or by a person who attended class with her.

Bradley instruction emphasizes the naturalness of childbirth, and instructors emphasize the value of good health care and nutrition during pregnancy, and avoidance of medication and other medical interventions during labor. Sometimes instructors are available as coaches, but classes are designed for couples, and it is usually assumed that the father will be the labor coach. The method relies on a very simple breathing technique. Rather than being taught to distract herself during labor, the mother is taught to concentrate on internal sensations.

Women find advantages in either method. Faith, who preferred the Bradley method, explained, "Their philosophy really helped me." Clara said, "I chose the LaMaze method because looking inward only makes me more tense, and I liked having so many choices for breathing technique." When you interview a childbirth instructor, it may be helpful to ask the following questions:

- *What method do you teach?* Not all advertisements state whether the teacher is a LaMaze or a Bradley instructor. The type of breathing used may be important to you. Faith was simply unable to breath deeply during her first labor, although she found such breathing very relaxing during her second labor. Women who experience dysreflexia when they breathe deeply might not want to spend time in a class which emphasizes this method. Or, you might want to make sure that you will learn a variety of techniques. Judi recalls a student who disliked practicing shallow breathing in class, but found this method most useful during labor, and was glad she had learned it.

- *What are the philosophy and content of the class?* Hearing the teacher explain class philosophy in her own words can give you the best sense of whether you would enjoy working with that teacher. Class content should include any topics of concern to you. In addition to childbirth methods, the list might include information about general relaxation methods, exercise, breast feeding, medical procedures and medication, cesarean delivery, fetal development, preparing older siblings for the birth, and emotional concerns of new parents.

- *How is the class organized?* How much time does the teacher allot for lecture, small group discussion, and practice? Is the mix comfortable for you?

- *How large is the class?* Some people prefer the intimacy of a small class, while others prefer a large class where they can meet more people, or feel that in a large class, students will ask more questions and make the class more informative. If you are concerned that the teacher cannot give individual attention to students in a large class, perhaps you can visit one of her current classes and see what it is like.

- *Do you make other information available?* Some people learn more if lecture and practice are reinforced by slides, video tapes, or printed materials.

- *Do you think you can find ways to adapt your class to my disability?* Many teachers will enjoy the challenge of helping you find alternative ways to exercise or give birth. Hilary's teacher was happy to help her try to find a position in which she could receive a spinal injection.

Emotional Concerns

In the first trimester, pregnancy is private; nobody knows but the people the mother chooses to tell. In the second trimester, visibly pregnant, women are confronted with curiosity, congratulations, and all manner of unsolicited opinions and advice—not only from friends and family, but from strangers as well.

Because of widespread ignorance about disability, many people respond to the sight of a pregnant, disabled woman with surprise and even rudeness. Samantha commented, "It was hard for strangers to connect a wheelchair with pregnancy." While Patricia and Arlene felt that people simply asked questions because they were curious, other women met with behavior that was clearly inappropriate. Corrine, who walks with a limp, was approached by complete strangers asking, "Aren't you afraid your child will be disabled?" Sharon recalled that when she went to the emergency room with an ear infection and asked whether the prescribed medication was safe in pregnancy, the doctor asked, "Do you know who the father is?"

Many people who are obviously stifling their question, simply stare. Heather recalled, "People stared a lot. Some people couldn't handle a pregnant woman on crutches with only one leg.... Don't let it bother you if strangers, friends, or family have difficulty understanding. Just do your own thing." Different women handled the staring in different ways. Sylvia spoke for many when she said, "How well I handled the stares and comments depended on my mood." Christina, who "just blocked out the stares," seemed to feel more uncomfortable than Portia, who said, "I usually get stares, so I didn't notice any difference when I was pregnant."

Some women enjoyed having a chance to disprove misconceptions about disability. Samantha explained, "I enjoyed shooting down people's idea that disabled people are asexual." Stacy liked to wear a T-shirt that said "Under

Construction," because she enjoyed seeing the shocked expression on people's faces, and Pam said, "When people stared at me I just stuck my stomach out further."

Other women simply did not let themselves be affected by strangers' reactions, like Faith, who said, "When strangers looked at me like I shouldn't be pregnant, I didn't care because I was just so elated."

Of course, women cared much more about the reactions of their friends than the reactions of strangers. These reactions may include fear for the pregnant woman, admiration of her courage, or simple support. While Paula said, "I enjoyed having people tell me what guts I had," Celeste complained, "I got tired of hearing people worry that I had too much to struggle with."

Quite often the chief concern women expressed was not related to their disability, but to the desire for emotional support that any mother-to-be feels. So, for example, Julie, who was not married, worried about how the people in her church would react, and was very happy when "they turned out to be a tremendous support." Arlene recalled, "It was nice to see my friends waiting to see what *I* wanted to do, whether I would have an abortion or have the baby. I knew they would support any decision I made." Sasha, who felt that her family was always fearful and over-concerned about her disability, said she felt "vulnerable and betrayed" when they were not supportive of her pregnancy.

The feelings women expressed about pregnancy, body image, and self-esteem closely paralleled those of many able-bodied women. For example, Sybil said, "I felt good about myself; all my life I wanted a baby," and Mary said, "I felt fulfilled as a woman."

Remarks about body image reflected typically contradictory feelings. Patricia, Roberta, and Jennifer all thought they were better looking when pregnant, and Jennifer added that she also liked having a reason to buy new clothes. Some women thought they were more attractive because their breasts were larger. Paula's comment was classic: "I had a special glow that all pregnant women have."

A few women expressed the well-known feeling that pregnancy makes a woman look "fat and clumsy." Sheila regretted "losing her figure," and Stephanie thought her "huge stomach and spindly legs looked ridiculous." Some women feel better if they find ways to enhance and enjoy their appearance, perhaps by buying or borrowing a pretty maternity blouse, or trying a new hair style. This is even more important for those women who feel that an attractive appearance is partial compensation for a negative body image. To a woman who says, "My body may not work right, but at least it looks good," losing her figure may be especially painful.

Also, feeling "as huge as a house and just as clumsy," as Heather did, reflects the reality that mobility is reduced. Like Paula, a woman who has been enjoying her pregnancy as a sign that her body can function normally, becomes frustrated when "things are even more difficult than before." Still, despite the problems with reduced mobility, the feeling that pregnancy represented normality was important to many women. Corrine remarked, "It's the first time my body worked; it was doing what it should." Christina said, "I felt better about myself, because I was experiencing something all women do."

Some found a new sense of kinship with other women. As Celeste said, "It felt good to be a part of the sorority." Many women enjoyed comparing notes with able-bodied women, like Margie, who said, "It was fun. I found my body doing what it should." However, women who had problems during pregnancy, like Laura, said, "Sometimes it was difficult being with women who had it easier." Sylvia, who had an unusually difficult pregnancy, remembered feeling jealous of other women.

For women who are experiencing problem pregnancies, a more serious problem than jealousy is fear for the baby. Heather, who had a threatened miscarriage, said, "Even though it was a positive experience, I was frightened. I kept wondering if my baby was moving enough." Dawn wished she could have found a support group for high-risk mothers. If you would like to find such a support group, you could try asking local hospitals with maternity units—especially those with high-risk facilities—children's hospitals, a genetic counselor, a United Way agency (which might refer you to a member organization), or a community mental health clinic. If there are no established support groups, you may get help with starting one.

Be sure to discuss your fears with your doctor. Even if what s/he tells you is not completely reassuring, your doctor can help you to keep your fears in perspective. Perhaps most important, s/he can remind you how to distinguish ordinary pregnancy discomforts from real danger signs.

While it is not easy to cope with the fear one feels during a problem pregnancy, it can be worthwhile. Leslie said of her miscarriage during her second pregnancy, "It is the end of all the dreams you've had. I went to a support group and I felt terrible for everyone in the class." Still, she decided to try a third pregnancy. She explained, "I always would have wondered if I could have done it. I knew I was ahead of the game if I tried. If I didn't try, I'd have no baby. If I tried, I'd have either a live or a dead baby; I knew I'd tried everything with the first and second. I did worry that the baby would be disabled if it was premature, but I was ready to take what came."

THIRD TRIMESTER

Office Visits

Office visits are more frequent during the third trimester. If your pregnancy is uncomplicated, visits are every 2 weeks until about the thirty-sixth week, and then they are weekly. These visits follow much the same routine as second trimester visits, including a urinalysis and measurement of weight, blood pressure, fundal height, and fetal heart rate. During your physical examination, your doctor may check your hands and feet for edema, and your legs for varicose veins. At the twenty-eighth week, your blood glucose (sugar) test may be repeated. This is a screening test for diabetes, and further testing is needed if results are not normal. Some visits may include taking a blood sample to test for anemia, or to aid in the treatment of pregnancy or disability complications (for example, tests of kidney function or of medication levels).

After the thirty-second week, your examinations will include palpation (feeling) of your uterus to determine the presentation of the fetus. If your doctor suspects that the fetus is not in a normal presentation, an ultrasound examination may be needed.

During the last few weeks of pregnancy, the cervix (opening of the uterus) may be manually examined to determine whether it has started to dilate. Your doctor will not necessarily examine your cervix; s/he must judge the risks and benefits. For example, if a woman has a placenta previa (see Chapter 7), her cervix must not be examined because of the risk of causing bleeding. However, women with spinal cord injuries may be examined as early as the twenty-eighth week, and certainly after the thirty-second week, because they have a higher risk of pre-term labor, and because those with injuries at or above the T-10 level usually are not able to feel labor contractions. You may notice a small amount of brownish or pink discharge a day or two after an internal examination. However, pink discharge is sometimes a sign that labor will begin soon, as is slightly blood-streaked mucus (bright red spotting is a danger sign).

As usual, you may discuss the results of any diagnostic tests that have been done. When you and your doctor discuss symptoms you have been experiencing, you may talk about the frequency and strength of Braxton-Hicks contractions. It is a good idea to discuss how you are feeling about the approaching birth of the baby, and how members of your family are reacting. Talk about your hopes and fears about what will happen during the birth, and what your previous experiences have been.

If you and your doctor have not already developed a "birth plan," now is the time. Table 6-2 is a sample birth plan, adapted from a plan prepared by a couple in one of Judi's birthing classes. Of course, your plan may contain different details—for example, you may want to have a warm bath available for the baby just after birth. To avoid misunderstandings later, ask your doctor what situations s/he thinks might make it necessary to depart from the plan. (For example, the plan in Table 6-2 mentions presence of friends, relatives, and siblings: Does the hospital limit the number of people who may be present? Require siblings to take a special class before attending the birth? Require people who will attend the birth to have their temperatures taken, so that the baby will not be exposed to illness?)

Below are some questions and issues you may wish to discuss during your office visit:

Table 6.2
Mark and Jolene's Birth Plan

We, the parents, realize that flexibility and a willingness to accept changes in our plan may be necessary. Following are our preferred options for a normal, natural labor and birth and for possible variations from the normal.

Labor
A. Husband be present throughout labor and delivery.
B. "Minishave" for episiotomy.
C. Freedom to walk and change positions while in labor and delivery.
D. Spontaneous labor—no induction or breaking of membranes.
E. Able to drink fluids—ice chips, juice, fruit popsicles.
F. Friends, relatives, siblings may be present.

Birth
A. Birth in labor bed if possible.
B. I would prefer no catheterization.
C. Episiotomy only if necessary, and *local* anesthetic for pain of episiotomy.
D. Spontaneous delivery with no forceps.
E. Mirror to watch birth.
F. Tape recording and photos of birth.

After Birth
A. Baby on my chest right after birth until cord is cut.
B. Bonding and breast feeding after baby is cleaned.

Baby
A. No glucose water given to baby.
B. Delay administration of eye drops.

In Case of Cesarean Birth
A. Husband present for moral support throughout delivery.
B. Father to hold baby and mother to see baby, if it is not in distress.
C. Mother allowed to breast-feed in delivery room if her and her
   baby's condition permit.

In Case of Premature/Sick Infant
A. Mother allowed to hold and see baby, if it is not in distress.
B. Father and mother involved as much as possible in care of baby;
   mother to express colostrum to feed baby.

If all goes well, we would also like to be able to celebrate with a "birthday cake.'

_____   _____
Parents' signatures, date   *Doctor's signature, date*

- *Can my husband and I continue making love?* This question occurs to many people, and often the answer is yes. If your doctor advises you to restrict sexual activity, s/he will give you a reason (for example, a woman who has placenta previa would be advised to avoid intercourse). If possible, ask this question when your husband is with you, so you can both hear the doctor's explanation and ask any questions that you might have.

- *I'm considering breast feeding my baby. Can you advise me about possible advantages or disadvantages?* In Chapter 9 we discuss some of the issues involved in this decision. Your doctor can provide information on how your medications might affect your baby, and insights on how breast feeding might affect your health. If a physical limitation such as poor hand control might be a problem, s/he can refer you to an occupational therapist.

- *How can I prepare my breasts for breast feeding?* Your doctor may have additional suggestions, and ideas for what to do if you have inverted nipples.

- *How will I know labor has started?* You may want to supplement the information in the next chapter, and what you learn in birthing class, by discussion with your doctor.

- *If I think I am in labor, when should I call you?* Ordinarily, women are told to call their doctors when contractions are 7–10 minutes apart, and last 45–60 seconds. However, your doctor may give you different instructions, especially if complications have been diagnosed.

- *What should I do if you are unavailable when I call?* Should you wait for a return call, or leave a message and go to the hospital?

- *When should I go to the hospital?* Ordinarily, women are advised to go to the hospital when contractions are 5 minutes apart, and last 45–60 seconds. A number of circumstances could modify this rule. For example, if you live very far from the hospital, you may need to leave home earlier in labor. Your doctor might advise you that if the "bag of water" breaks before you feel strong contractions, you should leave for the hospital without waiting. If your pregnancy is complicated in some way, you may need medical attention as soon as possible after labor begins.

- *Can you suggest a good pediatrician?* If your doctor is a family practitioner s/he can become your baby's doctor. Your baby must have a physical examination before s/he can leave the hospital, and while this can be done by a staff physician, you may prefer to have it done by the person who will care for him or her later. Give yourself plenty of time to find a pediatrician who works well with you, by starting to look 4–6 weeks before the baby is due.

- *What might happen in the hospital if my baby is affected by pregnancy complications or my disability?* For example, if you will need cesarean surgery, you will want to know how surgery and anesthesia will affect your baby. If there is a risk that your baby will develop heart problems, you will want to know what kind of treatment s/he will need, how long s/he will be in the hospital, and other information. In some cases, your doctor will arrange for a specialist to care for your baby, and will refer you to him or her for answers to your questions.

Medical Procedures and Diagnostic Tests

Rh Antibody Treatment

If a woman has blood that is Rh negative, and is exposed to the red blood cells of an Rh-positive fetus, she will develop antibodies to Rh-positive cells (she is "sensitized"). A woman can become sensitized during childbirth, ectopic pregnancy, miscarriage, or from placental bleeding during a first pregnancy. Sensitization is the same process as the development of immunity to disease after a vaccination.

When a sensitized, Rh-negative woman is pregnant with an Rh-positive fetus, her antibodies will attack fetal tissues. Prolonged exposure to these antibodies causes severe fetal illness.

If the blood tests which were done during the first office visit show that an Rh negative woman is not sensitized, then at the twenty-eighth week she is given an injection of Rh-immune globulin, which suppresses antibody formation and prevents Rh disease in the fetus. If she is already sensitized, amniocentesis will be performed regularly to measure changing levels of antibodies in the amniotic fluid. Pre-term delivery may be necessary if the level gets too high.

Because of these procedures, Rh disease and associated birth defects are increasingly rare.

Amniocentesis

Amniotic fluid can be tested to assess fetal lung maturity and possible fetal distress, as well as assessing the presence of Rh antibodies.

Measurement of the L/S ratio, the relative amounts of two chemicals, diagnoses fetal lung maturity. The appropriate L/S ratio reflects the presence of enough surfactant to keep the lungs from collapsing on contact with air. This test is important when pre-term delivery is being considered.

When there are signs of fetal distress, or in the case of post-term pregnancy, amniotic fluid may be examined for the presence of meconium (fetal wastes), which may stain or thicken the fluid. Meconium contamination may be an indication for immediate delivery. Tests of certain chemicals in the fluid also help assess fetal health.

Sonography

Ultrasound may be used to monitor fetal growth and activity, as well as being used as an adjunct to amniocentesis.

When growth retardation is suspected, not only is sonography used to assess the fetus' overall size, but specific body parts can be measured for more precise diagnosis. Sonography may also be used when there is concern that a post-term fetus will grow too large for vaginal delivery.

A "biophysical profile" is a study which produces scores for fetal heart tones, movement of muscles which will be used in breathing, flexion and extension of limbs, and the volume of amniotic fluid. This study can be used to assess the well-being of the fetus. Some physicians recommend its use for fetuses at risk of developing heart block (in mothers with SLE who have SS-A and SS-B antibodies).

Stress and Non-stress Tests

In a non-stress test, an external monitor is used to measure fetal heart rhythms. There are a number of indications for this test, which include the following:

- Pre-term labor
- Post-term pregnancy (perhaps the most common reason)
- Lack of fetal activity
- Signs of fetal distress
- Maternal complications, such as bleeding or high blood pressure, which might harm the fetus
- Multiple pregnancies
- Hydramnios (excess amniotic fluid)
- History of pregnancy complications

When Leslie experienced bleeding and pain after partial placental abruption, this test helped to determine that immediate delivery was not needed.

Non-stress testing may be repeated for continuing assessment of fetal health. Arlene, who had miscarriages in her first two pregnancies, said that during her third pregnancy "they hooked me up from time to time to see if she was healthy. There were never any problems." When there is a risk of fetal heart block, monitoring may be done as often as once a week from the twenty-eighth to thirty-fourth weeks, and twice a week from the thirty-fourth week to delivery.

In a stress test, monitoring is performed after uterine contractions have been stimulated by nipple stimulation or IV injection of oxytocin (a hormone which, in larger doses, induces or augments labor). This test evaluates how well the fetus would withstand the stresses of labor and delivery.

External Version

This term refers to a procedure for changing fetal presentation or position (*version* means "turning"). In recent years, many physicians have renewed the use of this procedure, which may help prevent some surgical deliveries. If the fetus is in a presentation which might make delivery difficult, the physician may attempt to manipulate it into a new position by pressing on the mother's abdomen. During the procedure, which is performed during the thirty-sixth or thirty-seventh week, sonography is used to locate the fetus, and an external monitor is used to assess changes in fetal heart rate. A medication is given to relax the uterine muscles, which can make the procedure more effective and also prevent contractions. The medication also reduces any discomfort caused by the procedure.

Physical Changes

For the most part, the physical changes of the third trimester are a continuation of processes that have begun earlier—growth of the breasts and uterus, increase in blood volume, and other changes. Some women find that they stop gaining weight, or gain weight more slowly. Many women do notice one change that is specific to the third trimester—a feeling of increased warmth. For women who have disabilities that impair circulation, the feeling of warmth may be welcome. Several women commented, "It was the first time I felt really warm when it wasn't summertime." If it *is* summertime, you may feel uncomfortably warm.

Increase in Blood Volume

The feeling of warmth may be caused in part by the continuing growth of the blood supply. In the third trimester, blood volume is 40% greater than it was before pregnancy. While this increase can contribute to such discomforts as edema and varicose veins, it also has positive effects. Many women noticed that, despite their increased weight, they did not have pressure sores and their skin condition was better than it had ever been.

Skin

Another skin change is "stretch marks," reddish streaks which may appear on the breasts, hips, or abdomen. Not every woman develops these marks when her skin is stretched by growth of underlying tissues, but some women's skin, like some pieces of elastic, does not have quite enough "give." This is purely a matter of individual difference, and while a little moisturizing cream can make you more comfortable if your skin is dry, there is no need to bother using expensive creams and exotic ingredients, which cannot prevent stretch marks. While the appearance of your stretch marks may bother you, remember that they usually fade after pregnancy.

Breasts

Your breast size may increase enough to make you uncomfortable. If you do not normally wear a brassiere, you may need to start wearing one during pregnancy so that your breasts do not bounce, ache, or become damp and sticky underneath (this may be the first time you have an "underneath"). If your disability makes it difficult for you to fasten a brassiere, try using an athletic brassiere that fastens in front or pulls on over your head; you can also fasten your brassiere in front, then turn it around. Replacing hooks with snaps or a strip of Velcro may also help.

Your breasts may become more sensitive to touch or temperature. For example, your nipples may contract painfully in cold water, or feel uncomfortable in the shower.

While colostrum usually does not appear until after delivery, it may appear during the last several weeks of pregnancy. Do not worry if you notice a few drops of clear, slightly yellowish secretion, or some dried material on your nipples. Simply rinse it away with clear water, or wipe it away with a damp washcloth.

Some women's nipples become sore during the first weeks of breast feeding, and women who are planning to breastfeed often try to toughen their nipples so that they will not be as sore at first. You can try the following suggestions:

- Cut holes in the cups of your brassiere, or wear a nursing brassiere with the flaps down, so that your clothing rubs against your nipples.
- Rub your nipples with a rough washcloth.
- Expose your nipples to sunlight or a sun lamp for up to 10 minutes, twice a day.
- Gently but firmly squeeze and turn your nipples between your fingertips.

Uterus and Cervix

Several changes occur in the uterus and cervix. The cervix, which begins to soften early in pregnancy, changes the most during the third trimester. Normally the cervix feels about as firm as the tip of your nose; by the end of pregnancy, it feels as soft as an ear lobe. The cervix may also begin to efface (retract into the uterus) at about the thirty-eighth week, and may dilate (open) as much as 2 cm. (about 3/4 inch) before labor begins. Dilation is a sign that labor may begin soon, and if your doctor does a vaginal examination and finds that your cervix is dilated, s/he will tell you. You may want to make final preparations for childbirth, such as arranging your transportation to the hospital or contacting a diaper service. A woman whose cervix has dilated may also notice a blood-streaked mucus discharge as early as 2 weeks before labor begins (this "bloody show" often does not appear until after labor has started). If you notice such a discharge, call your doctor and watch for other signs of labor, which are described at the beginning of Chapter 7.

Your uterus has been contracting continuously (but not regularly) since the beginning of pregnancy. These contractions are more noticeable by the seventh or eighth month, and they may be quite uncomfortable during the last few weeks. They often feel stronger during a second pregnancy than a first. They usually last about 30 seconds, but may last as long as 2 minutes. These contractions are called Braxton-Hicks contractions, practice contractions, or false labor. Besides exercising the uterine muscles in preparation for labor, Braxton-Hicks contractions may cause some effacement and dilation of the cervix. Many women take advantage of these contractions to practice the breathing and relaxation techniques they have learned in birthing class. At times, Braxton-Hicks contractions can seem very much like true labor.

If you do not feel practice contractions, you may not feel true labor. Women who have spinal lesions that could interfere with labor sensations may be admitted to the hospital in the thirty-eighth week (or earlier if there are signs of pre-term labor) to avoid the risk of unattended birth. However, there are signs of labor you can watch for at home, and it might be possible for you to rent a home monitor to detect labor (your doctor would advise you how often to check). You should discuss the alternatives with your doctor.

Some women, especially first-time mothers, may experience "lightening" 2–4 weeks before giving birth. The fetus drops lower in the pelvis, and the fundal height is lowered correspondingly. The mother's abdomen will look different, and she may find that she breathes more easily and/or has fewer problems with heartburn and indigestion. "Lightening" can also cause various discomforts, since pressure from the fetal head can cause urinary difficulties, perineal pain, backaches or groin pain, and mobility difficulties.

Faith said, "When the baby didn't drop in my second pregnancy, I was afraid I might need another C-section. I went to physical therapy, and used the standing table for half an hour, 3 times a week. The gravity helped; on the third day the baby dropped." Faith may have worried needlessly, because often, especially in repeat pregnancies, the baby does not become engaged in the pelvis until after labor has begun. Yet it is true that, when women remain upright during labor, gravity assists the baby's descent, and Faith's physical therapy may have had the same effect.

Joints
The gradual softening of joint tissues continues in the third trimester, contributing to the distinctive "waddling" walk of late pregnancy.

Pregnancy Discomforts

Breathing Difficulties
By late pregnancy, the growth of the uterus raises the diaphragm (the muscle used for breathing) about 4 cm. (1.5 inches). Many women feel short of breath after exercise. Others feel uncomfortable more of the time, like Faith, who could not talk without stopping frequently to take a breath. While some women, like Carla, simply noticed that their breathing was shallower, others, like Stephanie and Hilary, commented that breathing was actually painful.

Women who feel short of breath can experiment until they find a position which allows them to breathe more comfortably. Stephanie, who felt that her baby was positioned higher than other women's, said, "Her feet were constantly pressing on my diaphragm, and the only way I could relieve the pain was to lie down." Other women found that it was hard to breathe when lying down, but Sheila solved the problem by sitting up when she slept. For some women, difficulty in breathing while lying down poses special problems. Leslie, who had an incompetent cervix, needed bed rest to prevent miscarriage. She was advised to stay flat, with pillows under her knees, but felt short of breath when she lay in this position. Faith, who had difficulty breathing even in the first trimester of her pregnancies, found that she breathed most easily in a reclining position, and wished she could have afforded a reclining wheelchair. Women who breathe more comfortably in a reclining position could try to find out whether their medical insurance would pay for a reclining chair if the medical indications are explained by a physician.

Some women, like Faith, are more comfortable if they eat small meals. By doing so, they avoid adding the pressure of a very full stomach to the pressure of the uterus.

Sometimes special breathing techniques are helpful. Sylvia breathed more easily when she inhaled deeply through her nose, then exhaled through her mouth. If you cannot breathe comfortably in any position, ask your doctor if a referral to a physical or respiratory therapist is appropriate.

More severe problems may occur in women who have disabilities that ordinarily interfere with breathing—for example, women with myasthenia gravis, severe scoliosis, or spinal cord injury affecting the diaphragm. Besides having more difficulty with breathing, these women are more susceptible to respiratory infection. If breathing is very impaired, lowered oxygen levels can endanger both mother and fetus. Ask what symptoms require a phone call to your doctor's office. If you have not yet discussed this issue with your doctor, call him/her if you must pause for breath while speaking, or if you develop even mild symptoms of infection or other problems. Do not wait for an emergency! While some women only need testing or adjustment of their medications, others may need hospitalization. Your doctor must also look into the possibility that the problem is caused by pre-eclampsia. Even when breathing difficulties are not severe enough to threaten the mother's life, they can interfere with fetal development or cause pre-term labor.

A few women may find that breathing is easier in late pregnancy, like Portia, who commented, "The baby acted like a corset. The pressure made it easier for me to breathe and to cough."

Vaginitis

While vaginal infections may occur any time during pregnancy, none of the women we interviewed recalled having one before the third trimester. Women who are not pregnant can also develop vaginitis, but the hormone changes of pregnancy do increase susceptibility to infection. These infections should never be ignored—they not only cause discomfort, but they can be passed to babies during birth.

The discharge associated with vaginal infections is different from the usual thin, clear or whitish discharge associated with pregnancy. With the most common infection, called *candida, monilia,* or *yeast,* the discharge is thick and opaque; many people say it looks like cottage cheese. It has a mild but characteristic odor. Clara remarked, "I knew when I had a yeast because I recognized the smell." *Trichomonas* infections produce a thin, yellow-green, sometimes foamy, foul-smelling discharge.

Yeast organisms are always present in the vagina, but some conditions can cause them to multiply rapidly, causing discharge, mild to intense itching, irritation or burning, and redness. Women who experience signs or symptoms of infection should call their doctor. The doctor can then examine them and, if necessary, prescribe local medications—creams, gels or suppositories which are inserted in the vagina. Yeast organisms thrive in warm, moist conditions. So, women who keep their genitals clean and dry, and wear cotton rather than synthetic underwear, not only feel more comfortable, but are likely to heal faster and reduce the chance of re-infection. Some women find it is especially helpful to wear a skirt without any underwear during the day, and a nightgown rather than pajamas at night. Do not douche without a doctor's instructions.

Some antibiotics can increase susceptibility to yeast infection, and women who must use them should be alert for symptoms.

Symptoms of trichomonas include pain at the vaginal opening (especially during intercourse), itching, and irritation. Again, women who experience these symptoms should call their doctor, who can prescribe oral medication. Remember to ask your doctor about medication side effects. This infection is easily transmitted between partners, and it is a good idea to have your partner examined when you are. If he is also affected, you can avoid re-infection if both of you are treated at the same time.

Women who have reduced sensation may not be able to feel the irritation of vaginitis, so their attendants should check for discharge or redness when bathing them.

Heartburn and Related Discomforts

Heartburn is a type of indigestion which has nothing to do with the heart. It occurs when stomach acids are forced from the stomach into the esophagus (the "tube" leading from the throat to the stomach). Irritation of the esophageal lining causes a burning sensation. While this problem can occur earlier in pregnancy, it is most common in the third trimester, when pressure from the enlarged uterus is greater.

A related problem is "reflux," in which a small amount of food is forced back into the esophagus (the amount may not be great enough to be considered vomiting). Some women find that reflux is more likely to occur after fetal movement. To the mother, it can feel as though whenever she eats, the fetus responds to pressure from the stomach by kicking or stretching.

Many women feel uncomfortably full after meals, even when they are not bothered by heartburn or reflux. Using the following suggestions can help to avoid or reduce heartburn, reflux, and discomfort:

- Eat small, frequent meals, so you do not become over-full. Julie commented that this advice from her nutritionist was particularly helpful.
- Take small bites and chew and swallow slowly.
- Sip cool water to "rinse" the esophagus, relieving irritation and washing digestive acids back into the stomach. Liquids may also help by diluting stomach acids. Heather felt more comfortable when she sipped milk or lemon-lime sodas, but other women may find soda irritating. It is interesting that Sasha, who restricted her fluids, was the only woman with a spinal cord dysfunction who suffered heartburn.
- Avoid gaining excess weight, which can increase pressure on the stomach.
- Do not wear tight clothing.
- Bend at the hips and knees, not the waist, when lifting objects and tying your shoes.
- Change sleeping and resting routines, if necessary. Do not go to bed less than 2 hours after eating. Raise the head of the bed about 6 inches, or sleep with several pillows. If you must rest during the day, do not lie flat. Julie preferred to be propped up at a 45° angle, and said, "I wish I had a recliner."
- Avoid foods which seem to make the problem worse. You may need to avoid greasy foods, spicy foods, processed meats, chocolate, carbonated beverages, and other foods.
- Heartburn is another good reason to avoid cigarettes and coffee !
- Avoid stress during and after meals. Tension can make heartburn worse. Notice whether heartburn occurs when you are under stress, and try to find ways to solve the problem (for example, by changing your work schedule). Try playing soft background music while you eat to help you "slow down." Afterwards, take a few minutes to do some deep breathing or relaxation exercises (but do not lie down to relax).
- Exercise several times a day. Raise your arms straight overhead, clasp your hands a moment, then lower your arms to your side. This exercise temporarily relieves pressure, and may stimulate the fetus to change position. If you cannot do it independently, your husband or attendant can assist you.
- Do not use antacid medications without your doctor's recommendation, and be sure to avoid home remedies, such as baking soda. If these medications are not used properly, they can cause diarrhea or constipation (depending on the medication) and other problems.
- Try to avoid slouching, especially when sitting, as this increases pressure on the stomach.

Like vomiting, reflux can be a problem if it interferes with absorption of oral medications. Discuss the problem with your doctor. Perhaps you can adjust by taking medication between meals. If not, it may be necessary to take some medicines by injection.

Constipation

Remember, constipation refers to hard, dry stools and strain during bowel movements. Do not worry if bowel movements do not occur every day, as long as stools are soft and pass easily.

Constipation is a rather common discomfort during late pregnancy. Pregnancy hormones relax the muscles of the intestines, making digestion less efficient, and pressure from the enlarged uterus adds to the problem. Stress, some medications, and lack of exercise can make constipation worse.

Women who have a disability that causes constipation may have worse problems during pregnancy. Only two of our interviewees had impacted bowels, but women who are paralyzed should be aware that this can occur. This problem should be taken seriously, since pressure from impacted bowels sometimes causes breathing difficulties. Call your doctor right away to discuss whether you should use an enema, or go to the office or emergency room for disimpaction.

Iron supplements can be constipating, and several women commented that they reduced or eliminated their dose to relieve constipation. Iron is a very important nutrient so, rather than eliminating iron on your own, talk to your doctor about taking another type of iron, possibly even an injectable form.

Many women were helped by drinking plenty of liquids and eating foods rich in fiber (some fiber-rich foods are listed in the Appendix). Stacy and Stephanie found thay they had to use suppositories more frequently. None of the women mentioned using exercise to reduce constipation, but women who can walk may find that it helps. At least try changing position more frequently and, if you are able, use the exercise for relieving constipation described at the end of Chapter 5. Try resting your feet on a footstool to reduce strain during a bowel movement. Several women mentioned using various types of laxatives. However, use of laxatives can also cause problems, and you should discuss the problem with your doctor before using them. Your doctor can prescribe a stool softener if s/he has not done so already.

Sylvia's problems were different from those of other women. She explained, "I had an unpredictable bowel; it never responded to the suppository." At times, Sylvia had diarrhea, and often soiled while being transferred. She wore disposable underwear and tried to eat foods that would lessen the problem. Continuing diarrhea can be a serious problem, leading to dehydration. Women with this problem should start drinking plenty of clear fluids (to replace what is lost), and call their doctor.

Remember, too, that diarrhea can be a sign of labor. So, notice any other symptoms that accompany diarrhea and be sure to report them to your doctor.

Hemorrhoids

Hemorrhoids are swollen veins in the area of the anus. External hemorrhoids look like "blood blisters." They may be itchy or painful, and are especially painful during bowel movements. Sometimes they bleed, especially after a difficult bowel movement. Itching, pain, or bleeding of the anus can be caused by problems other than hemorrhoids, and should be discussed with your doctor.

Several factors can contribute to the development of hemorrhoids: pregnancy hormone may relax the walls of the veins, blood may pool in the lower body, or heredity may be responsible for weakness of the veins. Straining during bowel movements can also contribute to the development of hemorrhoids, or make existing hemorrhoids worse.

Because prolonged sitting can cause hemorrhoids, this problem may be worse for many disabled women. Stephanie commented, "I already had hemorrhoids. When I was pregnant, I had swelling all through the perineal area, and the hemorrhoids got worse."

Women who have hemorrhoids can use the following methods to reduce discomfort, and avoid irritation, infection, and constipation, since straining during bowel movements can make hemorrhoids worse (use suggestions presented in Chapter 4):

- Keep the perineum and anus clean. After each bowel movement, rinse with clear, warm water.
- Use white, unscented toilet paper.
- Ice packs or witch hazel compresses can relieve pain for some women. (Ice did not help Stephanie.)
- Warm compresses or warm soaks can help some women. If you cannot use a bathtub, use a sitz bath.
- Avoid prolonged sitting to the extent that your disability allows. Lie on your side, or lie or recline with your legs elevated to improve circulation.
- Use a cushion to reduce pressure when sitting. Some women use a special inflatable, ring-shaped cushion.
- Check with your doctor if you want to try medicated creams or suppositories, e.g., topical cortisone cream.

Varicose Veins

Varicose veins are swollen veins, like hemorrhoids, but the problem is in the veins of the legs. They have the same causes as hemorrhoids. The leg veins may be only slightly more noticeable than usual, or they may look like very swollen, twisting blue lines on the legs. They can be painless, mildly achy, or quite uncomfortable. Sometimes when the problem is severe, an embolism (clot) may develop in the varicose vein. Varicose veins usually improve after pregnancy, but may re-appear or become worse in later pregnancies.

Women who have varicose veins can minimize the problem as follows:

- Avoid excessive weight gain.
- Avoid prolonged standing or sitting. When sitting or lying down, elevate the legs to improve circulation.

- Do not wear tight girdles, tight pants, or elastic-topped stockings, which can interfere with circulation.
- Wear support stockings all day if your doctor prescribes support stockings. Put them on before getting out of bed in the morning, and take them off just before going to sleep.
- Exercise as much as your disability allows to encourage circulation. If you cannot exercise much, perhaps a physical therapist can provide passive exercise or massage to improve circulation.

Edema

Some swelling, especially in the feet, is quite common in the third trimester. Swelling of the hands is less common, but some women may need to remove their rings until the end of pregnancy. As we explained above, increased blood volume contributes to edema, and it has increased by 40% by the third trimester. When the walls of the veins relax, and the uterus increases pressure on the leg veins, pooling of the blood can occur, which may contribute to edema.

Various studies have found that from 33% to 75% of able-bodied, pregnant women experience edema. 55% of the women interviewed for *Mother-to-Be* had this problem. One might expect that mobility impairment would make women more susceptible to edema, yet there was no such pattern among interviewees. Sylvia had "minimum swelling;" Samantha said, "It wasn't as bad as I thought it would be;" and Stephanie commented, "I have always had edema, and it was just a little worse." However, Paula reported that she did not experience edema during her first pregnancy, before she was disabled, but did have edema during the two pregnancies occurring after she became disabled.

Normal pregnancy edema may cause enough swelling to make your wedding ring tight or your shoes uncomfortable. More severe swelling can be a sign of pre-eclampsia. Pam recalled, "The swelling in my feet was so bad, my doctor thought I might have pre-eclampsia, but found my blood pressure was normal." If you experience severe or sudden swelling, call your doctor.

It is also important to differentiate normal pregnancy edema from disability symptoms. When Renee was awakened by swelling and pain, she realized it might be rheumatic inflammation and reduced the pain by taking a hot bath.

Especially in warm weather, when swelling may be worse, cool soaks may make your hands and feet more comfortable. Resting with your legs elevated also helps. Raising your legs higher than your body is best, but some women's disabilities make it difficult. Julie remarked, "I used a footstool—it was better than nothing."

Several women felt that it was helpful to elevate their legs with pillows when they slept. Hilary felt better when she fastened her shoes more loosely. It may be worthwhile to buy inexpensive shoes that are more comfortable. Wearing elastic stockings helped some women. If you want to try them, first buy *one* pair and make sure it is not too hard to put them on and take them off.

Some women remembered taking diuretics and/or avoiding salt. For several years controlling edema in this way was not considered appropriate during pregnancy, but many doctors have started using this treatment again. You can expect to urinate more frequently if your doctor prescribes diuretics. If you have bladder problems, call your doctor but *do not* stop drinking plenty of fluids.

Urinary Problems

All women find that they have to urinate more frequently during the third trimester because of pressure from the enlarged uterus. Some begin to have problems with stress incontinence (loss of control when laughing, sneezing or straining). Very late in pregnancy, sudden fetal movements can also cause incontinence. Sometimes, the flow of urine is so sudden that the mother cannot tell whether she has urinated or her "bag has broken." In this case, she must call her doctor's office, find out whether her doctor wishes to examine her, and watch for other signs of labor.

Existing urinary problems may get worse but sometimes the reason for urgency or frequency is unclear. Marsha, who took a vacation in Hawaii late in her pregnancy, said, "I couldn't tell whether the problem was from the heat, pressure from the baby, or exacerbation of multiple sclerosis." Many women coped with frequency by making sure that they were never far from a bathroom. Some women who also had difficulty with bladder control stopped wearing pants or even underwear so that, when they reached a bathroom, they could use the toilet as quickly as possible. Since frequency can be a sign of urinary infection, it is also important to report this problem to your doctor.

Women who have catheters have additional problems, because their catheters may become obstructed by deposits of calcium crystals or pressure from the uterus. Sylvia, who has a suprapubic catheter, recalled, "I got a plugged catheter and I irrigated it twice a day. The problem was worse when I drank milk, so I got calcium from other sources." Because calcium is an important nutrient, Sylvia was wise to find alternative sources. Women who have catheters that are obstructed should not eliminate calcium from their diets without talking to their doctors or nutritionists about finding other sources. They can also ask their doctor about irrigating their catheters more often. Later in pregnancy, fetal pressure caused urine to leak around Sylvia's catheter, and her doctor re-inserted it at a different angle.

Some women, like Sara and Stacy, retain their urine, so they may need to use a catheter until they give birth. Stacy, who empties her bladder by manual pressure, said, "I can't empty my bladder completely. My obstetrician was concerned that if my bladder was full when I went into labor, it would interfere with the baby's descent. He inserted a catheter three days before the baby was born."

After Stacy's catheter was inserted, she found blood in her urine. Stephanie also noticed blood in her urine during the third trimester but, she said, "My doctor wasn't concerned" because the bleeding was caused by mechanical irritation from the catheter. Women who have catheters and find blood in their urine should not be too anxious, since the problem may be mechanical irritation, but they should still contact their doctors. Blood in the urine can also be a sign of bladder or kidney infection, and their doctors may want to examine them for other signs of infection.

Because urinary and kidney infections develop more easily during pregnancy, and are most likely to occur during the third trimester, women should be aware of signs and symptoms of infection. Understandably, many women hesitate to call their doctor when they experience frequency, because it is not always a sign of infection. During a regular office visit, ask your doctor what to do when you have urinary problems. Do not hesitate to call your doctor when there is more than one symptom. Take your temperature before calling, even if you do not feel hot, since your doctor will want this information.

Painful or Tingling Hands

Sometimes swelling is severe enough to create pressure on the median nerve, resulting in "carpal tunnel syndrome." This syndrome includes pain, tingling, and weakness in the wrist or hand, which makes it difficult to pick up objects. The syndrome is especially troublesome if the dominant hand is affected. Sometimes splinting helps to relieve discomfort.

In some women, postural changes during pregnancy, such as slumped shoulders, can press on certain nerves and cause numbness or weakness of the hands. Physical therapy may help.

If hand weakness is making normal daily activities more difficult, ask your doctor for a referral to an occupational therapist. While it is impractical to raise your hands overhead to relieve pain and swelling, you can try resting your hands on a pillow or tray placed on your lap. Some women find massage or cool soaks helpful.

Back and Leg Pain

Women who did not have back and leg pain during the second trimester, may begin to have problems during the third because of the increased weight of the uterus and fetus. The same methods that help to alleviate discomfort during the second trimester continue to be useful.

In this trimester, back and leg pain and leg cramps may have an additional cause—pressure of the uterus or fetal head against the sciatic nerve. This nerve runs from the sacrum (lower spine) down the entire length of the leg, and sciatic pain can be limited to the lower back and buttocks, or extend part-way or all the way down the back of the leg. Carla remarked, "The pain made it difficult to walk. If I had it to do over, I would use a wheelchair." It is possible that sciatica is felt as phantom pain. Heather said, "The first time I was pregnant, I had muscle cramps in my stump, back pain and phantom pain. I think it must have been my baby pressing on the nerve, because I didn't have any of these problems the second time."

Little can be done about sciatic pain beyond trying to reduce it with local heat, and finding comfortable positions when sitting and sleeping. Many women feel more comfortable using a footstool when they sit, and placing pillows under their knees when they are in bed. This avoids stretching the sciatic nerve.

Sleeplessness

Many women have trouble sleeping during late pregnancy because they must get up at night to urinate, and because it is difficult to find a comfortable sleeping position.

Loss of sleep is unavoidable to some extent, and you may need to make up for the loss by napping or resting during the day or, if that is not possible, scheduling fewer activities. Cheryl changed her working hours from full-time to half-time.

It is important to find a comfortable resting position. The cardinal rule is, *"Never lie flat on your back."* When you lie on your back, your uterus presses on large veins and this interferes with circulation. It may also interfere with digestion or cause back strain. Many women will also have trouble breathing in this position.

Most women cannot lie on their stomachs, either, but Patricia managed to do so by placing pillows under her breasts and hips.

Some women sleep more comfortably in a reclining or partially sitting position, propped up by pillows, while others are more comfortable lying on their sides. If you prefer sitting, you might wish to use an inexpensive backrest to avoid the discomfort of having pillows shift or slide out from under you. If you can afford it, consider renting a hospital bed. Pam and Sheila both said they wished that they had had hospital beds. Pam elaborated, "I couldn't lie on my left side because of my shoulder fusion and spinal curvature, and I couldn't stay on my right side for long because the baby was more to the right and the pressure was uncomfortable. Pillows on either side just didn't help much. A water bed might have helped with the pressure points, but it's too hard to move." (Also, women who normally enjoy sleeping in a water bed may find that it is too difficult to get in and out of one during late pregnancy.) If you sleep in a sitting or reclining position, it can be helpful to place pillows under your knees. Women with leg pain may find that this is the only way they can sleep really well.

If you feel better sleeping on your side, try to sleep on your left side, since this position is best for good circulation. Place pillows between your legs, or place the top (right) leg somewhat in front of the bottom leg, supported by pillows. Michelle pointed out that, while pillows can add to comfort, they also make it difficult to move around.

Sleep will come more easily if you are relaxed and comfortable at bedtime. Do not eat too close to bedtime. If you are having difficulty controlling your bladder, consider keeping a urinal under your bed, as Hilary did, wearing absorbent underwear, or using a waterproof mattress-cover, so that anxiety about having an "accident" does not keep you awake. Make sure your bedroom is at a comfortable temperature. Try taking a warm bath, or doing stretching and relaxation exercises, just before you go to sleep.

Mobility Difficulties

Even able-bodied women feel clumsier during the third trimester. Because their weight changes rapidly, their center of gravity keeps changing and it is difficult to adjust their sense of balance. This problem is worse for disabled women. It affects not only their ability to move from place to place, but a variety of daily activities such as bathing, dressing, and transferring. Besides using the suggestions below, you may need to consult an occupational or physical therapist.

Many women who did not use wheelchairs, or had only used them part of the time, started using them in the third trimester. Hilary recalled, "The first time I was pregnant, I used my prostheses up until the eighth month, when I fell. Then I started using a wheelchair, and it was so much easier that the second time, I started using a chair as soon as it began to be harder to get around."

Heather, Julie, and Christina all said that it became difficult to stand up from a chair or toilet. It may help to use a raised toilet seat, and use cushions to raise the seats of chairs, because this brings one's center of gravity forward. Julie sat on a high stool when she was not using her wheelchair. Women who are not comfortable with their legs dangling can use a footstool, or try to find a stool with a crosspiece between the legs, and use the crosspiece as a footrest. Instead of using a cushion, Heather "scooted" to the front edge of her chair, turned around, and pushed up. However, this should only be tried in a heavy, stable chair. Another possibility is to slide forward in your chair, then use a table edge or a friend's arm as support while you come to a standing position. However, adding firm cushions is the safest solution.

Dawn said, "Moving from lying down to sitting up was a big hassle." Getting out of bed can also be difficult. It is even difficult for able-bodied women if the bed is low. These problems are not so difficult if you have remembered to avoid lying on your back. It is easier to move to a sitting position if you are sleeping with the support of pillows or a backrest. It may help to have a piece of sturdy furniture next to the bed and use it as support. If you have been sleeping on your side, try putting your legs over the side of the bed first, then using another person's arm or an overhead trapeze for support as you come to a sitting position.

Getting in and out of the bathtub was difficult for most interviewees, regardless of their degree of disability. Besides the problems of maneuvering in a small space, changing to a standing position, and stepping over the side of the tub, it was difficult to keep their balance on the slippery surface. Some women solve the problem by getting on their hands and knees, then rising to a kneeling position, then holding a grab bar, or a sturdy chair placed next to the tub, while they come to a standing position. (The same technique can be used when you have been sitting on the floor.)

Most women avoided the problem of raising and lowering themselves by using a bath bench or chair. Heather found an inexpensive plastic stool at a variety store. She said, "If my husband wasn't home, I would drain the water from the tub, then sit on the side and grab the sink to get up."

Another solution is to use a shower, either standing or sitting on a bath chair. If you do not have a shower, you may be able to replace your tub spout with a spout that has a hand-held shower attachment.

To prevent falls, place non-skid material on the floor of your bathtub or shower. Heather used a piece of "indoor-outdoor" carpet.

Some women, like Pam, may decide to take sponge baths. Pam explained, "I couldn't sit in the tub without feeling like I might drown. I wished I had a shower or a completely tiled bathroom." Women who use wheelchairs often have much more trouble transferring to the bathtub when they are pregnant. Sheila said, "It was scary. I used more people to get me in and out of the tub."

The bathtub is not the only place where transferring is difficult, and many women find that they must also change their methods of transferring in other situations. Sylvia, who prefers a cradle transfer when she is not pregnant, could not use it during the last two months of pregnancy because it made breathing more difficult. She found that a pivot transfer was best for moving from her chair to her bed. Pam, who prefers to be grasped by the waist when she is lifted, said, "I worried that pressure from the belt my assistant used might hurt the baby, but my doctor reassured me that the baby would be okay."

Another problem that many women experienced was difficulty getting in and out of cars. Hilary used two methods, depending on whether she was using her prostheses. Hilary has no femurs, and her prostheses are somewhat like stilts. She said, "When I was wearing my prostheses, I got in the car about the same way a paraplegic does. I would put my crutches in the car, then sit down on the front seat. I scooted backward a bit, then grabbed my legs under the 'knees,' where my prostheses are attached, and used my hands to pull my legs in. When I wasn't wearing my prostheses, I would begin by taking hold of the steering wheel. Then I'd put my left foot in the car and, holding onto the wheel, I'd pull in my body and my right leg. At this point, I would be lying face down on the front seat. I pulled a little farther in, rolled over, and sat up. I rolled to sitting just the way an 11-month-old baby does it."

Julie's solution was to use pillows as aids. She explained, "The pillow made it easier for me to slide off the seat of my wheelchair. I would then push back toward the passenger door to swing in my feet. Sometimes I would get stuck lying flat on the seat. Then, if I was alone, I would use an extra pillow I kept on the passenger side for leverage."

Portia said, "I used a sliding board even when I wasn't pregnant, and simply stopped driving when I couldn't fit behind the steering wheel. Another problem was that my wheelchair was so heavy I needed help getting it in and out of the car. I usually tended to stay home more during the last three months (Portia had five pregnancies). Mostly I just went out with my husband." Carla, too, felt it was easier not to go out too often. She said, "I had my parents or my husband do the shopping."

Many women avoided going out because they were afraid of falling. Two of these were women who needed adaptive equipment to walk. Several women did fall during the third trimester, and they reacted to the experience in a variety of ways. Celeste said, "I only fell once. It could have happened to anyone. It wasn't bad; it felt like falling on a balloon." However, Julie said, "When I tripped over a rug, it really shook my confidence. I was afraid of falling again. I became much more cautious, and stopped work earlier than I had planned. I increased attendant care and limited my outside activities."

For some women, a good alternative may be to use a wheelchair for a few months. Using a wheelchair more of the time, or learning to use a wheelchair, may create some problems. Sara recalled, "Before I was pregnant, I only used a wheelchair for going long distances. I used crutches until the seventh month, then balance was enough of a problem that I decided to use a chair. Once when I was going over a curb it flipped backwards." Sara was the only person whose wheelchair flipped while she was pregnant. However, weight change can change the way the chair maneuvers. Some women felt that they might fall forward, especially when taking their chairs over curbs. If you must start using a wheelchair, use the following precautions:

- Avoid taking the chair over curbs.
- Use a driveway when you cannot find a curb cut.
- Hang filled sidepacks on the chair to improve stability.
- Have an anti-tipping device installed, or have the chair re-adjusted.

Loss of balance and the size of the pregnant abdomen make it difficult to do tasks which require bending forward, such as adjusting a wheelchair or dressing. Samantha pulled up her legs to put on her shoes, and Julie used a footstool. Faith's husband helped her put her shoes on. Women who are able to balance well enough (possibly while holding onto a support) might try stepping into loafers.

Athina had difficulty using her hands for such activities as writing and washing her face. Normally she stabilizes the hand she is using by placing her opposite elbow on her armrest and grasping her forearm. However, she could not use the armrest because she needed to sit further back in her wheelchair, and she also had trouble reaching across her abdomen. Perhaps installing a lap tray would have helped.

Julie developed joint pain if she stood too long, and sat on a high stool when doing things like washing dishes. Jennifer said, "Walking was easier than standing—I got uncomfortable when I stood still. So I just walked back and forth whenever I had to wait in a line."

Complications

Gestational Diabetes

Ordinarily, the pancreas produces insulin, which facilitates the transfer of glucose (sugar) from the blood stream to all the cells in the body. In women who have diabetes, the pancreas does not produce enough insulin, causing blood glucose levels to get too high. During pregnancy, a number of hormonal changes affect the body's use of insulin, and some women develop gestational diabetes.

Diabetes of pregnancy adversely affects both mother and fetus. Effects on the mother include a greatly increased risk of developing pre-eclampsia/eclampsia, increased susceptibility to infection, and possible difficulties in labor because the fetus grows unusually large. Possible effects on the fetus include birth injuries resulting from disproportion between a large fetus and the mother's pelvis, respiratory distress, metabolic problems, and birth defects.

Diabetes can be controlled by diet if is mild, but more severe cases must be treated with insulin injections. You will need to work closely with your doctor, and to have frequent blood tests to monitor the effectiveness of your treatment. Gestational diabetes usually disappears at the end of pregnancy, but some women who have gestational diabetes become diabetic some years later.

Pre-eclampsia/Eclampsia

Pre-eclampsia may begin or become worse during the third trimester. Signs that the problem is getting worse include the following:

- Sudden or excessive weight gain
- Puffiness of the hands or face
- Abdominal pain
- Persistent headaches
- Visual changes

Treatment for pre-eclampsia includes partial or complete bed rest, and medication may be prescribed to lower your blood pressure. You may be hospitalized, as Laura was. Discuss your feelings with your doctor if you are reluctant to go to the hospital. Perhaps you can rest well at home, but that is not the only concern. It may be necessary to closely monitor your blood pressure, or watch for signs that you need medication to prevent or control seizures.

Ultimately, the only "cure" for pre-eclampsia is delivery of the baby. Sometimes pre-term delivery is necessary. While delivery may be delayed until tests show that the baby's lungs have matured, increased blood pressure, signs of placental failure, kidney failure, or very severe symptoms may necessitate immediate delivery.

If convulsions occur, pre-eclampsia has become eclampsia. Warning signs are severe headache, difficulty breathing, blurred vision, or pain in the upper right area of your body, above the stomach. If you are in the hospital and experience any of these symptoms, ring for a nurse immediately. If you are at home, call your doctor but do not attempt to drive to his or her office or the hospital, since such pain is a sign that convulsions may occur soon. While you should tell your doctor if you have any of the above symptoms, be aware that some of them may not be caused by pre-eclampsia. For example,

Michelle's blurred vision was an MS exacerbation, and was not associated with any other symptoms of pre-eclampsia. Severe headaches are also caused by dysreflexia.

Disability Exacerbations

Possible exacerbations of each disability are discussed in Chapter 2. Some disability symptoms are most likely to be exacerbated in the third trimester because of the effect of normal pregnancy changes. For example, since uterine pressure on the lungs is greatest during this stage, breathing difficulties are more likely to worsen at this time. Myasthenia gravis, in particular, is more likely to be exacerbated in the third trimester.

Kidney impairment, which is associated with more than one disability, is of special concern. If kidney function worsens and no reversible cause can be found, such as infection or dehydration, pre-term delivery may be necessary.

Pre-term and Post-term Labor

Full-term labor is labor occurring 40 weeks after the estimated date of conception, which is the average length of pregnancy. Babies born about 2 weeks "early" or "late" are within the normal range of variation, and they are unlikely to differ from full-term infants in health or appearance. Often, labor only seems to be early or late when, in fact, the date of conception has been miscalculated. Therefore, pre-term labor is defined as labor occurring before the thirty-seventh week of pregnancy, and post-term labor is defined as labor occurring after the forty-second week. Sonography and, sometimes, hormone tests may be used to confirm diagnosis of pre- or post-term labor. The causes of pre-term labor include the following:

- Infections (such as urinary tract infection)
- Cervical incompetence
- Placental abnormalities (such as placenta previa and placental abruption)
- Chronic maternal illness (such as high blood pressure, kidney disease, and diabetes)
- Use of some illegal drugs
- Distension of the uterus by excess amniotic fluid or multiple pregnancy
- Structural abnormalities of the uterus
- Fetal death

Often the cause of pre-term labor cannot be identified.

Myasthenia gravis, systemic lupus erythematosus, and spinal cord injury represent an increased risk of premature labor. To some extent, the increased risk results from other complications associated with disability. For example, a woman who has SLE, but not pre-eclampsia or lupus flare, is less likely to have pre-term labor than a woman who does have these problems. Sylvia's episode of premature labor was caused by "dysreflexia and bowel problems" (Sylvia seems to have meant impaction). However, the relationships are not simple and predictable. For example, Sheila had persistent bladder infections throughout both of her pregnancies. During her second pregnancy, she used antibiotics more consistently and had less urinary discomfort, yet it was in this pregnancy that she had an episode of pre-term labor.

It is possible to have episodes of pre-term labor, yet not give birth prematurely (only 25%–50% of these episodes end in pre-term delivery). Treatment consists of bed rest and, sometimes, medications which suppress labor. Additional medications may be used to treat an underlying cause of pre-term labor (such as lupus flare, infection, or high blood pressure). If tests show the fetus' lungs are immature, the mother may also be given a medication (betamethasone) which speeds up fetal lung development, so that the baby will do better if s/he is born early.

In some cases, the condition causing pre-term labor may threaten the mother or fetus so seriously that pre-term delivery is the best treatment. (Risks must be balanced against the risks of induced or surgical delivery.) Tests such as kidney function tests or pulmonary (lung) function tests can help to determine whether pre-term delivery is appropriate.

If you are admitted to the hospital for treatment, it is important that someone familiar with disability be involved in your care, if only as an advisor to the obstetric staff. Sharon was hospitalized in her seventh month (the baby was born six weeks early). Her muscles stiffened, and spasms became more frequent, because she was not given enough physical therapy. A consultation with a rehabilitation specialist might have prevented this problem.

Because spinal-cord-injured women are more likely to give birth prematurely, it is often advised that they enter the hospital at least two weeks before the "due date," or earlier if the cervix is effaced and dilated. This precaution is especially important for women with injuries at or above T10, who cannot feel labor contractions, and still more important for women with injuries above T-6, because of the risk that dysreflexia will occur during labor.

One of the hazards of pre-term labor is that the mother will not know that she is in labor. Leslie recalled, "My contractions were one-sided, and I was in labor for 16 hours without realizing it. I thought I had the flu. I didn't know what was happening until my bag of water broke."

Signs that labor may be starting are described in detail at the beginning of Chapter 7. Briefly, they include the following:

- Contractions which do not disappear with rest or change of activity (unlike Braxton-Hicks contractions)
- Contractions increasing in frequency and intensity
- Lower back pain
- "Bloody show"
- A sudden gush of fluid, followed by another gush after about an hour (the bag of water breaking)
- Diarrhea or indigestion

With spinal cord injury, symptoms may also include the following:

- Internal discomforts feeling like indigestion or the need to have a bowel movement
- Dysreflexia symptoms
- Muscle spasms or clonus

The problem associated with some post-term pregnancies is that the fetus grows so large that delivery is difficult. As a result, mother or infant may be injured during delivery, or cesarean delivery may be required. In other post-term pregnancies, the aging placenta begins to function poorly, and fetal growth is retarded. Other changes may cause fetal distress.

If you appear to have a post-term pregnancy, your doctor must consider the possibility that the date of your last menstruation was miscalculated. You may have had ultrasound examinations earlier in pregnancy which confirmed the length of your pregnancy. If not, sonography or amniocentesis may be done at this time. Stress or non-stress tests and/or a biophysical profile may be used to assess the well-being of the fetus. Labor may be induced if the cervix is effaced and the fetus engaged.

Fetal Development

The fetus grows dramatically during the third trimester, from about 13 inches in length and 1 3/4 pounds in weight at the end of the twenty-fourth week, to 20 inches in length and 7 pounds in weight at the fortieth week. The appearance matures as fat is deposited under the skin, the hair and nails continue to grow, and the size and tone of the muscles increase. Only the mother can feel fetal movement during much of the second trimester. Now, as movement gets stronger, she knows that the fetus will not stop moving just when she has invited other family members to "come feel the baby kick."

During the last few weeks of pregnancy, when there is less room for the fetus to move, it may seem less active. If the amount of fetal movement changes gradually, you do not need to worry, but if you feel any concern, you certainly should bring it up with your doctor. A sudden increase or decrease in fetal activity may be a sign of fetal distress.

While the nervous system continues to mature even after birth, development during the third trimester is significant, as the brain continues to grow, and reflexes such as thumb sucking, and responses to light and sound appear. Some time during the third trimester, parents will notice that at times a little lump appears on the mother's abdomen where the fetus stretches a limb and, if they press the lump, the fetus reacts by pulling away. "Chase the baby" becomes an enjoyable game.

The immune system is also maturing. But even at full term, the immune system is immature, and passive immunity conferred by the mother is an important protection. As a result, premature babies are more susceptible to infection than full-term babies. Because breast feeding provides some antibodies to the infant, it is important to feed premature babies with breast milk if possible.

Lung development is a special concern during this trimester. Inability to breathe, or difficulty breathing, are the chief threat to the survival of premature babies. By the end of the seventh month, the alveoli (bubble-like sacs at the surface of which oxygen is transferred to blood cells) have formed, as well as the system of blood vessels in the lungs. However, a baby born at this time will still have respiratory difficulties because the lungs are not producing surfactant, a chemical which prevents the alveoli from collapsing on contact with air. S/he can survive with intensive care, but chances of surviving and avoiding complications are improved as surfactant production increases later in pregnancy. So, when doctors delay treating complications with pre-term delivery, or attempt to suppress pre-term labor, the primary reason is that they are trying to allow time for the lungs to mature.

Emotional Concerns

Some important concerns in the third trimester are the following:

- Changes in sexual relationships
- Unhappiness about increased dependence
- Anticipation and fear about childbirth and motherhood

Most women experience some change in their sexual relationship when they become pregnant. Many couples experience a new sense of freedom, particularly during the first trimester. Many people feel more sexual desire and make love more frequently since they do not have to worry about contraception. However, pregnancy discomforts can reduce desire. A woman who feels nauseated or short of breath simply does not feel "sexy." Later in pregnancy, when uterine contractions become noticeable, orgasm can cause uncomfortable contractions which feel somewhat like menstrual cramps. Cheryl recalled, "It was difficult because it (uterine contractions) caused more muscle cramps."

A problem many couples encounter in the third trimester is difficulty finding a comfortable position. The problem may be worse for disabled women, whose choices may be limited by lack of mobility even when they are not pregnant. Heather said, "It was awkward. We tried different positions, but it was most difficult during the seventh and eighth months." Sheila said, "After the seventh month it was just too uncomfortable." Dawn felt that the problem was not one of awkwardness, but a "full" feeling that made insertion difficult. Possibly this problem arises for women whose babies are "engaged." Some women found that side-lying or sitting positions gave them more room to maneuver.

Some couples worry that lovemaking will harm the fetus or stimulate labor. There is almost never any need to worry, but if there is any doubt in your mind, do not hesitate to ask your doctor. S/he has answered similar questions hundreds of times, so there is no need to be embarrassed. You may be advised to avoid intercourse if you or your partner has an infection, or if you have signs or symptoms indicating a risk of pre-term labor. Christina and Leslie were both advised to avoid intercourse when it became clear that they were at risk for miscarriage. If you must avoid intercourse, remember that you can show affection in other ways. Sylvia recalled, "We couldn't have sex in the last month because the baby was lying too low. We found other ways to satisfy the sex urge. Oral sex was a nice substitute."

Sometimes a couple's concerns have a more emotional basis. For example, a woman who feels that she looks less attractive may want to avoid nudity, even though she wants the reassurance of tenderness and romance. Either partner may become uncomfortable with physical intimacy as she or he wonders how a new baby will affect the marriage. Try to set aside time to discuss these feelings. Sharing them can deepen and enrich your relationship and prevent misunderstandings, and there may be fewer chances to share feelings later when a new baby is absorbing your time and energy. Many couples feel it is helpful to join a support or discussion group for prospective parents. They may talk about anything from infant-care tips to ideas for coping with interfering in-laws, depending on how the discussion group is structured. As couples become comfortable with each other, they may discuss sexual relationships. It can be reassuring to learn that what you are feeling, whether it is increased desire or a complete loss of interest, is felt by others.

As a woman becomes slower and clumsier in late pregnancy, she may find that she has to depend more on others to do everyday tasks like carrying groceries. This dependence can be especially frustrating for women with disabilities. For some women, the problem even causes a strain on their relationships. Pam felt that one reason she and her husband separated was that he was burned out from giving her extra help in late pregnancy. These women may need to find ways to get extra help. Perhaps a social worker can arrange for home help or additional attendant care which is not ordinarily available. Other women are upset that pregnancy affects independence skills which were developed during years of hard work. It can help to take the attitude that if you are in control of a situation, you really are independent. For example, if you must ask someone to shop for you, make out a detailed list so that you know you will have the groceries you want. Most important, remember that your situation is temporary, and ask a good friend to remind you, "When you think you're at the end of your rope, tie a knot and hang on!"

Feelings about the impending birth intensify during the course of the third trimester. While some women enjoy pregnancy so much they wish it would last forever, others feel like Arlene, who said, "I was waiting for it to be over, so I could have my normal body back." Many women fantasize that the baby will be born a week or so early, although in a first pregnancy it is somewhat more likely to be born a few days later than expected.

Some women fear the birth process even though they are eager for the pregnancy to end. Patricia said, "I had an x-ray so I knew I could have a vaginal birth. I had two emotions at the same time. I was relieved that I didn't have to have a C-section, but I was apprehensive about labor and delivery. I kept trying not to think about how scary and painful labor might be." It really does help to discuss these fears in birthing class, and to women who have already had children. You will see that often a labor which includes "scary and painful" moments is still a worthwhile experience.

Another common feeling is a mixture of fear and anticipation of motherhood. Stacy remembered, "I was acting confident outwardly, but inside I was apprehensive." If you have never had children, and you watch the mother of even a young baby, it is easy to wonder, "How does she change a diaper so fast when he squirms like that? How does she know that one cry means he's hungry, and another cry means he's wet? How will I ever do it?" Of course, the answer is that she learned from experience and you will, too.

Meanwhile, you will start noticing babies wherever you go—in the same aisle at the grocery store, standing in line with you at the bank. Many pregnant women notice that they start exchanging a special, secret smile with strangers pushing strollers. They start remembering lullabies and bedtime stories they had not thought of for years. Shopping for baby clothes, having a baby shower, and trying to choose a name all contribute to the feeling that, "Yes, I really will have a baby...soon!"

CLOSING COMMENTS
. . . .

Each pregnancy is unique, even the different pregnancies of one woman, and uncertainty about what may happen from day to day can make nine months seem like a long time. Both anticipation of motherhood and frustration with pregnancy discomforts can intensify the feeling that each week lasts a month. But even when it seems impossible to wait one more day, there are milestones that make the whole experience worthwhile. Most women with disabilities treasure the feeling that their bodies are functioning well, doing what only women can do.

In this chapter, we have not provided a road map to pregnancy (that is impossible), but pointed out the landmarks and offered the tools that will help each woman make her way. Pregnancy is a preparation for parenthood in more ways than one. Independent effort, cooperation with others, flexibility and practical ways of solving problems, and the ability to relax and enjoy momentary pleasures, all are needed to get the job done. These same tools are useful when the goal is in sight, as we will explain in the next chapter.

7 MOTHER AT LAST— LABOR AND DELIVERY
· ·

THE COURSE OF LABOR
· ·

Like pregnancy, labor progresses in a series of well-defined stages, one of them subdivided into phases. These stages are defined by changes in the condition and activity of the uterus. The length of time that each will last varies substantially for different women.

The uterus is a pear-shaped, muscular organ, with the neck of the uterus—the cervix—extending into the vagina. In Stage I of labor, the cervix becomes effaced (thinned) and dilated, as it is pulled back into the uterus until the opening at the center (the *os*) dilates from 0 to 10 cm in diameter. At the end of Stage I, when the cervix is fully effaced and dilated, the interior of the uterus is continuous with the vagina.

Stage I progresses through three phases. By the end of the early phase, also called *prodromal labor* or *latent labor,* the cervix is completely effaced and the os has dilated to 3 cm in diameter. By the end of the active phase, the cervix has dilated to 7 cm. The phase during which the cervix dilates from 7 to 10 cm is known as transition because it is the turning point between Stage I and Stage II. In Stage II, the function of uterine contractions changes from opening the cervix to squeezing out the baby. This stage is completed with the baby's birth. During Stage III, uterine contractions expel the placenta from the uterus. Finally, Stage IV refers to the first few hours

233

after childbirth. During this time, bleeding from the area where the placenta was attached should stop, and uterine contractions begin to close the cervix and return the uterus to its pre-pregnant size. The uterus continues to return to normal during the postpartum period, which is discussed in Chapter 9.

Signs and Symptoms of Labor

Before we describe the many physical changes women experience during labor, we want to make a few general comments.

Many childbirth educators avoid the old-fashioned phrase "labor pains." Instead, they use the term *contractions,* because the processes of labor and delivery are accomplished by rhythmical contractions of the uterine muscles. For many, if not most, women these contractions *are* painful, yet educators hesitate to describe them as such for fear of causing unnecessary anxiety. Because anxiety and tension can increase sensitivity to pain, many childbirth educators try to avoid overemphasizing the painfulness of labor.

On the other hand, women who have read books or taken classes in which the painfulness of labor is minimized are sometimes unpleasantly shocked to find that coping with labor contractions is more difficult than they had expected. For some women, labor is *very* painful. In some cases, labor was the most severe pain they have ever experienced. However, if we do not know what other pain these women have experienced, the comparison is not very meaningful.

It cannot be emphasized enough that labor is a very individual experience. Some women said it was easy. Sasha said, "On a scale from 1 to 10, labor was a 5 or 6." Disabled women who have had painful injuries or surgeries might well agree with Sasha's assessment.

What a woman feels during labor depends on many factors outside of her control, including the position of the fetus, its size in proportion to her pelvic opening, and how long labor lasts. Symptoms other than pain are also unpredictable. For example, the pain of excessive muscle stretching, including uterine stretching, often causes nausea. Clara, who falls frequently and becomes nauseated whenever she strains a muscle, was sure that she would be nauseated during labor, but she was not.

The breathing and relaxation exercises taught in prenatal classes help many women to cope with labor pain and minimize the use of medications. We believe it is worthwhile for every woman to learn these techniques, which can also be used to cope with pain in the years to come. Yet, while women who give birth without using medication often feel joy and a sense of pride, women who have unusually painful labors should not be disappointed in themselves if they need pain medication.

Having acknowledged that labor hurts, we will not dwell on that fact. For the rest of this chapter, we will use the term *uterine contractions.*

Stage I

Early Phase

It is not surprising that women wonder, "How will I know I'm really in labor?" There are a great variety of signs and symptoms of early labor, many of them quite subtle. Weeks before labor begins in earnest, women may experience Braxton-Hicks contractions ("practice" contractions) that are surprisingly strong. Often, a woman in the last few weeks of pregnancy is told during a prenatal visit that her cervix is already slightly dilated. As she hears other women's stories, she learns that the sensations of early labor may not be what she expects. When Leslie was in the early phase, her contractions caused a dull, cramping feeling that she thought might be the flu. She remembers saying jokingly to her sister, "I'm probably in labor and too dumb to know it." Then she called her doctor and found out it was no joke!

Some women with disabilities may experience some atypical symptoms, and many women who have disabilities that involve the loss of sensation may not have the experience they expected. The sensory nerves to the uterus are between T-10 and T-12, so women who have injuries that are below T-10 will feel labor, while most women with injuries higher than T-10 usually do not feel labor (those who do may have incomplete lesions). Samantha was sure she would feel labor contractions despite her disability. She had been experiencing Braxton-Hicks contractions, and her midwife told her that her cervix was slightly dilated. However, she never felt early labor. It began while she was sleep, and she suddenly woke up in the transitional phase (some able-bodied women have had similar experiences). Other women were surprised when they *did* feel labor contractions. After we describe the common signs and symptoms of early labor, we will describe other signs and symptoms that some disabled women have experienced.

Of course, a good way to answer the question, "Am I in labor?" or even the question, "What is this discomfort I'm experiencing?" is to do what Leslie did. Call your doctor, midwife, or hospital and describe whatever is occurring. Experiencing any of the signs and symptoms we describe is certainly reason for a call, but any unusual or uncomfortable symptoms also merit a call to the doctor.

For some women, the first sign of labor is a "bloody show"—leakage of blood-tinged mucus. The cervical os contains a plug of mucus which becomes dislodged as the cervix dilates. Sometimes a few tiny blood vessels break as the cervix dilates, and the mucus plug has a pinkish or brownish stain or a few streaks of blood. Intercourse or a vaginal examination may result in some blood spotting about 48 hours later, but otherwise, a show of brown or pink mucus is usually a sign that labor will begin soon. "Soon" means some time between a few hours and 2 weeks. However, *bright red spotting* is a danger sign that should be reported to the doctor immediately.

Of course, bloody show may also appear with the first noticeable contractions. Carla remembers being awakened by "a crampy feeling," then finding the bloody show.

Thinner fluid flowing from the vagina may be amniotic fluid. Between 10% and 20% of labors begin with rupture of the amniotic membrane (also called the "bag of water breaking"). Sometimes there is an uncomfortable sensation of pressure before the membrane ruptures. Jennifer felt as if she needed to have a bowel movement, and her bag broke while she was on the toilet.

Sometimes it is hard for a woman to be sure what is happening. The amniotic fluid may come out in a slow leak or a sudden gush. If the flow is sudden, it may feel like a loss of bladder control. Also, there are times when a pregnancy is near full term that sudden fetal pressure on the bladder really does cause a loss of control. When fluid is leaking through a small tear, she may find that the flow is more continuous when she lies down: when she stands or sits, the baby's head presses against the cervix and can block the flow. Since the amniotic fluid is constantly replaced, one sign that the membranes have ruptured is another sudden gush of fluid about an hour after the first one.

If there is a sign that the membranes have ruptured, whether a slow drip or a sudden gush of fluid, it is time to call the doctor—do not wait to feel labor contractions. Your doctor can do a simple test to determine if there is amniotic fluid in the vagina, and s/he needs to know what time the membranes ruptured. For most women whose first sign of labor is the breaking of the bag, contractions start within 12 hours. Your doctor will need to examine you for two reasons:

1. S/he will need to make sure that the baby's head is well engaged in the pelvis. If not, there is a chance that the umbilical cord, no longer supported by amniotic fluid, will slip down into the cervix. Then, later in labor, uterine contractions might press the baby's head against the cord, compressing it and interfering with the fetal oxygen supply.

2. The uterine environment is open to infection once the membranes have ruptured. It is important that contractions begin promptly because of the danger of infection to mother and/or baby. The doctor or midwife may watch for signs of infection by taking the mother's temperature or checking vaginal secretions for bacteria. If contractions have not begun within 24 hours, it may be necessary to induce labor. (We will say more about induction in the section, "Medical Procedures.")

Besides noting what time the membranes rupture, check the color of the fluid before calling the doctor. It should be a clear, pale yellow fluid. Cloudiness and brownish or greenish staining can be signs of fetal distress, and mean you should call your doctor immediately.

For most women, the sensation of contractions is the first sign that labor has begun. Some women feel contractions intensely even in the early phase; there is no doubt in their minds that labor has begun. Others have mild contractions at first, and it can be difficult to recognize them for what they are. Julie, who had not attended a birth preparation class, was thrown completely off guard. She "thought labor would be like in the movies with women screaming and pushing," so she thought her discomfort was the after effect of a fall in the eighth month of her pregnancy. Early contractions felt like gas pains to Portia and Sasha. Contractions that feel like gas pain or indigestion are sometimes accompanied by diarrhea. Patricia and Carla both said the sensation was "like menstrual cramps, only it hurt more."

Some women notice that their discomfort starts in the lower back, then spreads to the abdomen. Other women in early labor keep feeling as if they have to urinate, but do not produce more than a few drops; others feel a backache. Another occasional subtle symptom of early labor is change of mood—not knowing quite what bothers her, a woman becomes more irritable, short-tempered, or humorless.

As contractions continue, it may become more obvious that labor has begun. Portia commented that with her second child, as with her first, "it was impossible to tell labor pains from gas pains at first.... I needed it to go on longer to make sure it was labor." Stacy thought she "was having Braxton-Hicks contractions," but realized it was labor when "they didn't go away, they just intensified."

One sign that labor has begun is that cramping sensations do not stop. Try getting up, moving around, and possibly taking a shower—if contractions continue, labor has begun.

Another way to make sure labor has begun is to time contractions, using a watch with a second hand. In false labor, contractions commonly occur at irregular intervals and last for varying amounts of time. In true labor, contractions are more likely to occur at increasingly regular intervals which gradually grow shorter. (So, in false labor the intervals may be 10 minutes, 6 minutes, 15 minutes; in true early labor, the intervals may be 30 minutes, 30, 35, 30...25, 27, 25, 25...15, 15, 15). In true labor, it is more likely that each contraction will last the same amount of time—at least 45 seconds, with contractions gradually becoming longer as labor progresses. In timing contractions, it is important to note the time each contraction *begins*. An example of a written record is shown in Table 7.1

In this example, if the woman called her doctor at 9:00, it would be enough to say that contractions are "about 11 minutes apart." By 9:50, contractions last the same amount of time, but are much more closely spaced. Transition may be approaching, and the mother, who may have called her doctor or midwife to say that her contractions are 5 minutes apart, should be on her way to the birth center or hospital. Remember that this pattern is common, but does not describe what happens to *every* woman. One of

TABLE 7.1
CONTRACTION CHART

Beginning of Contraction	End of Contraction	Duration	Spacing
8:40:30	8:41:20	50 sec	
8:51:20	8:52:10	50 sec	10 min 50 sec
9:01:10	9:03:00	50 sec	9 min 50 sec
.			
.			
.			
9:45:00	9:45:45	45 sec	
9:50:00	9:50:50	50 sec	5 min

Note: "Duration" refers to the length of time of the contraction. "Spacing" refers to the time between the beginning of one contraction and the beginning of the next contraction.

Judi's students recalls that her first noticeable contractions were 5 minutes apart, and contractions continued to be 5 minutes apart throughout labor. "Expect the unexpected" certainly applies to the birthing experience!

It may be difficult to time contractions, because a contraction becomes more intense as it continues. A woman who does not feel her contraction at first may be recording contractions from peak to peak, not from beginning to beginning. That is probably what happened to a student in one of Judi's birthing classes whose contractions seemed to be lasting only 30 seconds, just 2 hours before she gave birth. To avoid this kind of confusion, the mother-to-be or a friend can rest a hand on her lower abdomen, and wait to feel the first tightening or hardening of her uterus.

Women with spinal dysfunction may experience labor differently. Those who have injury at the T-10 level or higher often cannot feel labor contractions as such. Women who have some internal sensation, such as the ability to feel bladder fullness, fetal movements, or Braxton-Hicks contractions while pregnant, may feel something during labor, but *what* they will feel cannot be predicted. Stephanie, who "didn't expect to feel it that well" and thought "the sensation would be sufficiently dull to take the edge off," was surprised when "it hurt more than I expected." Sharon described a feeling of "pressure." Sheila said that when her second child was born, she felt "an uncomfortable tightening" and was able to time her contractions, although she did not feel contractions with her first child.

Women with spinal dysfunctions may need to be alert for other signs or symptoms of labor. Sheila remembers that the night before she knew labor had started, she felt an urge to urinate every 20–30 minutes, but never did pass much urine. However, her amniotic membrane ruptured in the morning, and then she realized she was in labor. Looking back, she realizes that her urges to urinate must have been a response to labor contractions. Sheila remembers that just before her water broke, she looked down and noticed that "my stomach had an odd, lopsided shape." Sharon, too, commented, "I saw my stomach stick out, then fall."

In the last weeks of pregnancy, a woman with spinal cord dysfunction can respond to internal discomforts such as pressure, a feeling like indigestion, a feeling as if she needs to have a bowel movement, or a recurring need to urinate, by watching her abdomen to see if it seems to be tightening and relaxing. If she is able to, she can rest her hand just below her navel and feel for tightening or hardening, or she can ask her spouse, friend, or attendant to check. Since some women never do feel labor, we suggest that women with spinal dysfunction make a habit of looking or feeling for contractions a few times a day during the weeks preceding their due dates.

For some women, dysreflexia (which can occur in woman with lesions above T-6) symptoms are a sign that labor has begun. When a labor contraction increases pressure inside the uterus, they experience the same changes caused by pressure in a full bowel or bladder: blood pressure rises, accompanied by symptoms like sweating, headache, or muscle spasm. For Sheila, the experience was slightly different with each birth. With her first child, she had an excruciating headache; she lay down to rest, and when she sat up, her ` membrane ruptured, fluid gushed out, and her headache disappeared. With her second child, the change was less dramatic; there was no gush of fluid, but a slow, steady leak accompanied by a milder headache. For Sylvia, however, the first sign of labor was unusually intense leg spasms. Other surveys have found that women with spinal cord dysfunction sometimes experience increased leg and ankle spasms or clonus during labor.

Variations in Early Labor One variation from the pattern we have been describing is back labor, in which the mother feels constant lower back pain, which becomes worse—often excruciating—during contractions. Clara, who had back labor with her first child, said, "I could never tell when a contraction was starting because the pain was continuous; it just never seemed to let up." Renee had back labor the second time she gave birth. She said, "It was more painful than the first time....Contractions went from peak to peak." Back labor is often, but not always, caused by malposition of the fetus. The fetal head compresses the spinal nerves, rather than pressing against the cervix. This causes pain which does not stop at the end of a contraction.

When we discuss ways that women can cope with labor, we will also discuss how to cope with the unusual discomfort of back labor.

A second variation is *precipitate labor.* Early labor usually begins with contractions as much as 20–30 minutes apart. As the interval approaches 10–20 minutes, it becomes clear that early labor has begun. Early labor lasts several hours, and active labor begins as the interval between contractions approaches 5–10 minutes. In precipitate labor, the whole process of labor is much shorter, lasting less than 3 hours. Contractions in this type of labor are intense from the beginning, and may be only 5 minutes apart. Some labor seems precipitate because the cervix has been gradually dilating for several days, and the mother first notices contractions when she is close to transition. Otherwise, precipitate labor results from low resistance in the birth canal or unusually strong contractions. The cervix may dilate very quickly—Clara's cervix dilated from 2.5 to 10 cm in diameter in 20 minutes.

Precipitate labor can present problems for both mother and fetus. The sudden, intense sensations may make it very difficult for the mother to adapt to labor and use breathing techniques to cope with her pain. If the cervix, vagina, or perineum are firm and resistant to strong contractions, there may be tears or, in rare cases, uterine rupture. If these tissues are soft or well stretched, the mother probably will not experience complications, but a resistant birth canal may cause trauma to the baby's head. Another problem is that very strong contractions, without much relaxation between them, may interfere with blood flow in the uterus, and thus with the fetal oxygen supply. A few women who have precipitate labor may experience injuries, and the baby may be born suddenly (and even fall out and be injured if the mother is standing), so they may need attention at any moment. If a woman first becomes aware of labor because she experiences intense, closely spaced contractions, she may be starting a precipitate labor and should call her doctor or midwife right away. She should not be alone.

A third variation is *dysfunctional labor* (also known as *dystocia*), which includes any labor that progresses too slowly. Labor is dysfunctional if the early phase lasts more than 20 hours for a woman having her first child, or more than 14 hours for a woman who has had at least one child. Maternal exhaustion and increased risk of infection are just two of the problems presented by dysfunctional labor. There are several possible causes for dysfunctional labor, as we explain below, and appropriate treatment depends on the nature of the problem.

While early labor contractions usually are not very painful, they can be strong enough to keep a woman from falling asleep. She may become so exhausted from lack of sleep, that even mild contractions are unbearable.

Active Phase

A physical examination is often the only way to confirm that a woman is in the early phase of labor. Yet many women in the early phase hesitate to call their doctor or hospital. Some are afraid they will be told, "You're not really in labor—better go home." Others prefer to wait before dealing with the possibility of medical interventions. By the time a woman is in active labor—the phase in which the cervix, already effaced, dilates from 3 to 7 cm across—she really does need to see her midwife or doctor, and she should not hesitate to call. She probably *will not* hesitate either, since most women experience increasingly intense and frequent contractions as active labor begins. Stephanie, commenting on the difference between early and active labor, said, "*That's* when my husband started asking me if I wanted something for the pain." Jennifer said, "My husband knew it was time to go the hospital because I was looking distressed and doubling over with each contraction."

Most women are advised to call their doctor or hospital when contractions are 5 minutes apart (from beginning to beginning). These contractions commonly last between 45 and 60 seconds. This guideline worked well for Stacy and Patricia, but Clara commented, "With my first baby I went to the hospital when my contractions were 5 minutes apart, and they found I'd only dilated to 2 cm." Another common sign of active labor is mucus dripping from the vagina.

It is also common for women in active labor to become more sensitive. As women find themselves concentrating more and more on their own sensations, some are literally unable to see anything that is not right in front of them, and are oblivious to sounds and conversation around them. Others are just the opposite—irritated by bright lights, noise, laughter, or anything else that distracts them from their effort to stay relaxed. In addition, many women need more and more emotional support.

In the active phase, most women start using the breathing and relaxation techniques they learned in childbirth class. (There are always exceptions—Judi remembers one student who did not need to breathe differently, even during contractions.)

If the early phase is prolonged, sheer fatigue can make it more difficult for a woman to relax and concentrate on appropriate breathing during active labor. On the other hand, when a woman has a vaginal examination and is told that she is finally in active labor, the boost in morale can give her a fresh burst of energy.

The active phase of labor lasts approximately 4–5 hours. As in the early phase, an unusual position of the fetus can cause back pain, or even slow the progress of labor. ("Position" describes which way the fetus is facing in relation to the mother's body. "Presentation" describes which part of the fetus is next to the cervix; in *vertex presentation,* the head would emerge first, and in *breech presentation,* the buttocks would emerge first.) Sometimes the fetus spontaneously changes to a more favorable position during this phase. However, if the active phase lasts too long, or if the fetus' position does not change by the end of the active phase, intervention will be considered.

Transition Transition is the part of the active phase when the cervix dilates 7–10 cm. It has some specific signs and symptoms. While a vaginal examination may be needed to verify that a woman is in early or active labor, a woman who experiences signs or symptoms of transition can probably expect to be ready to push very soon. Here are some common symptoms of transition:

- More intense and frequent contractions
- An urge to push
- A sensation of rectal pressure (as if one has to have a bowel movement)
- Nausea, vomiting, belching or hiccups
- Trembling—either all over or just in the legs
- Chills or hot and cold flashes
- Drowsiness
- Heavy perspiration
- Emotional changes
- Muscle cramps or clonus

Occasionally a woman will experience one of these symptoms before her cervix is dilated to 7 cm. Some women do not notice any real difference during transition, like the student of Judi's who commented after her cervix was fully dilated, "So that was transition? Boy, that was easy!" However, most women will experience one or more symptoms.

Women with spinal dysfunction, and the medical personnel attending them, should remember that many transition symptoms are similar to those of autonomic dysreflexia—extreme fear and anxiety, sweating, markedly increased heart rate, and goose bumps. If these or other symptoms of dysreflexia occur (such as headache and nasal congestion), staff should be prepared to respond by measuring the woman's blood pressure and giving appropriate medication. Ideally, the obstetrician and a specialist familiar with spinal cord dysfunction will discuss appropriate medication *before* labor begins.

Transition is a difficult time for many women because contractions are spaced so closely together. Typically, contractions are 1–3 minutes apart and last 60–90 seconds. So, for example, if there are 2 minutes from the beginning of one contraction to the beginning of a second, and the first contraction lasts 90 seconds, there is only a 30-second rest period between contractions. When Samantha talked about this phase of her third labor, she said, "The contractions were right on top of each other—unlike my other labors, where I seemed to have some space between contractions. It was *very* intense." Samantha's remark is especially significant because her third labor occurred *after* her injury. We want to emphasize again that it is very difficult to predict what labor will be like for women with spinal cord dysfunctions.

Many consider the true hallmark of transition to be a strong urge to push. Childbirth attendants are usually on the alert for this symptom.

Jennifer remembers asking a nurse who had just checked on her, "When should I call you?" and the nurse replied, "When you feel like pushing." This urge, or sometimes a feeling of rectal fullness, is caused when the fetal head presses against the rectal nerve. The sensation is not mild, by any means. When Michelle said, "I needed all my concentration not to push," and Stacy said, "My need to push was too strong to control," they were both voicing very common reactions. Yet it is very important not to push before the cervix is fully dilated, and some of the breathing techniques practiced in birthing class are specifically designed to help women who are not quite ready to push. Some women will be told not to push because there is a *cervical lip*. When the cervix is completely effaced around most of its circumference, but one segment is still thick and distinct from the uterus, the thick segment looks like a lip. This lip of tissue could become bruised, swollen, or torn from the pressure of the fetal head if the mother starts pushing too soon. Only when the lip is drawn back into the uterus is the cervix fully dilated.

Half of the women with spinal cord injuries experienced an urge to push. Possibly more women could have felt the urge, but some of them had been given regional anesthesia to prevent dysreflexia. Sara, whose spinal cord dysfunction is caused by a tumor, may have felt the urge to push without recognizing it. She recalled, "I felt like I had to go to the bathroom, but nothing happened." Sasha was given general anesthesia while in transition, and does not remember if she experienced the urge to push. Since most studies of pregnancy in women with spinal cord dysfunctions involve very small numbers of women, the frequency for experiencing the urge to push cannot be compared to the frequency for able-bodied women. However, able-bodied women may not feel the urge to push, either, if the fetus is not in position to press against the rectal nerve during contractions. So, when a woman with spinal cord injuries does not feel the urge, fetal position, rather than spinal dysfunction, may be responsible.

Sheila had an unusual reaction to the pressure of the fetal head—her legs became numb. She said, "Usually I can do a standing pivot transfer to get into the car. But I couldn't do it then. My legs went numb and they were limp as spaghetti."

Most of the other symptoms of transition are as variable for disabled women as they are for able-bodied women. Even muscle spasms were not very prevalent—they only occurred in four labors.

For many women, the emotional reaction to transition is even more dramatic than the physical reaction. Women who are coping with the intense sensations of this stage can become irritable, very sensitive to distractions, and quite uninhibited. Michelle was annoyed by the smell of apple juice in her room, by being touched, by the sensations of her identification bracelet, and by cloth against her skin—"I didn't want any clothes on and that was a surprise because I'm usually so shy." Patricia was equally uninhibited about expressing the frustration and fear that can occur during this phase—"I can remember wondering when it would be over. I was really frustrated that I couldn't push, and I kept thinking that they were lying to me. I usually don't let strangers see me cry or see any sign that I'm in pain. But this time I *wanted* them to know I was in pain. I didn't care who saw me cry, and I cried."

Stage II—Delivery of the Baby

Progress during the first stage is described by how much the cervix has dilated. Progress during the second stage is described by how far the baby has moved down relative to the ischial spines, the protruding points on the pelvis. (The space between the ischial spines is also called the pelvic outlet. It is the opening in the bony ring through which the baby must pass.) When the baby's head is 1 cm above the ischial spines, it is at the "-1 station." Level with the spines is the 0 station, 1 cm below the spines is the +1 station. At the +3 station, the baby's head is in the vagina. At the +5 station, the baby is *crowning* (the top of the head is emerging), and the baby will soon be born. A woman in Stage II labor may be told that her baby's head is (or is not) engaged; when the baby's head is engaged, the widest part of the head is between the ischial spines.

Stage II lasts an average of 50 minutes for women having their first baby, and 20 minutes for women who have previously given birth. This average represents a great deal of variation, and while some women deliver their babies with just a few pushes, others may need to push for a few hours. Intervention will be considered If Stage II lasts more than 2–3 hours.

For many women, the beginning of Stage II is a welcome relief: now, instead of having to resist the urge to push, the mother is encouraged to bear down as uterine contractions push the baby through the pelvic outlet and the vagina. The frustration of transition comes to an end when, as Patricia said, "It feels good to push." Effective pushing feels comparatively pleasant to many women. It is comparable to the relief of finally going to the bathroom after having to wait. Patricia's frank comment, "It's just like taking a shit," reflected a very earthy experience.

Other sensations during Stage II are caused by the stretching of the soft tissues of the cervix, vagina, and perineum as the baby descends. Women feel sensations of stretching or even tearing, or of burning and stinging. Unusually severe pain may be a sign that something is wrong. Leslie had a laceration of the cervix and uterus, and she said, "It felt like I was torn apart. I have a very high pain threshold—I was able to drive myself to the hospital with a ruptured ectopic pregnancy, but this pain was worse." Leslie did wonder whether her pain was intensified by her fear that something was wrong with her baby, who was born prematurely. Often, the burning, stretching sensation is strongest when the top of the baby's head begins to stretch the perineum (the skin and muscle between the vagina and anus).

At this point, women may need to stop pushing while the skin stretches, but breathing through contractions at this time is often less difficult than during transition.

How a woman feels during Stage II is affected by how long she has been in labor and how long she has to push. Clara contrasted the births of her two children: "The second time, it felt like a torpedo going through me. I wasn't even aware I was pushing; I just knew another entity was going through. The first time, I had to push an hour and a half. The doctor yelled at me to push harder when I thought I already was pushing hard. I don't remember a physical sensation so much as feeling inadequate." Christina, too, felt the exhaustion that is common for women who have labored more than 12 hours, then have to push for another 15 minutes or more. She remembers thinking, "I can't go on."

Yet delivery may not be any more difficult for a woman with disabilities than it is for an able-bodied woman. Mary said simply, "It was easy; it only took 10 minutes." Paula's doctor, who was worried because he had never had a patient with postpolio syndrome, stayed with her during her entire labor, and told her afterwards, "There wasn't any resistance; it was easier than the average delivery."

Some women with spinal dysfunctions do not feel pushing contractions as such, but are able to follow instructions to bear down during Stage II. Sharon, who had felt no urge to push, said her baby crowned after three or four pushes, and then delivery was completed with forceps. She said, "I could have pushed better if I'd been able to use my stomach muscles." Sheila, who was able to push with her second child, said, "I didn't feel different with the pushing, but I could feel the baby slip down." Both Stacy and Samantha did some pushing before their attendants tried pressing on their abdomens in an attempt to make it more effective.

It is true that the flaccid stomach muscles of paraplegic and quadriplegic women may not be helpful for voluntary pushing. On the other hand, the stomach muscles also do not resist fetal descent because they are flaccid. In some women with spinal cord injury, the abdominal muscles spasm during labor, possibly massaging the uterus and assisting labor. We suspect that the strength of the stomach muscles is less important to the outcome of labor than the strength of uterine contractions. Some able-bodied women also have difficulty giving birth, and their difficulties are clearly related to weak or uncoordinated uterine contractions. The effect of spinal cord dysfunction on uterine contractions is not consistent; all four women with spinal cord injury had longer, stronger, and more frequent contractions than what is usual. What is most important is that these women and their physicians should be aware that they may well be able to give birth vaginally, often without assistance.

One special concern of disabled women at this stage is the transfer from a labor room to a delivery room. If the hospital permits women to labor and deliver in the same room, it may be helpful to take advantage of this policy.

Otherwise, it is a good idea to let the woman's attendant show the hospital staff how she normally transfers. Usually, a woman needs to stop pushing while changing rooms, and will not have any spare energy for explaining how she needs to transfer.

Muscle spasms are also a concern during this stage. Sometimes able-bodied women suffer muscle cramps during Stage II, but women with disabilities may suffer more severe cramps or actual clonus. Labor-induced cramps may provoke clonus in women who have disability symptoms that usually include muscle spasms. The intensity of these spasms will vary. Whereas Sylvia said, "I had some spasm when I was pushing, but so much was happening I didn't notice," Sara said, "With the second labor, I wasn't pushing very long when the muscle spasm started. The spasm made it hard to keep my legs open, so they put me out." Among the women we interviewed, two women with spinal dysfunction and one with cerebral palsy experienced spasms during Stage II.

Women may experience very intense physical and emotional reactions once the baby is born. Physical reactions are typical fatigue symptoms, as might be expected after the hard work of labor and delivery. They include trembling, uncontrollable shaking, fatigue, or a feeling of intense cold.

Emotional reactions can depend on what is happening. Sharon, whose son had to be taken to an incubator, thought the coldness she felt after delivery was intensified by her loneliness, adding, "My sister wasn't there and I needed someone to share the experience with." Sasha, who had to wait several hours to see her daughter, said, "I felt robbed....I was a basket case. But it felt so powerful when they finally put her in my arms."

Other women felt excited, relieved, and amazed at their accomplishment. Celeste had been haunted during her first pregnancy by the fear that she would give birth to a dead baby; she simply could not believe that the baby on her chest was really hers. With her second child, she was less anxious during pregnancy and when the baby was born, "bonding started right away. I remember how nice and warm the baby felt."

The baby must be examined and given some basic care before it is given to the mother. An Apgar Score will assess the baby's well-being (see Table 7.2), and a physical examination will help to determine gestational age (whether the baby is pre- or postmature). Mucus will be suctioned from the baby's nose and mouth, and it will be wiped clean and wrapped in a blanket. Before the baby leaves the delivery room, it will be given an identification bracelet, blood will be removed from the umbilical cord or heel for testing, the stump of the umbilical cord will be clamped and bandaged, and in many states, medication will be put in its eyes to prevent blindness from infection by vaginal bacteria.

Holding the baby is difficult for some disabled women. Even if they are not tired or shaking, they may feel insecurely balanced on the narrow delivery table, or fearful of dropping the baby because of poor hand control. A

TABLE 7.2
APGAR TEST

	Score		
	0	**1**	**2**
Appearance (color)[a]	Blue or pale	Body pink, feet and hands blue	Whole body pink
Pulse (heart rate)	Absent	Less than 100 beats/minute	More than 100 beats/minute
Grimace (response to irritation of sole of foot)	None	Grimaces ("makes a face")	Strong cry
Activity (muscle tone)	Limp	Some movement of limbs	Active movement
Respiration (breathing)	None	Slow, uneven	Good, crying

[a]For babies who are dark-complexioned at birth, the assessment is based on their lips, nailbeds, and the soles of their feet.

Note: The Apgar test is a quick examination to assess the newborn's general well-being. It does not diagnose subtle health problems. The test was devised by Dr. Virginia Apgar, and the letters A-P-G-A-R stand for the five factors which are evaluated.

Apgar evaluation is done 1 minute after birth, and repeated 5 minutes after birth. A low score at 1 minute means the baby needs resuscitation. A low score at 5 minutes means the baby has a higher than average risk for health problems in the weeks after birth. A score of 7–10 means the baby is normal or only slightly depressed. A score of 4–6 means the infant is moderately depressed. A score of 0–3 indicates severe depression; the infant will need resuscitation. The great majority of babies score 7–10.

little help from the father or nursing staff can assure that the first moments after birth will be joyous ones.

Stage III—Delivery of the Placenta

For most women, this stage is brief and mild. Sometimes, when women are encouraged to stimulate Stage III contractions by nursing their newborns, the extra stimulation makes contractions more painful. (These contractions also tend to be stronger after a second birth than after a first.)

Stage III generally follows closely after Stage II. The placenta may slip out, or the mother may be told to give a few more pushes. Contractions sometimes stop just after birth, then begin again about 5 minutes later. While the placenta usually separates within 3–5 minutes after birth, up to 30 minutes may be allowed for its expulsion. The amount of time allowed depends on the mother's condition, especially on the amount of uterine bleeding. If the placenta is not delivered promptly, or part of the placenta is retained in the uterus, some intervention may be necessary. However, if the placenta has separated from the uterine wall, only minor intervention is likely to be necessary, such as hand pressure on the fundus (top of the uterus).

Stage IV—Postpartum

Stage IV is generally uneventful, a time for resting quietly. In this stage, the function of contractions is to begin the process of restoring the uterus to its pre-pregnant size and shape. Some of these contractions may be uncomfortable, but usually they are not as painful as the contractions of labor and delivery.

If a woman had an episiotomy, it will be repaired during this stage. If she did not have anesthesia during labor, the doctor will inject a local anesthetic before starting the repair. Women who are paralyzed, but do not have complete loss of sensation, may want to remind the doctor to give them an injection. Stacy's obstetrician assumed that, since she was paralyzed, she had no perineal sensation. Stacy said, "Boy, those stitches *hurt*."

The mother will be encouraged to urinate at least once within a few hours after giving birth. If she is in a birth center with an early release program, she must urinate before she goes home. If the bladder or urethra were irritated or injured during labor, and urination is difficult, this problem must be diagnosed and treated.

METHODS FOR COPING WITH LABOR DISCOMFORTS

A variety of methods have been developed to help women feel as comfortable and relaxed as possible during labor. The methods we describe in this section are nonmedical. Pain medication and anesthesia, and their advantages and disadvantages, are included in the section entitled "Medical Procedures."

Not every method is useful in every situation. For example, most women will not have back labor, and will not need to use our suggestions for coping with it. The same woman may find light massage relaxing during one phase of labor, yet annoying during another phase. Many women find that a method which helped during one labor does not help during another, like Faith, who said, "With my first baby it really helped to have a focal point, but the second time I didn't use it." Still, nearly every woman will probably use at least one of these methods some time during her labor.

The best approach is to become familiar with our suggestions and be ready to use whatever coping method feels comfortable. It is also helpful to pack the labor kit described in Table 7.3; not every item will be used, but what is used will be appreciated! Pack the labor kit a few weeks before the due date—nobody wants to be searching for socks and a mirror when it is time to leave for the hospital! (As an extra reminder, items that belong in the labor kit will be in *ITALICS* when they are mentioned.)

Most techniques for coping with labor can be included in one of the following categories: breathing techniques; other relaxation techniques; and relief of particular discomforts, such as cold feet or chapped lips.

Breathing properly helps the mother to relax and get enough oxygen for the hard work of uterine contractions, and also helps the fetus withstand the stress of labor. Relaxation techniques are every bit as important as other techniques for maintaining comfort. A woman who is tense or frightened is more sensitive to pain. The mother's fear and tension can affect uterine contractions and, indirectly, the baby's blood chemistry. When relaxation techniques are effective, they can help the mother avoid using pain medication, or use less, so that she will not have to worry about side effects.

Breathing techniques are most useful when they have been practiced in advance. A number of different techniques should be practiced, so the mother is ready to try an alternative method if one is not useful. We suggest that women practice every possible technique, because a method which is uncomfortable for a woman who is not in labor may feel different when she is. Judi recalls a student telling her that a breathing technique she had disliked in class was very helpful when she was in labor. Since it is best to learn breathing techniques in a class, where they can be *demonstrated,* not just *described,* and where the instructor can help with practice, we will not describe breathing in great detail. When we suggest using a breathing technique during a specific phase, such as transition, we do not want to imply the technique should be used only during that phase, but that it is most likely to be helpful then. Some women prefer to use the breathing suggested for the early phase all through Stage I, while others need to use transition breathing before they are in transition. As with other coping methods, a woman in labor should use whatever type of breathing helps her feel that she is relaxed and in control.

Many coping methods can be used by the mother without assistance, while others can or must be used with a coach's help. The coach can practice before labor by going to birthing classes with the mother, learning and

TABLE 7.3
LABOR KIT

Item	Purpose
Copies of medical information forms	If hospital misfiles this information, it won't have to be given all over again
Handouts on labor from birthing class	Reminds coach of coping methods
Stopwatch or watch with second hand, pen, paper	Timing and recording contractions
Money, including several coins	Coach's snacks, phone calls
Bag lunch or snacks	Food helps coach during long labor, coach may need to stay with mother
Massage items	Powder and body oil, bonger, tennis balls, rolling pin for back labor
Focal point objects	Objects to focus eyes on to aid in relaxation (see text)
Spoon	For feeding ice chips
Washcloths	Help keep mother cool, wipe away sweat, help with massage
Breath spray	Freshen dry mouth or stale breath
Chapstick	Moisten dry lips
Sour lollipops	Sugar keeps up mother's strength, sour more refreshing than sweet, mother cannot choke on lollipop
Paper bag	Mother can breathe into bag if hyperventilating
Mirror	To let mother see birth
Glasses	Contact lenses shouldn't be worn during labor
Tape recorder, tapes, and headphones	Relaxing music or hypnosis tapes
Warm socks	To warm mother's feet if **cold**
Camera	Birth pictures
Telephone list	People to call after birth

Note: Pack all items 2–3 weeks before due date (except perishable food items).

practicing breathing techniques with her, giving her massages, and so on. Yes, the mother must breathe for herself, but if she feels tired or overwhelmed by her sensations, the coach's practical and emotional support are very important. Other relaxation techniques can be used while the coach is taking a break, or while the mother is waiting for him/her to arrive.

One of the coach's most important jobs is timing the mother's contractions, using the *STOPWATCH* from the labor kit. As the labor falls into a regular rhythm, the coach can help the mother breathe by letting her know she is doing a good job, signaling that a contraction is about to start, and letting her know when a contraction may end. Sometimes a labor contraction feels like it will last forever. The coach can reassure the mother by telling her, "You're halfway through now....It's going to end in 15 seconds...10...5." Emotional support is also important. Corrine said, "My husband hadn't had any birthing classes, but his presence was calming." Sharon said, "I didn't need a coach, but it was good to have my sister there, even though we were just laughing." Stephanie thought both aspects of a coach's job are crucial. "He helped me breathe, he timed my contractions, he helped me decide about pain medication." The coach can also help the mother communicate with medical staff. For example, sometimes the mother is so intent on her labor that she does not hear something a nurse says, but when her coach repeats it, she responds to the familiar voice. Or the coach may tell a doctor or nurse, "She'll answer your question in a minute, she just started a contraction."

A coach who is familiar with disability can also help by letting medical staff know about the mother's special needs. People who are very skillful at helping in childbirth may not have much experience with disability, and the coach may need to show them how to help the mother transfer, or remind them to help her change position to prevent pressure sores. Some coaches have an easy time. Jennifer's husband, who had been expecting a long labor with many "trials and tribulations," said that her 5-hour labor was really "boring." For other coaches, especially those who assist in a long or difficult labor, the job can be very tiring. Christina and Michelle made sure they had enough support by arranging for two coaches. Michelle said, "My husband gave me emotional support, and my labor coach helped me to relax between contractions, which was especially important." Christina said her second coach helped her husband to be more effective because "my husband was anxious and my friend had had a baby and knew what to expect." Coaches can give each other rest room and snack breaks, or work together in helping a severely disabled woman change positions.

Stage I

The coping methods commonly suggested for the early phase in particular are eating, enemas, and mild exercise.

Eating

The advantage of eating lightly during early labor is that food may help to keep up the mother's strength if the labor is long. However, if surgery and general anesthesia become necessary later in labor, the mother is at risk for coughing up and choking on any food remaining in her stomach. If the mother wants to eat, she should get the doctor's permission, and then eat *lightly*—something like gelatin, broth, or apple juice.

Enemas

In the past, laboring women were automatically given enemas when they entered the hospital. This practice is now much less common. Medical experience has shown that fecal material in the bowel will not inhibit labor, and proper care eliminates any risk that the baby will get an infection from feces.

Some people feel that enemas speed up labor. Stacy said, "It really helped my labor progress. After the enema, I went from 2.5 to 7 cm really fast." But Stacy's labor might have speeded up anyway. In addition, medical evidence shows that, on average, women who have enemas labor just as long as women who do not have them. A better reason for having an enema is for comfort. An enema early in labor assures that a bowel movement will occur while it is still relatively comfortable. Also, many women feel more comfortable about pushing if they are not worried about fecal material coming out with each push. Women who have had problems with constipation may be concerned about having one last bowel movement before they give birth, because they may not have a bowel movement for a couple of days afterwards. Women who are concerned about constipation can ask if their doctor thinks it is advisable to have a prepackaged Fleet enema ready to use at home when labor begins.

Women who have problems with dysreflexia should *not* use an enema, since the pressure of the enema might cause an episode.

Mild Exercise

Standing up and walking around are also very helpful during early labor. Standing helps labor to progress because gravity helps to maintain the pressure of the amniotic sac (or the fetal head) on the cervix. Mild exercise can help keep up the mother's spirits, but she may want to stop and lean on her coach or a piece of furniture during contractions. Walking is also helpful in later phases, but as labor intensifies, many women will prefer standing still or sitting instead of walking around. Clara's husband reminded her, "I *knew* you were in labor when you started refusing to move at all." Michelle and Renee also felt it was unpleasant to try to walk while in labor. Carla, by contrast, usually does not like to walk, but said, "I needed to walk during labor." Marsha could not walk but, "standing was less painful. I stood up and held onto a chair. My husband stood either behind me or at my side for support. I sat down in the chair between contractions."

If labor slows down, medical staff will certainly encourage the mother to get up and walk around, so that gravity can make contractions more effective.

In every phase of labor the mother should be encouraged to go to the bathroom about once an hour. Then, instead of walking aimlessly, she has a specific place to go which is a short distance away. She can change position from standing, to sitting, to standing again. An empty bladder is more comfortable and less susceptible to injury. In addition, the mother's ability to urinate is an important sign that she is not becoming dehydrated.

Breathing Techniques

Labor breathing methods help a woman to relax in the early and active phases because they help her focus on slow, rhythmical movement. Continuous rhythmical breathing gives her a sense of continuity between the times when the uterus is contracted and when it is relaxed. Cheryl said proper breathing was "the most important technique" she used to stay relaxed. Julie, who had not taken childbirth classes and was taught how to breathe by her nurses, still found that these methods made her "successful in handling contractions."

The two most useful breathing techniques for Stage I labor are *deep chest breathing* and *"ah-hee" breathing*. Some women begin with deep chest breathing, and change to "ah-hee" as labor sensations intensify. Others are more comfortable using one technique throughout Stage I.

For most women, the most useful technique for the early phase is slow, deep breathing, called deep chest breathing by some birth educators and abdominal breathing by others. The mother inhales slowly through her nose, and exhales slowly through her mouth. She breathes so deeply that her abdomen and ribs visibly expand when she inhales.

Deep chest breathing is combined with the *cleansing breath,* an especially deep in-and-out breath with which the mother begins and ends each contraction. The cleansing breath is useful for a number of reasons. The extra-deep breath gives the mother a boost of extra oxygen. Early in labor, when a regular rhythm of contractions is just starting, the mother can take a cleansing breath to signal to the coach that a contraction is beginning or ending. Later, when contractions are occurring more regularly, the coach can tell the mother to take a cleansing breath when the contraction is about to begin. That is better than telling her, "Your contraction is about to start," which may cause her to tense up. Reminding her to take a cleansing breath helps her to do what she must do to stay relaxed.

An alternative to deep chest breathing is *vocalization*. With this variant, the mother takes a deep breath, then breathes out with a slow, deep groan. For many women, the sound provides an auditory focal point, especially when other people in the room join in vocalizing (the effect is somewhat like the chanting heard during some religious ceremonies). Others simply find vocalizing more comfortable than other ways of pushing, like Stephanie, who said, "Groaning got me down more."

Another alternative to deep chest breathing is a somewhat shallower breathing which some birthing instructors call *ah-hee breathing*. Because this breathing is somewhat more rapid and shallow, the mother needs to concentrate to keep from breathing increasingly faster, and more shallowly. A good way to stay in control is to whisper "ahhhhh" while inhaling, and "heeeee" while exhaling. Another way to avoid hyperventilating during ah-hee breathing is to pause for one count between the "ah" and the "hee." The coach may have to remind the mother to slow down, especially if she starts feeling dizzy or nauseated, or if her hands and feet tingle (symptoms of hyperventilation). If the mother hyperventilates, she can breathe into a PAPER BAG until her symptoms disappear. Although this type of breathing requires concentration, many women prefer it. Faith said, "I had a hard time relaxing in my first labor and I couldn't deal with deep breathing." However, Faith preferred deep breathing during her second labor. Priscilla said she found "slow breathing helpful" early in labor, and "ah hee at the end also helpful." Ah-hee was the only method Clara liked. She explained, "I find it difficult to relax. I found it difficult to take a deep breath. I found ah-hee took all my attention, which I liked because I was able to focus on the breathing instead of the pain or the effort to relax."

For women whose spinal cord injuries are high enough to make deep breathing difficult, ah-hee breathing may be a useful alternative. If the labor nurse is worried because this shallower breathing seems to be happening too early in labor, the coach can explain that it is an adaptation to disability.

Relaxation Methods

Some women will start using relaxation techniques during early labor, especially if it is prolonged, yet still more women start using relaxation methods by the time they are in the active phase. Most of these methods involve either physical relaxation or visualization.

A Comfortable Position One of the best ways to help keep muscles relaxed is very simple—finding a comfortable position. A number of positions may be useful during labor. It is best to change position approximately every 45 minutes, both to maintain comfort and to help labor progress. Women can try the following positions:

- Standing
- Kneeling

- Getting on hands and knees
- Sitting upright
- Sitting partly reclined (back at a 45° angle to bed)
- Side-lying

Sitting and standing may help labor progress by taking advantage of gravity. Women who are more comfortable lying down need to remember to lie on their left sides. This assures that the uterus does not press on major blood vessels, interfering with the oxygen supply to the baby. Side-lying will be more comfortable with the legs bent, the top (right) leg slightly forward, and a pillow between the legs or under the right knee.

Sitting, reclining, and side-lying are especially useful for women with disabilities. Women who have difficulty changing positions should consider practicing with attendants or coaches beforehand so that when they are in labor, position changes can be made smoothly during the breaks between contractions. Samantha recalled, "I had my best friend and husband help me change positions. They helped me to sit up and to turn onto my side." Sharon can usually turn onto her side by herself, but she felt she "needed to be careful because of the epidural catheter that was placed in my back in case I got dysreflexia" (to administer medication), so she got help for turning onto her side. Heather needed help because the IV in her arm (explained below) made it difficult to change position.

For some women, an ordinary hospital bed was helpful. Stacy grasped the hand rails to help herself turn. Using the controls of the bed, a woman can get into a comfortable seated position, or move to a reclined position as a first step toward a side-lying position. Heather mentioned that her most comfortable position—reclining—was still more comfortable with a pillow under her amputated leg.

When Faith had her third child, she labored sitting in her wheelchair. She explained, "My husband was sick and he couldn't help me transfer, so it was easier to just stay in my chair till I went to the delivery room. When they needed to do an exam, I just went over to a bed and somebody propped my legs up on the side of the bed."

When a woman is resting in a comfortable position, she can use specific methods of muscle relaxation. Again, it helps to practice these methods before labor begins. When practicing, the mother should try relaxing in different positions that she might use during labor. Some people recommend practicing as much as 20 minutes daily to develop real skill in relaxation. Michelle "had a special coach who I had practiced with. She would find where I was tense and help me get that part of my body relaxed."

Progressive Relaxation One method of learning to relax is known as progressive relaxation. In this method, the pregnant woman practices relaxing as a response to muscle tension. She practices by first tensing, then relaxing, one part of the body (for example, her right arm), then progressing to another, until her whole body is relaxed. This can be done alone or with the help of a coach. One should not tense the limb strongly, just slightly enough to increase awareness of those muscles and make it easier to consciously relax. Some disabled women, especially those with cerebral palsy, may find this technique too difficult. For some, it is simply impossible; once the limb is tense, it takes so much energy and concentration to relax that another relaxation method is obviously better. For others, tensing one limb will cause the other limbs to become tense and possibly spasm.

Touch Relaxation Another relaxation technique is touch relaxation, in which the coach uses touch rather than words to communicate with the mother. The coach's touch calls the mother's attention to a part of the body she needs to relax. The coach can touch an area that looks tense, such as the shoulders, or, as with progressive relaxation, move slowly and systematically from one part of the body to another. Moving slowly is important for this technique to be effective. The coach's hands must be *warm,* since a touch from a cold hand is likely to startle the mother and make her tense her muscles. The appropriate touch is light; the coach simply rests a hand gently on, for example, the woman's arm, until s/he sees or feels the tense muscles relax. This method will probably work better if it has been practiced beforehand, so that it has become a habit for the woman to relax at her coach's touch. Still, some women, like Jennifer, Renee, and Michelle, simply do not like to be touched during labor, and would not like this method. For some women, a light touch is unpleasant but firm massage is enjoyable. For others, touch relaxation is wonderful. Hilary's disability made it very difficult for her to be given a spinal injection. Her husband's verbal suggestion and gentle touch helped her to relax, and she takes pleasure in recalling his touch on her forehead and neck.

Effleurage is a variety of touch relaxation in which the abdomen is gently patted in circular fashion. For some women, effleurage helps by bringing their attention to the surface of the body, away from their contractions. A woman can use effleurage on herself. Few of the women interviewed for this book tried effleurage; none liked it. Renee explained, "It was very distracting." Yet many of Judi's students have found effleurage very helpful. It is certainly worth trying.

Autogenic Training Another relaxation method is *autogenic training.* With this method, a woman tells herself, or her coach tells her, to think of her body, or a part of her body, as feeling warm and heavy. Or, the suggestion may be, "Your arm is very light, it's floating." Either suggestion can help a woman to feel more relaxed. Sometimes this method works well in combination with touch relaxation.

Visualization Techniques   Visualization techniques differ from other relaxation methods in that they concentrate the woman's attention on something outside of herself. One such technique is use of a *FOCAL POINT*. A focal point is anything a woman can focus her eyes on as an aid to concentration. Some people like to use a picture that helps them think of their labor in a positive way, such as a picture of a dilated cervix or a baby. Some women are very choosy about the focal point. Faith brought along two pictures and when she did not like one, she had her coach take it down and hang up the other. For other women, any focal point will do. Stacy said simply, "concentrating on an object helped," and Marsha said, "I stared at the wallpaper." Clara invented a focal point on the spot during her second labor—"I suddenly remembered watching my LaMaze teacher moving her finger back and forth like a pendulum during breathing exercises. I started moving my finger the same way. Watching it helped me control my breathing even though my labor was so intense."

Judi has noticed that many women hold their husbands' hands during labor, and one partner is always squeezing. The hand-holding may be working as touch relaxation, or as a kind of tactile focal point.

Using a focal point does not always help. Renee commented, "In my first labor, focusing on the baby was helpful, but during the second labor I was in too much pain to focus." Faith, who had used two focal points in her first labor, found during her second labor that she needed to concentrate on herself rather than an outside object. The best plan is to pack an emotionally satisfying object in the labor kit, and to be flexible about whether to use it.

Visualization uses imagery to assist relaxation. Imagining a relaxing situation can help a person to relax. For example, a woman can imagine that she is at the beach, resting on soft sand, feeling the sun's gentle warmth on her skin as her limbs grow heavier. A woman can privately imagine such images, or her coach can verbally paint a word picture, talking softly and slowly.

An alternative that some women enjoy is using images of effective labor. For example, her coach can tell her, "Your contractions are working on your cervix. Your cervix is opening wider and wider, like a rose blooming."

If she wishes, a woman can try playing a recording of a relaxation *TAPE*.

Hypnosis   Hypnosis and self-hypnosis are similar to visualization, with imagery or a focal point used to achieve a trance state. Hypnosis does not work for everyone, but when it does work, it can effectively help a laboring woman stay relaxed and in control. Hypnosis is a skill that must be taught by a trained professional. Sometimes the professional will help in preparing a *TAPE RECORDING* that can be used during labor. Clara said, "I never could do self-hypnosis. It's much more successful when my husband hypnotizes me. We had several sessions with a professional who taught us how....My first labor was very long. After 24 hours I felt very discouraged and I was losing control. My husband was able to calm me down. He was able to hypnotize me and I stayed in control for the rest of the labor and delivery—another 8 hours!"

Music *MUSIC* can also help a laboring woman to relax. Faith made a point of saying, "It really promoted relaxation during my second labor." Music may help in more than one way. Rhythmical music may help a woman to control her breathing; music can serve as a focal point; music can create positive feelings in a way similar to visual imagery. Some studies have shown that women who listened to soft music while they were laboring, seemed better able to relax and feel positive about their labor afterwards. An added advantage is that quiet music may also help birth attendants to relax. It could be useful to play soft music while practicing relaxation before labor, and then bring the same music in the labor kit. Some women like to use *HEADPHONES* to screen out distracting noises, but others feel too isolated when they use headphones.

Massage and Acupressure When using massage and acupressure, the coach works more actively to help the laboring woman. In massage, the coach gently but firmly kneads the tense area. Good places to massage are the feet, hands, neck, shoulders, and back. The neck and shoulders are especially important, since many people tense these areas when under stress. Massage can also help with muscle cramps. When using massage with a disabled woman, the rule is, "Go for the cramp."

The person giving the massage should have warm hands, and should be alert to the woman's feedback as to whether the massage is too firm, too gentle, or just right. Massage can be given more gently as the tense area relaxes.

The coach can use massage aids from the labor kit. *POWDER* or *CORNSTARCH* can be used to reduce friction. (Talcum powder is less likely to cake on contact with body moisture. Cornstarch will cake, but some people prefer it because it has no odor.) Some people prefer the dry, silky feeling of powders, others like the gliding feeling of a massage lubricated with *MASSAGE OIL* or *HAND LOTION*. Oil or lotion will soothe dry skin, too. If the coach's hands are getting tired, or s/he is disabled, a *MECHANICAL MASSAGE AID* such as a vibrator, rolling pin, or a "bonger" can be helpful. (A "bonger" is a hollow rubber ball on a flexible metal blade set into a wooden handle. The coach gently taps—"bongs"—the tense area with the ball.) Do not rely only on a vibrator, because the buzzing sound may annoy the mother.

To help with thigh muscle cramps, which often occur during transition, squeeze the front of the thigh with both hands. To help with calf cramps, place the hands just below the knee, one on each side of the leg, and apply pressure. Another way to relieve a calf cramp is to bend the foot upward at the ankle, keeping the leg straight, and hold it until the cramp is gone (see Figure 7.1). Do not massage the cramping calf muscle, or it will feel sore for a while after the cramp is relieved.

Some women get more relief from acupressure than from massage. Our descriptions of pressure points are approximate. The coach will need to try several spots in a small area, continuing to press one spot when the woman says, "That's it!" First try going slowly down the spine, pressing with the thumbs about one inch to each side of each vertebra (the little bumps of the spine). This works well with the woman lying on her side, or sitting in front of the coach. Next, the coach can find the point that relieves tension in the neck and shoulders. The point is on the back of the neck, between the shoulders. The woman can lean her head slightly forward, resting her forehead on the coach's hand for stability, while s/he gently presses the thumb of one hand and the first finger of the other hand on different points up and down the neck until the right spot is found. Other pressure points are in front. Gently press along both sides of the hairline and the soft areas near the temples, working from the center of the forehead around to the back of the head and down toward the collarbones. Finally, a technique which may relieve pain during active labor and transition involves placing the fingers firmly on top of the head, with the thumb on the bridge of the nose, then gently pressing with the thumb. These techniques can also reduce pain and promote relaxation when practiced during pregnancy.

Warm Showers or Baths Warm showers or baths can also aid in relaxation. Water baths for labor have been used in Russia, France, and England. There has been concern that laboring in water increases the risk of infection, but studies in France have not shown any connection between water labor and infections. In the United States, practices differ widely. In some hospitals, whirlpool baths are being installed in labor suites, while in others, the nurse has to get a doctor's permission to let a laboring woman take a shower.

A warm water bath may help a woman relax partly by dilating surface blood vessels and increasing blood flow to muscles. Also, women seem to feel that contractions are less painful when they labor in warm water, perhaps because they feel relaxed. Those who favor laboring in water theorize that contractions which are less painful will be more efficient. Some midwives feel that women who labor in water have shorter labors, while others feel that a warm bath or shower simply makes labor more comfortable. A warm shower helps to relieve the discomfort of back labor. The shower works best when the water flows directly onto the lower back.

Only two of the women interviewed tried using warm showers. Clara was enthusiastic: "I found the shower incredibly relaxing. It really helped. I'll never forget how good it felt." Michelle disliked the shower because walking and standing were too uncomfortable for her. She might have been more comfortable with a chair in the shower, which some hospitals will provide.

Laboring in a warm bath could have additional advantages for women with disabilities. Warm baths relieve muscle spasms, and women who are having problems with spasms may be helped by moving to a tub. Laboring in a bath can help women with arthritis avoid excess stress on their joints. Women who are paralyzed will not have to change position as often. For some women, transferring to and from a slippery shower or tub may be too complicated or even risky. To use a bath safely, the woman must be able to sit independently or she could slip under the water.

Methods for Relieving Symptoms

Back Labor or Backache Whether a woman has true back labor, in which the pain is caused by the pressure of the fetal head against the spinal nerves, or simple muscle pain, the following techniques can be helpful.

The coach can place his or her thumbs in each of the dimples on either side of the lower back, just above the buttocks, and press firmly and steadily. If the pressure is helping, the mother will say so. The only disadvantage of this method is that the coach's hands and arms may get tired.

Some women are helped by constant pressure on the lower back. The coach can rest his/her palms on the back, and lean gently. Or, the coach can press a sock stuffed with two *TENNIS BALLS* against the mother's back. When the coach gets tired, try having the mother sit in a chair, place a *ROLLING PIN* or a soft drink can against the chair, and have the mother lean back so that the rolling pin presses against her back.

Some people like to use a hollow, plastic rolling pin filled with water. Some prefer the relaxing effect of hot water, while others, including women with MS, usually prefer the numbing effect of cold water.

The coach can also give firm massage, possibly using a *VIBRATOR* or a *BONGER.*

Sometimes a change of position relieves back pain. Renee got on all fours with her knees on a beanbag and her head on a pillow, so that her buttocks were higher than her head. She said this position "eased the pressure." During her first labor, Priscilla used a position between kneeling and being on all fours. Her knees were supported by a beanbag and she faced the bed and held onto the rail. She said, "When I got into this position, the baby was sunny-side-up" (the face, rather than the back of the head, was toward the front of Priscilla's body) "but getting in that position helped the baby to turn, and that relieved the back labor." The change of position undoubtedly eased delivery as well. Women who cannot kneel or get on their hands and knees can try lying curled up (lie on the *left* side, not the right). Either of these positions makes it easy for the coach to apply lower back pressure.

Dry Mouth or Thirst Labor breathing is mouth breathing, so a mother may easily get a dry mouth or chapped lips. Use *CHAPSTICK* from the labor kit to soothe chapped lips. For a dry, cottony feeling in the mouth, use

BREATH SPRAY, or give the mother a *SOUR LOLLIPOP* or ice chips to suck—whichever she prefers. (It is important to have a lollipop rather than a loose piece of candy, which might cause choking if the mother gasps at the beginning of a contraction.) Of course, ice chips are best for thirst.

Nausea Nausea is most likely to occur during transition, but some women become nauseated at the end of a long early phase. Ice chips are often helpful. Sylvia said, "The ice chips helped so much they kept a tray nearby so I could get them easily." Faith found that ice chips helped, and having her face wiped with a cool, damp *WASHCLOTH* also felt good. Some women will vomit, so a basin should be kept nearby (the hospital will provide one).

Muscle Cramps Muscle cramps are most likely to happen during transition. Besides massaging the cramped muscle, the coach can try holding and bracing the leg. Bracing is especially useful for the very severe cramps and/or spasms some disabled women experience. Cramping may be less likely if range of motion exercises are used throughout labor to help keep muscles loose. Christina had severe leg spasms during transition and her three coaches took turns helping her. One coach would hold each leg while the third coach rested. Clara's worst spasms occurred during Stage II. They were so strong that her second coach could not hold her leg, but her husband managed by bracing Clara's foot against his chest and using both hands to turn it outward (see Figure 7.1).

Faith found a very original way to relieve muscle spasms. During one of her labors, she spent part of her time kneeling against a beanbag. She said, "Leaning against the beanbag was very comfortable. Then I started having spasms—my legs jumped with every contraction. We spread a sleeping bag on the floor and I got on all fours on the sleeping bag. The pressure on my knees stopped the spasms." Faith's method might not work for all women, but is worth trying if other methods of relieving spasms have not worked.

Hot and Cold Flashes Flashes are most likely to happen during transition. If a woman is cold, cover her with a light blanket. Sometimes a laboring woman's feet are especially cold, so *WARM SOCKS* come in handy. If she is hot, wipe her face and body with a damp *WASHCLOTH* to cool her.

Sleepiness Sleepiness is most likely to happen during transition. Labor coaches used to be taught not to let a laboring woman sleep, in case she would feel disoriented and panicky when awakened by contractions. Now the trend is to let a woman doze because the rest may refresh her.

Anxiety Sometimes a woman expresses her fear directly, and sometimes her inability to follow directions will be a sign that she is feeling afraid or

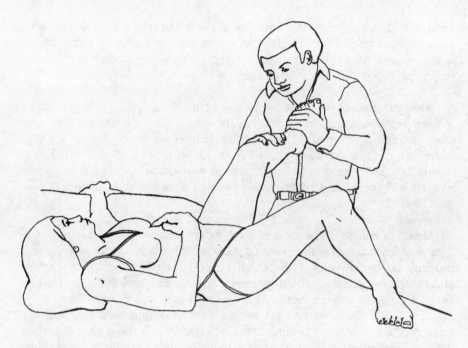

FIGURE 7.1. Birth position in which a spasming leg is being supported.

out of control. These feelings are more common during transition. Wait until a contraction ends before helping her calm down. Some women are helped by a simple remark like, "You'll be able to push soon," or, "You're in transition now and you'll feel better soon." It also helps to concentrate on just *one* contraction at a time. Tell her that breathing will help her feel better, and help her to breathe rhythmically by giving her instructions or breathing with her. As she gains a sense of control by controlling her breathing, she really will feel better!

Urge to Push Often a woman will start to feel like pushing during transition, but must avoid pushing while she waits for the cervix to dilate completely. Also, a woman may need to stop pushing briefly during Stage II, for example, to slow the descent of the baby and give the perineum time to stretch. A woman can avoid pushing by blowing out short puffs of air during contractions. Michelle said, "It was like blowing out a candle." It is impossible to bear down while blowing. (Some readers may like to pause and try it!) If the urge to push becomes irresistible and the mother stops blowing and starts pushing again, the coach can try leaning closely and blowing in her face. Just as breathing in rhythm with the mother helps with deep chest breathing, blowing in her face may remind her to blow. For some women, the coach's closeness is a signal that, "I won't leave you alone until you do what you need to do." Clara recalled, "I knew the only way my husband would get out of my space was for me to start blowing."

Stage II

Methods for coping during Stage II consist of finding a comfortable position and using appropriate breathing techniques.

Finding a Comfortable Position

Sitting with the back supported, squatting, and getting on the hands and knees can all be useful during this stage. Sometimes a woman will be encouraged to sit on a toilet to push. This method is very useful when the baby gets stuck at the +2 station, which can happen when the baby's head is large in comparison to the pelvic opening. When the woman sits on the toilet, gravity helps her with pushing. Also, pushing out a baby feels much like having a bowel movement, and sitting on the toilet often makes the pushing feel more familiar and comfortable.

Once the baby is at the +3 station (head in the vagina), a woman can try any of several positions while she pushes the baby to +5 (crowning), and then gives birth. She may try squatting, lying on her side with her upper leg in the air, sitting partially reclined (her back at a 45° angle) with her legs supported by stirrups or held out to the side, seated in a birthing chair, or lying on her back on a delivery table, with her legs raised, spread, and supported by stirrups. Some women lie on the delivery table while resting between contractions, then sit up with the coach's help while pushing.

There are advantages and disadvantages to using a delivery table. Some women feel restricted by the stirrups, others appreciate the help in keeping their legs supported and separated. Because lying on the back is not a good position for laboring, women may not be taken to the delivery table until the baby is crowning. However, moving then is a nuisance, especially for women with mobility problems. Some hospitals have modified delivery tables, with moveable handles. When the woman pushes, she presses down on the handles, partially sitting up. Pushing in this way may be more effective. Other hospitals provide birthing chairs, which offer the advantages of sitting up during labor, and supporting the woman comfortably with her legs well spread. Delivery tables and birthing chairs are more comfortable for birth attendants than the ordinary beds available at home births and alternative birth centers. When a woman is laboring or pushing in an ordinary bed, her attendants are likely to get backaches or sore knees from bending or kneeling, though they may be more comfortable if they sit on the bed with her.

A woman's disability will influence her choice of position. Squatting is not feasible for many disabled women—some will be unable to balance, while others must avoid the stress on their joints. Using a birthing chair may help a woman use a position similar to a squat, and sitting on a toilet also has many of the advantages of squatting.

For many disabled women, side-lying or partially reclined positions work well. These women may also need help holding up their legs. Heather, who did not deliver vaginally, still needed a nurse to hold her stump during a pelvic examination. Sheila "preferred someone holding my leg. It was more comfortable." Christina used a delivery table, but could not use the stirrups because she cannot bend her knees. Instead, two nurses helped, each one holding one of Christina's legs out to the side. Sharon used the stirrups part of the time, and had her legs held by nurses part of the time. Other women found the delivery table and stirrups helpful or even comfortable. Women who got leg spasms from using stirrups during prenatal examinations probably should avoid using them during labor.

Samantha, who gave birth at home, sat more comfortably when her husband was behind her and she could lean on him for support. She held her thighs and someone else supported her lower legs.

Celeste chose a side-lying position because she has difficulty spreading her legs. When she lay on her side, a nurse held up her top leg and the delivery went well (Figure 7.2).

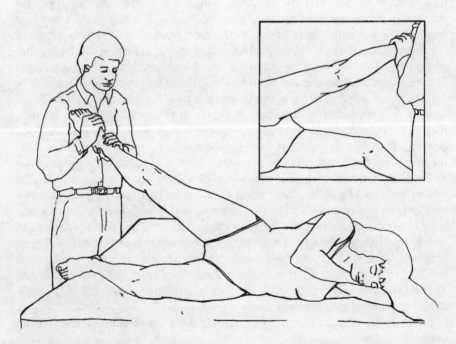

FIGURE 7.2. Side-lying birth position for women who cannot use stirrups or spread legs widely.

Breathing Techniques

Two kinds of breathing may be used during Stage II: the Valsalva maneuver and gentle pushing. The two methods begin in the same way: One breathes in deeply through the nose, then breathes out through the mouth, then breathes in through the nose and holds her breath.

For the Valsalva maneuver, the mother continues to hold her breath while bearing down. The mother feels her throat close, and is then able to create maximum air pressure on the uterus.

For gentle pushing, the mother slowly lets out a little air as she bears down. The sensation of letting out just a little air is like talking while holding the breath. The woman may quietly say "eeeeeeee" as she pushes down (she will feel pressure in her throat as she pushes out the sound).

Some birth professionals favor gentle pushing because they worry that doing the Valsalva maneuver may increase the rise in blood pressure that occurs during contractions, while others do not believe there is a problem. A woman may practice one type of pushing in birthing class, then be shown another by her labor nurse. She may prefer the method the nurse shows her. If not, her coach can explain, "She's comfortable with the way she's pushing now because that is the way she practiced in birthing class."

Sometimes it is necessary to stop pushing during Stage II. If a woman can avoid pushing during a few contractions, her perineum can stretch more slowly and she may be able to avoid an episiotomy. Or, if the umbilical cord has wrapped around the baby's neck, the mother may need to stop pushing while the doctor or midwife slips the loop of cord over the baby's head, or suctions mucus from the baby's mouth and nose. If the mother needs to stop pushing, she can "blow through" the contraction in the same way she did during transition. For some women, contractions will come very close together. For others, there will be time to rest between contractions. They may use deep chest breathing while resting.

COMPLICATIONS OF LABOR

. . . .

Complications of labor are variations from the normal course of labor which threaten the well-being of the mother or the fetus. The rarest complications are not described here.

Pre-eclampsia

This pregnancy complication was explained in the previous chapter. Pre-eclampsia may be characterized by extremely high blood pressure, which is dangerous to both mother and fetus. In addition, it can progress to eclampsia during labor, and the mother may experience convulsions, possibly leading to coma. Besides treatment with medications to lower blood pressure, and other emergency measures, surgical delivery may also be necessary.

Prolongation or Arrest of Labor

Insufficient Contractions

One cause of prolongation or arrest of labor is weak or uncoordinated uterine contractions. It is not always possible to determine the cause of insufficient contractions. Sometimes excessive or poorly timed doses of pain medication weaken contractions. A rigid cervix may also cause prolonged labor, since uterine contractions cannot dilate the cervix if appropriate changes in the cervical tissue have not occurred. If the cervix is not rigid, then contractions may be stimulated by induction or augmentation, as described below in the section on "Medical Procedures."

Fetopelvic Disproportion

Labor will also be prolonged if the size or shape of the pelvic girdle does not allow the fetus to pass through. This condition is known as fetopelvic disproportion. The problem may arise from the mother's individual anatomy, the presentation or position of the fetus, or the size of the fetus. The most favorable (and most common) fetal presentation is the *occiput anterior* (crown of the head first, fetus facing the mother's spine). Other presentations include *posterior presentation* (fetus facing front of mother's body), *brow presentation* (forehead first), and *breech presentations* (other parts of the body first, most commonly buttocks). Abnormal presentation is a problem because the presenting part of the fetus does not fit well into the pelvic outlet.

Scoliosis or congenital hip or pelvic deformities can cause fetopelvic disproportion. Dangers of this complication are maternal exhaustion, uterine injury, or fetal distress (defined below).

Placenta Previa and Premature Placental Separation

The placenta is normally attached to the uterine wall in the upper part of the uterus. In fewer than one half of one percent of pregnancies, the placenta implants low in the uterus, with part of it over the cervix. *Placenta previa* may block the descent of the fetus, or the placenta may begin to tear away from the uterine wall as the cervix dilates. If the placenta separates from the uterine wall, maternal blood loss and fetal hypoxia (lack of oxygen) and distress can be problems. Sometimes, bleeding without pain is the first sign of placenta previa. Surgical delivery may be necessary if the placenta covers more than 30% of the fully dilated cervix. If placenta previa is less extreme, there may be a trial labor, during which the fetus is monitored and preparations are made to treat hypoxia and blood loss.

Premature placental separation, which is also called *placental abruption* or *abruptio placentae,* is a separation of the placenta from the uterine wall before the fetus is delivered. If blood does not escape through the cervix, then severe pain or fetal distress may be the first signs of placental separation.

Umbilical Cord Compression

Multiple pregnancy, fetopelvic disproportion, displacement of the umbilical cord by premature rupture of membranes, and other conditions may lead to compression of the umbilical cord between the fetus and the uterine wall. If, as usually happens, compression of the cord is brief and intermittent, there may be no harm to the fetus, but prolonged or continuous compression may cause hypoxia and distress. Fetal distress is often the first sign of cord displacement and compression.

Fetal Distress

Labor is always somewhat stressful to the fetus. However, the fetus is usually well able to tolerate some stress, reacting with moderate changes of heart rate. During contractions, the uterine muscles squeeze the blood vessels supplying the placenta, reducing the flow of oxygen to the fetus. Interference with the oxygen supply leads to hypoxia—a lack of oxygen. Prolonged or extreme hypoxia can cause brain damage or even death. The fetus is also stressed by the pressure of uterine contractions on its body, and pressure on its skull as contractions press the head against the cervix, then the vaginal wall, and then the perineum.

When severe stress occurs, it can become distress. One symptom of distress is extreme change in heart rate (the heart may beat either more quickly or more slowly). Change in fetal heart rate can be diagnosed by auscultation (listening with a stethoscope) or electronic monitoring. Scalp blood sampling can differentiate between stress and distress if there is any question about the accuracy of diagnosis by monitoring. These procedures are discussed below in "Medical Procedures."

Other signs of fetal distress are extreme fetal activity and meconium staining of the amniotic fluid. Meconium is a tarry material, somewhat like feces, in the fetus' digestive tract. Passage of meconium is reason for concern because it is a sign of hypoxia. Also, the fetus may aspirate meconium, which is harmful.

Treatment of fetal distress can range from simply having the mother breathe oxygen, to emergency surgical delivery.

MEDICAL PROCEDURES
. . . .

In the section entitled "Methods for Coping with Labor Discomforts," we described simple, practical ways a woman or her birth attendant(s) can relieve the discomforts of labor. Other procedures can be performed by medical staff, although many of them cannot be done without a doctor's instructions. These procedures are considered below in four categories: general care of the mother, including routine diagnostic procedures; special diagnostic procedures; interventions that affect the course of labor; and pain relief.

Some of these procedures are routine, while others are used for specific reasons and have advantages and disadvantages which will be explained.

General Care

Enemas
In some hospitals, a laboring woman may be offered an enema shortly after admission. Advantages and disadvantages of enemas were discussed in the section on coping with Stage I labor.

"Prepping"
The entire genital and anal region is washed, and in some hospitals, the genital hair is clipped short or shaved. (If only the hair in the perineal area is removed, the procedure is called a mini-prep.) The washing may help to prevent infection, by removing germs that could be introduced into the vagina during a manual examination. Later, if an episiotomy becomes necessary, or if the perineum tears, it will be easier to keep the area clean and comfortable if the hair is short. While shaving removes hair more completely, it is more uncomfortable if the skin is nicked, and it becomes itchy when hair grows back. Also, a nick could in itself lead to infection. Many women prefer to clip their own hair at home a few days before the due date, to avoid the discomfort of having this done during labor.

Introduction of an Intravenous Line
An intravenous line is a very fine plastic tube inserted into a vein in the hand or, less commonly, the arm. The IV may be used to introduce medications, as we discuss below. In many hospitals, and in alternative birth centers, IVs are only used for specific reasons, not as a matter of routine.

Some women with disabilities must have an IV because they need to receive medications continuously, and labor interferes with the absorption of oral medications. For example, women who have myasthenia gravis must have an IV in place during labor.

In general care, the IV would be used to give the mother nutrient and/or electrolyte solutions to maintain her strength and comfort. (The nutrient is dextrose, a type of sugar, and electrolytes are salts. Either is dissolved in sterile water.)

If a woman has been vomiting, an IV may be the best way to give her fluid and nutrients, since she may need to replace fluids lost from vomiting. Or, a woman who has been laboring a long time without eating or drinking may need an IV to replace fluids and electrolytes and to help her feel stronger. Women in these circumstances may welcome an IV despite the disadvantages.

Sometimes it is suggested that an IV should be inserted in order to be prepared for giving medications or replacing fluids lost through sudden, unanticipated bleeding. However, it is reasonable to delay starting an IV until medications are needed.

An IV has a disadvantage because it reduces a woman's mobility. The plastic tube is attached to a bottle or bag hanging from a tall pole. Even though the tube is taped against the skin so it cannot be dislodged easily, the woman is somewhat more restricted in her movements. For example, if she wants to turn onto her side, or lie down from sitting, she must do so without lying down on the IV line. Also, if she wants to get up and move around or go to the bathroom, she or her coach will have to push the pole along.

While the inconvenience of an IV may be minor for able-bodied women, it is more of a problem for women with disabilities. Clara, who has hemiparesis, commented, "I'm really glad I didn't need an IV when I was in labor. Whenever I have surgery, they have to put the IV in my unaffected hand, because it's too hard to get a good vein on the other side. Then it's really hard for me to change position." Heather, who did have an IV during labor, said, "It was difficult to move. I was off balance." A woman who uses a wheelchair will need to avoid the IV line while transferring. Many women with disabilities are likely to be much more comfortable if they are not routinely given an IV.

Although the sensation from an IV is hardly noticeable, some women are bothered by having one more thing that distracts them from coping with labor sensations.

Some people are concerned that a laboring woman who has an IV may be given medication without her knowledge. This concern is resolved by good communication. The doctor or nurse can tell the mother what solutions are in the IV bag, or the mother or her coach can ask or look at the label.

Catheterization

If a woman has difficulty urinating, and if her bladder is becoming too full, a fine plastic tube (catheter) may be inserted into the urethra (which leads from her bladder to the outside of the body). This tube is inserted so urine may be removed. Any discomfort involved is balanced by the reduction in discomfort from an over-full bladder. An over-full bladder may interfere with descent of the fetus, or it can be injured when it is compressed by the descending fetus.

In some situations, it is best to insert a catheter without waiting for the bladder to fill. Some physicians recommend routinely catheterizing laboring women who have spinal cord injuries above the T6 level to prevent dysreflexia.

Routine Diagnostic Procedures

At regular intervals, the midwife, nurse, or doctor checks the mother's pulse and blood pressure. They may palpate her abdomen at times, to determine the position and presentation of the fetus. A stethoscope may be placed against the mother's abdomen to check fetal heart rate. Occasionally, the mother is examined internally. In the early phase, this examination is done to determine effacement and dilation of the cervix. In the active phase, it is done to assess the descent of the fetus. Sometimes, the internal examination must be done during a contraction; then the contraction will be more uncomfortable. The coach must be especially attentive and supportive at the time. To avoid causing infection, internal examinations are kept to a minimum, especially after the amniotic membrane has ruptured. The mother's temperature may be taken if she has symptoms of fever, or if much time has elapsed since her membranes ruptured.

Special Diagnostic Procedures

External Monitoring

External monitoring measures the fetal heart rate (FHR) and the frequency and duration of uterine contractions. Various patterns of FHR give information about how the fetus is affected by the stress of labor. Changes in the frequency and duration of contractions provide information about how well the uterus is functioning.

External monitoring may be done for a variety of reasons. When a woman arrives at the hospital, she may be monitored for a short time to establish a "base line"—that is, to learn how her fetus normally responds to contractions. Then, if the monitor is used again later in labor, the pattern of FHR can be compared with the earlier pattern. Problems that arose during pregnancy, such as pre-eclampsia or twin pregnancy, are among the reasons why external monitoring may be started as soon as the mother arrives at the hospital. Sometimes external monitoring may be necessary during the course of labor. For example, monitoring may be necessary if labor is not progressing well, or if abnormal fetal heart tones were heard during a routine examination. Monitoring is also necessary when labor is induced or augmented (see below). External monitoring has the advantage of providing more information than the routine methods described above, and it is noninvasive.

Two measuring devices are held against the mother's abdomen by plastic belts. One device, the tocotransducer, is pressure sensitive and records uterine contractions. The other, an ultrasound transducer, senses and records fetal heartbeats. Since the resulting recording shows FHR in relation to the contraction pattern, it is useful in determining how well the fetus is tolerating labor.

Monitoring the rate of contractions gives useful information about the progress of the labor, although it is only partial information. Also, the external monitor can help the labor coach. Instead of continually checking a stopwatch, s/he can concentrate on the mother, only glancing at the recording occasionally to see if a contraction is about to begin. The mother may appreciate the help in knowing when a contraction will begin. On the other hand, some people find that the coach becomes fascinated by the monitor and neglects the mother!

If the monitor shows the FHR is abnormal, the doctor can consider other diagnostic procedures, or take steps to resolve the problem. When the recording shows that the baby is doing well, the reassurance may help the mother to relax and cope with labor contractions.

Sometimes the belts the mother must wear are uncomfortable and need adjustment. This discomfort, like any other, may cause difficulty in coping with labor. Another problem is that the mother must lie still, because sudden movements interfere with the recording of the FHR. Frequently, the mother is instructed to lie supine (on her back), since it may be possible to get better recordings in this position. However, the mother must change position occasionally, because lying supine can in itself cause problems. The weight of the uterus resting on major blood vessels can interfere with blood flow to the uterus, reducing the amount of oxygen available to the fetus and slowing its heart rate. In these situations, if the mother changes position to her left side, the FHR may return to normal. Disabled women who have spinal deformities that make it difficult or impossible to lie supine, may need a pillow or other support, or may need to use another position.

Patience and good communication can reduce the discomforts of external monitoring. The mother and medical staff can work out a schedule which permits her to adjust or remove the belts, move around, or change position from time to time. If shifts change while the mother is in labor, her coach or advocate may need to remind the new staff of whatever arrangements have been made. Medical staff will check the monitor frequently. If they are delayed, and the mother has moved or changed position while waiting, they should be told so they will know that some changes in the recording may have been caused by the mother's movements.

Some birth professionals and consumers have expressed concern that the increased use of fetal monitors may have contributed to the recent increase in the rate of cesarean surgery. They worry that inaccurate diagnosis of fetal distress has led to unnecessary surgery in some cases. Yet, in other cases, external monitoring has certainly led to a correct diagnosis that might not have been made otherwise. Also, there are other factors contributing to the increase in cesarean surgery. (We will discuss this issue in *Chapter 8*.) Generalized studies of the use and misuse of electronic monitoring cannot determine whether electronic monitoring is appropriate in a *particular* situation, or what to do if the monitoring seems to show a problem.

These concerns can be addressed one at a time. First, parents and medical staff can discuss whether electronic monitoring is appropriate. Electronic monitoring will not automatically lead to other medical procedures. The advantages of other procedures can be considered if and when they are suggested. If the need for monitoring was not discussed before labor began, the mother or her coach should not hesitate to ask medical staff any questions that come to mind. For example, why do they recommend it, or can it be discontinued or interrupted.

An external monitor should not be used with women who have spinal cord injuries at or above the T6 level, since the pressure of the belt could stimulate autonomic dysreflexia. Instead, they can be examined periodically with a Doppler device, or monitoring can be done internally.

Internal Monitoring

Internal monitoring consists of two procedures: measuring FHR, and measuring the strength of uterine contractions. To measure FHR, an electrode is inserted under the fetal scalp, then attached to recording equipment.

The device for measuring the strength of uterine contractions is an intrauterine pressure catheter, which is a tube filled with fluid that is threaded through the cervix. During uterine contractions, pressure on the amniotic fluid places pressure on the fluid in the tube, which is connected to a pressure sensor attached to a recording device. In dysfunctional labor, the pressure catheter may be used to measure the strength of uterine contractions. It may also be used when labor is induced or augmented. If uterine contractions are too strong, medication may be reduced or discontinued.

When an internal fetal monitor is used, the mother can move somewhat more freely than with an external monitor, since her movements will not affect the recording of the FHR. This method gives more accurate information than external monitoring. In addition, the intrauterine pressure catheter gives information that cannot be obtained any other way.

However, there are disadvantages to these procedures. There is a small risk that the fetal scalp will be injured or infected by the electrode. There is also a risk that the tip of the pressure catheter will injure the placenta, or that the electrode or catheter will introduce infections. However, these risks are small with good sterile technique and skillful procedure. Still, it is because of these risks that internal monitoring is often reserved for specific indications (see "Amniotomy" below).

Internal monitoring is only possible if the cervix is partly dilated and the amniotic membranes have ruptured. Otherwise, an amniotomy (artificial rupture of membranes) will have to be done. The advantages and disadvantages of amniotomy are discussed below.

Ultrasound

As we explained in the previous chapter, ultrasound is a method for obtaining images by bouncing sound waves off the object under study. During labor, ultrasound examination can be used to determine the location of the placenta and the baby's presentation. Such an examination helps to determine whether augmentation of labor is appropriate (see below).

Fetal Scalp Blood Sampling

Changes in FHR may leave doubt about whether or not the fetus is in distress. In these situations, a small sample of blood may be removed from the fetal scalp for analysis. The amount of oxygen and carbon dioxide in the blood, and its acidity or alkalinity, are measured. Sometimes these measurements are repeated.

By helping the physician to monitor the fetus more accurately, scalp blood sampling can help to assure that emergency procedures are performed only when necessary.

Amniotomy

Some medical texts suggest that amniotomy can be used in evaluating fetal well-being. If labor has been protracted, or FHR is abnormal, and membranes have not ruptured spontaneously, amniotomy may be done so that the amniotic fluid can be examined. Meconium stains in the amniotic fluid are a sign of fetal distress, while blood stains are a sign of premature placental separation, which is dangerous to both mother and fetus. In either case, the fetus may have to be delivered quickly, perhaps surgically.

As explained above, amniotomy may be done as preparation for internal monitoring. However, amniotomy can be dangerous if the fetal head is not well engaged. When the head is not engaged and the amniotic fluid escapes, the umbilical cord may slip down into the space between the fetal head and the pelvic opening. Then, with each contraction, the cord can be compressed between the head and the pelvic bones. This compression can interfere with fetal blood circulation.

There are disadvantages to amniotomy even when there is no risk of cord compression. The fluid-filled membrane no longer cushions the fetal head during contractions, so fetal or maternal tissues may be injured as the fetal head is driven harder against the cervix. For the same reason, amniotomy may increase the pain of contractions, although the incision is not painful in itself. Patricia told us, "I had an amniotomy because the doctor said it would hurry up labor, but it didn't improve the pain—in fact it got worse." (Patricia never said whether her labor progressed more quickly after the amniotomy. In her mind, the increased pain was most significant.) On the other hand, the amniotic membrane often ruptures spontaneously early in labor, without harm to the fetus or the mother. After the membrane ruptures, the fetal head can mold better, easing passage through the pelvic outlet.

The strongest argument against amniotomy is that it opens a pathway for infectious organisms to enter the uterine cavity. When the membranes have ruptured, naturally or artificially, the risk of infection increases after 24 hours. So, amniotomy starts a clock that cannot be turned back. On the other hand, if there is concern about fetal distress, it may be important to deliver the baby soon. A woman who is worried about amniotomy might ask her doctor, "Will the risk of infection mean that we can't let the labor go on as long as we would otherwise?" If the doctor believes that there is a limit to how long labor may continue—out of concern for either the fetus or the mother—the risk of infection is not the most important consideration.

The use of amniotomy to alter the progress of labor is discussed below.

Interventions in Labor

Amniotomy

Sometimes, amniotomy is performed in an attempt to shorten labor. However, studies have yielded variable results about its effectiveness, and authors of medical texts disagree. Amniotomy may speed up labor for some women, but cannot be relied on for this effect. However, if induction or augmentation of labor are already being considered, it may be worthwhile to try amniotomy. Even if it does not stimulate labor, it can serve as preparation for the internal monitoring that is necessary when labor is augmented. Again, the question to ask is whether amniotomy will shorten the time that labor may be allowed to continue.

Amniotomy worked well for Michelle, who had a dysfunctional labor. Because women with MS are very susceptible to fatigue, Michelle's obstetrician was worried that continued labor would lead to exhaustion and worsening of MS symptoms. After 2 1/2 days of labor, her doctor performed an amniotomy, and the baby was delivered 5 hours later.

Induction and Augmentation of Labor

Induction of labor is artificial stimulation of uterine contractions when labor has not begun spontaneously. Augmentation is stimulation of uterine contractions after labor has begun. It is used when contractions have started and then stopped, or when contractions are weak.

Labor may be induced to treat some pregnancy complications which were discussed in the previous chapter. Labor will also be induced if contractions do not begin soon enough after amniotic membranes have ruptured. In this instance, induction can be seen as a preventive measure, since surgical delivery may be considered if the baby is not born within 24 hours of membrane rupture. However, it has become routine practice at many institutions to allow labor to continue for up to 36 hours after rupture of membranes. As of this writing, medical researchers are seeking to develop means of predicting the likelihood that infection will develop after membrane rupture.

Labor must not be induced or augmented unless specific criteria are met. At least one indication for induction must be present (for example, fetal postmaturity), and there must be no contraindications (for example, breech presentation). In women with spinal cord injuries at or above T6, the longer, stronger contractions of induced labor seem to increase the risk of an episode of dysreflexia. The medical staff must be prepared to differentiate dysreflexia symptoms from pre-eclampsia symptoms, since these conditions are managed differently. Ideally, a specialist will be available. The mother should tell staff immediately if she has dysreflexia symptoms, and expect to have her blood pressure measured frequently, during contractions, as well as between contractions. She may be given medications for control of her blood pressure, or regional anesthesia.

Prostaglandins and oxytocin are synthetic versions of body chemicals which naturally induce labor contractions. The use of prostaglandins is controversial, but they may be used to "ripen" the cervix. An unripe cervix is long, firm, and unyielding, while a ripe one is relatively shorter and softer. The cervix must be ripe before contractions can safely be induced. To ripen the cervix, a prostaglandin gel or suppository can be applied locally. Local prostaglandins work slowly, so the woman usually receives one application at bedtime and a second in the morning. While prostaglandins do not harm the fetus, they may cause nausea, vomiting, or diarrhea in the mother. Sometimes, the dose of prostaglandins which ripens the cervix will also stimulate uterine contractions.

Oxytocin is used to induce labor after the cervix has ripened either spontaneously or after the use of prostaglandins. It is given intravenously, in a gradually increasing concentration. When a maximum concentration is reached, or effective contractions have begun, the oxytocin is then given at a steady rate. Medical staff monitor contractions carefully to make sure the uterus is not being overstimulated. If contractions become too strong, the oxytocin should be reduced or discontinued—the remaining oxytocin will disappear from the mother's blood within an hour. If contractions are very uncomfortable, the mother or her coach can ask about reducing the dose of oxytocin. The flow of oxytocin may also be interrupted to assess whether contractions continue spontaneously. Sometimes oxytocin administration fails to induce labor. Induction may be tried again after a day or two, depending on the circumstances, or surgical delivery may be necessary.

Intravenous oxytocin is also used for augmentation of labor—that is, for stimulating contractions that have weakened or stopped after labor has begun. Just as there are specific indications for induction with oxytocin, there are specific indications for augmentation. It must be determined that the contractions were not false labor, and other conditions must be met as well. For example, augmentation must not be done if the mother has certain health problems.

The advantages of induction and augmentation are that, by shortening labor, they may prevent infection, maternal exhaustion, or fetal distress. Successful augmentation of labor can prevent the need for surgical delivery.

When labor is induced, contractions may be strong from the beginning, rather than gradually increasing in intensity as in most spontaneous labors, so the laboring woman may not have the same opportunity to adapt gradually. Oxytocin stimulation tends to produce longer, stronger contractions than are typical in spontaneous labors, possibly making it more difficult for the mother to cope. Reactions vary. Corinne said of her second labor, "The labor pains were very bad. They were worse than the first labor." However, Mary said, "I expected it to be more traumatic than what I experienced."

The longer, stronger contractions of augmented labor have a greater potential for causing fetal hypoxia than spontaneous contractions do.

Attempts to stimulate labor cannot be continued indefinitely, however. Whether labor is stimulated or spontaneous, forceps, vacuum extraction, or surgical delivery may be used to speed up delivery before the mother becomes too fatigued, or the fetus becomes too distressed.

Fourth-Stage Medication

Oxytocin or other medications may also be used after the placenta is delivered, since stimulating contractions can help to reduce bleeding at the site where the placenta was attached.

Episiotomy

An *episiotomy* is an incision (cut) in the perineum, the skin and muscle between the vagina and the anus. The perineum needs to stretch to allow the baby to emerge from the mother's body. Often a midwife or doctor tells the mother to stop pushing and blow through a few contractions so that the baby's head will press on the perineum more gently, allowing more time for it to stretch. The birth attendant may try to help the perineum to stretch by massaging it between contractions. If it appears that the perineum cannot stretch enough, and if it is likely to tear instead, the doctor will perform an episiotomy. An episiotomy may also be done to speed up delivery if the fetus seems distressed, or to prepare for the use of forceps.

One advantage of doing an episiotomy is that it may shorten the second stage somewhat. However, the primary reason for this procedure is to prevent tears, especially tears extending into the rectal cavity. The cut may be smaller than a tear would be, and it is easier to repair an episiotomy, which is a clean cut, than a tear, which has jagged edges.

The disadvantage of an episiotomy it that the vaginal area will hurt much more during the weeks following birth than it would if there were no cut or tear. Walking, sitting, urination, or bowel movements may be quite uncomfortable. And, like any cut, the episiotomy may become itchy or infected.

Clara recalls that she wanted an episiotomy during childbirth. "When I had my second baby, the labor was fast and intense, it felt like a train going through me. I remember my husband started to tell the doctor, 'We were hoping to avoid an episiotomy,' and I said, 'Never mind that! Just get this baby out!'" Later, Clara felt some regret, because the incision was sore, and walking and getting in and out of the tub were difficult.

Michelle wanted to avoid an episiotomy because she worried about blood loss. While she was pregnant she tried to prepare her perineum by massaging it frequently, and when the baby crowned she "did a lot of blowing and making noise," working hard to avoid pushing. She was pleased that she had only a small episiotomy with little blood loss.

Sometimes women who have episiotomies are disappointed. They wonder, "Did I really need the episiotomy? What if the doctor had allowed more time for my perineum to stretch? If there had been a tear, would it have been smaller than the episiotomy?" Such questions can never be answered. What can be helpful is knowing that the episiotomy was not done as a matter of routine, but in response to individual needs.

If no anesthesia was given before the episiotomy became necessary, it is done at a moment when pressure is numbing the perineum, or after a local anesthetic is injected. If the incision was made without anesthesia, medication will be injected before it is repaired.

Forceps Delivery and Vacuum Extraction

A doctor can assist birth by gently pulling the baby from the vaginal canal with forceps or a vacuum extractor.

There are several types of forceps. In general design, all types are like a pair of tongs with curved, blunt blades. The inside of the curved blade is designed to fit the side of the fetal head, while the outside curve fits the contours of the mother's body. Before forceps are used, an episiotomy may be done, and local or regional anesthesia may be administered. The blades of the forceps are placed one at a time, then locked together, and a gentle pulling motion is used to assist the baby's birth. "High" forceps procedures, in which the fetal head has not reached the pelvic floor, have been replaced by surgical delivery, which is much safer for both mother and baby. In "low" forceps procedures (also called outlet forceps), the fetal head is visible at the vaginal opening.

A vacuum extractor is essentially a cup attached to a suction device. The cup is placed over the baby's scalp and, once some skin has been drawn into the cup by suction, further suction and the doctor's gentle pulling on the device, done in time with uterine contractions, help to draw the baby from the birth canal.

Forceps or vacuum extractor may be used if it appears that uterine contractions are not strong enough to expel the baby. Shortening the second stage in this way may prevent maternal exhaustion or fetal distress. Forceps or vacuum extraction may also help to prevent injuries to the fetus or mother when the perineum is unyielding and episiotomy alone does not assist birth.

The use of forceps and vacuum extractors each has some advantages. Some types of forceps may be used to alter the position of the fetal head, whereas the extractor can only be used for pulling. The vacuum extractor is less likely to cause pain or injury to the mother. Each instrument may cause characteristic types of fetal injury (the most common and most minor are facial bruises from forceps and scalp bruises from the extractor). The doctor must carefully weigh the risks of using the instruments (which can be minimized by skillful use) against the risks of allowing labor to continue. Vacuum extraction has replaced the use of forceps in most metropolitan hospitals.

Pain Relief

A variety of analgesics, anesthetics, tranquilizers, and occasionally sedatives, may be used to assist a woman in coping with the discomforts of labor and delivery.

Analgesics and Sedatives

Sedatives may be offered to help a woman sleep during a prolonged early phase. Sometimes sedatives help to determine if a woman is experiencing Braxton-Hicks contractions or true early labor. If contractions have stopped by the time she awakens, it is assumed that she was having Braxton-Hicks ("practice") contractions. If contractions continue, with effacement and dilation of the cervix, then it is hoped that she will be refreshed from her rest and better able to cope during the remainder of labor and delivery.

Sometimes tranquilizers are used to increase the effectiveness of analgesics, which lower pain perception as well as induce relaxation or even drowsiness. These may be given intravenously or by injection. Some women find the relaxing effects of these medications helpful, like Cheryl, who was given Demerol (an analgesic) when her cervix was 5 cm dilated. She said, "I didn't ask for it but it was offered because I was having really hard contractions. That one shot helped me get through labor without any more medication. It was really helpful—I almost fell asleep." Other women dislike the drowsiness, and find that it makes coping more difficult. Clara was given first morphine (an analgesic), then Seconal (a sedative), in an attempt to help her sleep during protracted labor, and she said, "I kept waking up between contractions, completely confused."

Other women are helped by the pain-reducing effects of analgesics. While some women find relaxation and breathing techniques adequate, others do not, like Stephanie, who said, "I gave up on the breathing. I needed something else. I had other pain going on besides—similar to a phantom pain—and the Nisentil was able to dull the pain." (That particular medication, Nisentil, is no longer available.)

Each type of pain medication has specific advantages and disadvantages. Sometimes analgesics cause increased restlessness, rather than relaxation. Some women will have negative reactions, such as nausea, vomiting, or lowered blood pressure, to specific analgesics. Clara was given morphine to help her sleep and to determine whether labor had really begun; instead of sleeping, she suffered a long bout of nausea and vomiting. If analgesics are administered too early in labor, they may interfere with the development of strong, effective contractions. On the other hand, if they are administered too late in labor, the newborn may be sleepy, and suckling or breathing may be depressed.

Anesthetics

Unlike analgesics, which alter pain perception, anesthesia blocks all sensation in the affected area, making it completely numb (except that some pressure sensation sometimes remains). Local, regional, or general anesthesia may be used.

Local Anesthesia The most common local anesthesia is a *pudendal block,* in which the anesthetic is injected through the vaginal wall into the pudendal nerve, numbing the vagina and perineum. It is useful for blocking out the pain of forceps, episiotomy, and episiotomy repair.

A paracervical block is a procedure that numbs the lower uterus by injections of anesthetic near the cervix. While it effectively reduces uterine discomfort, it is used less and less because this form of anesthesia can easily affect the fetus. Priscilla chose a paracervical block because she was worried about spinal anesthesia. She said, "My leg went numb. It was my good leg. Psychologically it was one of the scariest moments. It lasted 40 minutes and it seemed like an eternity." In a subsequent labor, Priscilla chose to use analgesics in early labor and was much more satisfied.

Regional Anesthesia For *regional anesthesia*, medication is injected into the fluid surrounding the spinal cord (spinal anesthesia) or into the epidural space surrounding the spinal cord (epidural anesthesia). The *dura* is a membrane surrounding the spinal nerves and cerebrospinal fluid. For spinal anesthesia, a small, hollow needle is used to inject anesthetic through the dura into the cerebrospinal fluid. For epidural anesthesia, a relatively larger needle is inserted into the *epidural space,* a narrow "potential space," rich in blood vessels, which surrounds the dura. A thin plastic catheter is threaded through the needle, then used for intermittent or continuous infusions of anesthetic into the epidural space. Regional anesthesia may not block all sensation.

Either epidural or spinal anesthesia may be used for surgical delivery. However, spinal anesthesia is rarely used in labor. We will say more about the differences between spinal and epidural anesthesia in the following chapter on cesarean birth.

Regional (usually epidural) anesthesia can be used during long or difficult labors to increase the mother's comfort considerably. Roberta said of her epidural, "It was nice. Then my husband could enjoy my labor."

Regional anesthesia may cause a drop in blood pressure. While the lowered blood pressure may be treated in most women, regional anesthesia is usually avoided in cases of placenta previa, severe pre-eclampsia or eclampsia, or severe fetal distress. Some physicians emphasize that regional anesthesia may benefit the infant by reducing maternal stress and indirectly assuring a good fetal oxygen supply. However, others note that regional anesthesia may prolong labor, either by altering the pattern of uterine contractions or by affecting the mother's ability to push.

A woman's disability can affect the choice of appropriate pain medication. Regional anesthesia may be used to prevent dysreflexia in women with spinal cord injuries at T-6 or higher. Epidural anesthesia is preferable to spinal anesthesia because it is slower to take effect and blood pressure changes are monitored and controlled more easily. Women who have progressive neurological disorders, such as MS, are often poor candidates for regional anesthesia, while women with stable disorders, such as cerebral palsy, may be given regional anesthetics. Spinal deformities, such as scoliosis, or inability to flex the spine, can make it difficult to administer regional anesthesia. Arthritic changes in the spine, or the enlarged vertebrae sometimes associated with cerebral palsy, also might make it difficult to administer regional anesthesia.

Saddle block refers to anesthesia which numbs a very small area—the area which would be in contact with a riding saddle. The injection is given at the same site used for cesarean anesthesia, but a smaller amount of anesthetic is used. Often the injection will be given while the mother is in a sitting position, but some anesthesiologists prefer to have the mother lie on her side, so they can avoid "puddling" of the anesthetic in the sacral area.

General Anesthesia *General anesthesia* was once common during vaginal delivery, and two of the women we interviewed were given such anesthesia. This type of anesthesia is now reserved only for some abdominal deliveries. General anesthesia will be described in the next chapter.

Nonpharmaceutical Pain Reduction

Transcutaneous electrical nerve stimulation, or TENS, is a method for decreasing pain by electrical interference of nerve impulses to the brain. TENS has been used by physical therapists in treating certain types of muscle pain, especially chronic lower back pain. Many women with cerebral palsy will be familiar with its use in relieving muscle cramps. Recent studies show that TENS can be useful in controlling the pain associated with labor, especially back pain.

The TENS unit consists of electrodes attached to a hand-held, battery-operated device. For controlling labor pain, two pairs of electrodes are placed alongside the lower spine. In this placement, TENS stimulation blocks pain in the uterus, cervix, and perineal region. The electrical stimulation creates a moderate tingling sensation. The unit can be operated continuously, or the mother or her coach can turn it on at the beginning of a contraction, and off at the end.

The use of TENS does not appear to have side effects for the mother or the infant. Apgar scores of babies whose mothers used a TENS unit are comparable to those of babies whose mothers did not. When a TENS unit affects a fetal monitor reading, auscultation (listening with a stethoscope) may show that, while the TENS may have affected the monitoring device, it has not affected the fetal heart rate.

While use of TENS is not widespread, and it is not completely effective in controlling pain (for example, it is more helpful for back pain than lower abdominal muscle pain), it may be useful to use with other methods. When TENS can be used effectively, it has the advantage of avoiding or reducing the side effects of medication.

CLOSING COMMENTS

We would like to close our discussion of labor and delivery with a few suggestions for women with disabilities and their physicians.

First, supportive medical staff and good communication are vital if the mother is to have a satisfying childbirth experience. Certainly this is true for all women, but special care must be taken with disabled women who, like other laboring women, will be very sensitive to the attitudes of the people around them. Sylvia contrasted the "reassurance" of nurses who were experienced with disability with the "curiosity" of those who were not. Celeste recalled that when she gave birth, "There were a lot of people around, because they hadn't seen a disabled woman's delivery. They were expecting difficulty in the delivery process. They also didn't know what to expect when I delivered in a side-lying position." While some women might be oblivious to such onlookers, others would be disturbed. Some women felt that a nurse's inexperience with disability is less important than a supportive attitude. Leslie, however, recalled that, "When my nurse was frightened and unsure of what to do when my blood pressure went up, it made me more scared."

Women with disabilities also worry that they will be over-treated. It is very important for a disabled mother to understand the reasons for everything that happens. Julie, who was unable to spread her legs, clearly understood the need for surgical delivery and was satisfied that her treatment was appropriate. Faith, on the other hand, felt that she had a surgical delivery "because my doctor was freaked out by my disability." She was never given a clear explanation of the reasons for her surgery, and was dissatisfied with her treatment.

The expectant mother can take steps to ensure that she will have good relations with staff during childbirth. Like Sharon and Sylvia, she can make a point of meeting medical staff beforehand so she feels comfortable with them. She can work with her physician to assure that staff have information about her special needs. She can bring a coach or advocate who is prepared to provide information about her disability.

Finally, we anticipate that, as growing numbers of women with disabilities decide to have children, there will be an increase in research on the interaction of disability with pregnancy and childbirth. While we have attempted to provide a comprehensive survey of current knowledge, we are well aware that important new information could develop at any time. We encourage women and their physicians to seek new information which can help them make pregnancy and childbirth a positive experience.

8 ANOTHER WAY OF BIRTH— CESAREAN DELIVERY

Giving birth by cesarean is not inevitable for women with disabilities, but it is quite common. In our small sample, 14 of 36 women (39%) experienced at least one cesarean delivery. This figure is less startling when one considers that in recent years the rate of cesarean deliveries for all American women has risen to 20%–25%.

This increase in the rate of cesarean deliveries has led to concern and even controversy among medical professionals, consumer advocates, and the public. Clearly, a major factor in this increase has been concern for the well-being of the infant. It is certainly reasonable to ask whether this concern has been given too much weight in comparison to concern about the effect of surgery on the mother. The best approach cannot be one of "taking sides," as if women, infants, and health professionals were in warring camps; the best approach is to develop useful guidelines for individualized decision-making. As the medical profession seeks to reduce the frequency of all cesarean deliveries by re-evaluating the need for surgery in specific situations, the rate of such deliveries among disabled women will probably change.

Deciding whether a cesarean delivery is appropriate is like balancing an equation. On one side of the equation are the undesirable effects of surgery. On the other side are the undesirable effects of allowing a problem pregnancy or a difficult labor to continue. In some situations, the mother may be having no difficulties, but there are reasons to believe cesarean birth will be safer for the baby; in such situations, concern for protecting the mother's welfare and that of the baby must be balanced.

283

The special concerns of disabled women can affect any part of the balance—the effects of surgery, the effect of labor on the mother, and the effect of labor on the infant. This is true even when the need for surgery does not arise from disability. But it is important for the individual woman to be assured that the fact of her disability has not been weighed too heavily. Some of Faith's disappointment that her first child was a cesarean birth stemmed from her belief that her doctor overreacted to her disability. The mother is entitled to a clear explanation of the reasons for surgery, whether it was planned or unplanned. The explanation must differentiate between obstetric indications (pregnancy-related reasons which might also apply to an able-bodied woman) and disability indications (reasons based directly or indirectly on disability).

DISABILITY INDICATIONS FOR CESAREAN BIRTH

As shown in Table 8.1, there is a broad range of reasons that women with disabilities might need surgical delivery. For some women, disability leads to surgery in a very direct way. For example, severe spinal curvature, or a problem such as Julie's inability to spread her legs, make vaginal delivery physically impossible. Athina and her doctor agreed that, considering her breathing difficulties and muscle weakness, it might be hard for her to cope with the stresses of labor. Athina also worried that if her disability caused a prolonged labor, her baby might be injured.

For other women, disability only indirectly leads to surgery. For example, Sybil had a cesarean because her bladder had been removed before she was pregnant, and her doctor was concerned that remaining scar tissue might cause problems during labor. Sometimes surgery is scheduled because there is concern that a pregnancy complication will exacerbate the disability or cause a permanent medical problem if the pregnancy is allowed to continue. For example, Dawn had always had urinary problems, and when she developed a kidney infection, there was serious concern that she could be permanently affected.

While women with disabilities are more likely than others to have cesarean sections, the decision for any woman, in any category of disability, will depend on individual circumstances. Laura and Leslie illustrate this point well. They both have SLE: women with SLE often have difficult pregnancies, and miscarriages are frequent. Laura's surgery was probably an indirect result of her disability, for blood tests showed that her placenta was not functioning, possibly because her disease was causing rejection of the placenta. Leslie, however, also had many disability-related complications, but needed surgery for an obstetric reason—the fetus was in a transverse presentation.

FIGURE 8.1
REASONS FOR CESAREAN BIRTHS AMONG INTERVIEWEES

Name	Disability	Reason for Cesarean
Athina	Spinal muscular atrophy	Not strong enough for labor
Arlene	Arthrogryposis	Lordosis and pelvic deformity
Carla	Familial spastic paresis (symptoms identical to cerebral palsy)	Dysfunctional labor
Dawn	Dystonia	Kidney infection
Faith	Friedrich's ataxia	Dysfunctional labor
Heather	Hip dysplegia and scoliosis	Pelvic deformity
Hilary	Femoral hypoplasia syndrome	Pelvis too small[a]
Julie	Juvenile rheumatoid arthritis	Unable to abduct (spread) legs
Laura	Systemic lupus erythematosus	Loss of placental function (disability-related)
Leslie	Systemic lupus erythematosus	Fetus in transverse presentation
Pam	Postpolio syndrome	Pelvic deformity and spinal curvature
Portia	Postpolio syndrome	Fetopelvic disproportion and dysfunctional labors
Sybil	Spina bifida	Previous surgery (bladder removal)
Stephanie	Spinal cord injury	Fetopelvic disproportion

[a]Because of her disability, Hilary's pelvis was too small for delivery of even a small baby.

OBSTETRIC INDICATIONS FOR CESAREAN BIRTH

In Chapters 6 and 7 on pregnancy and labor, many of the problems that can lead to surgery are reviewed. The following sections are concerned specifically with the indications for cesarean delivery.

Fetopelvic Disproportion

This condition is responsible for a large percentage of cesarean deliveries. The fetus cannot pass through the birth canal, either because it is unusually large *(macrosomia),* or because the mother's pelvis is too small *(pelvic contraction)* or abnormally shaped.

Both macrosomia and pelvic contraction can be difficult to diagnose, even with ultrasound examination. Usually the diagnosis cannot be made until there has been a trial of labor.

Spine and hip deformities can lead to disproportion. Among the women we interviewed, seven of the 14 who had cesareans said that fetopelvic disproportion was the cause, and five mentioned spine or hip deformities: Arlene, lordosis; Pam, scoliosis; Heather and Hilary, small, misshapen pelvis; and Julie, spinal curvature. (Julie also needed the surgery because arthritis in her hips prevented her from spreading her legs widely.) Portia and Stephanie simply stated that their babies were "too big" and did not mention any relationship to disability.

More frequent diagnosis of fetopelvic disproportion has contributed to the general increase in the cesarean birth rate. The medical profession's effort to reduce the frequency of cesarean deliveries will include discussion of when this diagnosis is appropriate. It is reasonable to seek a second opinion to confirm a diagnosis of fetopelvic disproportion.

Placenta Previa

This condition is present when the placenta is lower in the uterus than the fetus, thus blocking the opening of the cervix. It may be discovered during an ultrasound examination following painless bleeding during labor. If such bleeding occurs, ultrasound examination is necessary because an internal pelvic examination could cause serious bleeding. When a large portion of the placenta covers the cervix, it will tear away from the uterine wall as the cervix dilates. The mother will then be in danger of bleeding to death, and the fetus can suffer brain damage or death from hypoxia (lack of oxygen).

Abruptio Placentae

Abruptio placentae, or placental abruption, refers to a separation of the placenta from the uterine wall before birth. Signs include bleeding and pain (in contrast to the painless bleeding of placenta previa). The dangers are the same as with placenta previa.

Fetal Position or Presentation

Some positions and presentations are always indications for surgery. For example, *transverse presentations* which do not change to breech or vertex presentation early in labor are dangerous to both mother and fetus, and surgery is required (see *Chapter 7*). Other presentations may or may not require surgery and must be evaluated on an individual basis.

The increasing use of cesarean surgery for breech presentations has contributed to the overall increase in the rate of cesarean births. Although breech presentation sometimes leads to fetopelvic disproportion, concern for the welfare of the infant is the main reason for cesarean delivery of breech babies. Techniques for vaginal breech delivery can be difficult, and infants can be injured or suffer hypoxia during such deliveries. Because cesarean delivery is often safer, obstetric training has included fewer opportunities to learn techniques of vaginal breech delivery. Lack of training in these techniques has reinforced the trend toward surgical delivery in breech presentations.

The medical profession's effort to reduce the rate of cesarean deliveries may lead to an increase in the number of vaginal breech deliveries. Improved techniques of diagnosing fetal distress can help in deciding which mode of delivery is more appropriate in any one case.

Previous Cesarean Surgery

A large proportion of cesarean deliveries are repeat surgeries. However, the old rule, "Once a C-section, always a C-section," is no longer true. We will explore this issue more thoroughly later in this chapter (see "Vaginal Birth After Cesarean Section").

Soft Tissue Abnormalities

Abnormalities such as uterine tumors or uterine deformity are rare. However, an unusual shape or position of the uterus is sometimes associated with congenital deformity.

Insufficient Contractions

Weak or uncoordinated contractions lead to a prolonged or arrested labor. When labor is prolonged, careful judgment is needed in deciding whether it is appropriate to allow time for labor to improve spontaneously, to stimulate labor, or to resort to the use of forceps, vacuum suction extraction, or surgery. While it is important to allow an adequate trial of labor to assure that surgery is necessary, it is also important not to increase the risk of fetal distress by delaying an inevitable surgery.

Fulminant Pre-eclampsia/Eclampsia

Surgery usually prevents the worst cases of eclampsia, in which the mother suffers convulsions or coma, endangering the lives of both mother and fetus.

Postmature Fetus

If pregnancy continues past the due date, tests will be done to be sure that the placenta is functioning. If the placenta is aging and the fetus could suffer malnutrition or other problems, labor may be induced. If inducing labor is not safe, surgery will be necessary.

Fetal Distress

This usually occurs when an inadequate placenta does not supply the fetus with enough oxygen. Distress may also arise from mechanical problems, such as placental abruption or a short umbilical cord. It may be possible to relieve fetal distress by having the mother change position, or by giving her oxygen and/or fluids.

If signs of distress persist, an emergency cesarean may be needed to prevent neurological or other damage, or death of the fetus.

As the rate of cesarean deliveries has increased, the percentage of surgeries performed after a diagnosis of fetal distress has also risen. Often, infants delivered in these circumstances seemed completely healthy, with good Apgar scores. These facts have raised the question of whether fetal distress is often wrongly diagnosed. Some critics argue that increased use of fetal monitoring has led to mistaken diagnoses of fetal distress, indirectly causing many unnecessary surgeries. The relationship between use of fetal monitors and surgery rates is not a simple one. For example, results can be affected by the the amount of experience a hospital staff has with fetal monitors, the use of fetal monitoring in high-risk cases, and other factors. Also, a newborn's healthy appearance may not mean that a diagnosis of distress was necessarily incorrect. Improved technology, such as fetal blood sampling, will help to resolve concerns about accurate diagnosis of fetal distress.

Maternal Isoimmunization (Rh Disease)

If the mother and infant have different blood types, the mother may develop antibodies which destroy fetal blood cells. A severe antibody reaction can cause illness, disability, or death of the fetus. If fetal illness is diagnosed, surgery may be necessary even if the fetus is not full term.

Genital Herpes

The increased incidence of herpes has contributed to the overall increase in cesarean deliveries. If the mother has an active herpes infection during labor, there is a high risk that the infant could become infected during vaginal birth. If it is the mother's first episode of herpes infection, the baby's risk of infection is very high, and a cesarean delivery is clearly necessary. The risks with recurrent infections are far less, and many obstetricians will explain the risks to the parents and give them the choice between vaginal and cesarean delivery. Most parents choose cesarean delivery because herpes infections are very dangerous to babies, often causing blindness, nerve damage or death.

Some books about childbirth suggest that tests for herpes infection be performed after the thirty-sixth week. However, the current practice is to watch for *active lesions* at the time of labor.

Some Maternal Illnesses

Illnesses such as severe kidney problems and some types of diabetes can indicate the need for cesarean delivery.

Cord Prolapse in Early Labor

If part of the umbilical cord protrudes through the cervix, the cord will be compressed each time a contraction drives the fetal head against the cervix. Pressure on the cord will then interfere with fetal blood circulation. Cord prolapse is unusual, but when it occurs, surgery is almost always necessary.

ADDITIONAL CONCERNS OF WOMEN WITH DISABILITIES

Even when cesarean delivery is being considered for purely obstetric reasons, disabled women have special concerns. These relate to both sides of the balance—concern for their babies' welfare and concern for their own welfare.

A woman with disabilities has additional reasons to feel concerned about preventing neurological problems or other injuries to her baby. Caring for an injured or disabled child is always a difficult task. For a disabled mother, however, the task can be especially difficult, as she may not have the physical resources to care for the child nor the financial resources to pay for additional attendant care. A relatively independent woman may worry that she will become dependent on others for help with her child. In addition to such realistic concerns, many women with disabilities are emotionally inclined to fear that their children will be disabled. In circumstances where some women may wish to wait a little longer, a woman with disabilities might think it is more reasonable to go ahead with surgery.

Yet disabled women must also consider how surgery or anesthesia will affect their own well-being. A major concern is that recovery from surgery may be more difficult for a woman with disabilities. The most obvious problem is the effect of abdominal surgery on mobility, for a woman's ability to change position, transfer, or walk can be affected. The effect will be brief for some women; for others, it will last for weeks. Heather said that with her first child, "It took 24 hours before I could get my balance. The first day I just sat on the side of the bed." With her second child, Heather was able to use her crutches the same day she had surgery. Carla was more seriously affected: "It was difficult to move. My mobility was shot. It took almost 6 weeks before I could walk holding onto the wall."

Mobility limitations also influence other aspects of recovery. Women who cannot exercise may be more vulnerable to emboli (blood clots in the veins), and to constipation, which is a common problem after abdominal surgery. Women with breathing difficulties may be more vulnerable to respiratory infection. For example, even though Athina's nurses encouraged her to cough and to do breathing exercises immediately after surgery, she had to spend some time in the intensive care unit as a safety precaution.

Women whose disorders are exacerbated by fatigue—for example, women with SLE or MS—face a difficult choice when labor is prolonged. Either the fatigue that follows protracted labor or fatigue associated with surgical recovery could contribute to a flare-up of symptoms.

While it is impossible to generalize about the effects of cesarean surgery on disabled women, it is clear that surgical delivery will not necessarily be safer or easier for the mother than vaginal delivery. It is important to remember the strong possibility that recovery may be more difficult for a woman with disabilities. Both the emotional and the physical aspects of recovery can pose a challenge.

WHAT HAPPENS DURING CESAREAN BIRTH

Preparation

Whether cesarean birth is planned or unplanned, the preparations for surgery are essentially the same. Preparations for a planned surgery simply proceed at a slower pace.

For a planned surgery, the mother is admitted to the hospital in advance of the scheduled time, usually the same day. Blood and urine tests will be done while she is in her hospital room, and her abdominal hair and some of her pubic hair may be shaved while she is in her room. The anesthesiologist will visit her to ask questions about her medical history, explain what will happen during anesthesia, and describe possible side effects of anesthesia.

The anesthesiologist may ask for information that is already in the medical records, but it is important to answer carefully, so that the anesthesiologist can make sure s/he has the correct information. Julie's experience shows how important it is to try to have complete medical records available to the current doctor, to remember as much as possible, and to provide as much information as possible. When Julie had her child, she had a rare allergic reaction to her anesthetic. Somehow, she never mentioned this to a surgeon she saw some years later. Fortunately, the anesthesiologist assisting this surgeon had also assisted Julie's obstetrician. He recognized Julie, partly because her reaction to the medication was so unusual, and he had never forgotten her. If the anesthesiologist had not known Julie, she might have been given the same anesthesia, and her reaction might have been stronger than the first, possibly fatal.

When surgery is unplanned, blood tests will be done when the mother is admitted to the hospital, whether she is in labor or has troublesome symptoms such as pain or bleeding. The anesthesiologist will talk with her in the labor room or the operating room. If there is an emergency, the conversation will be brief.

Other preparations will include washing the mother's abdomen and upper thighs, applying an antiseptic to these areas, and covering the areas around her abdomen with sterile drapes. (If the antiseptic is applied before anaesthetics are given, it may feel cold.) An intravenous (IV) line and a urinary catheter will be put in place. The catheter is a thin rubber tube in the urethra which drains urine from the bladder. It may be put in after anesthesia is started. Women who have general anesthesia will be given an endotracheal tube after they are unconscious; the tube keeps the throat from becoming obstructed, assuring proper breathing.

Anesthesia

Either regional or general anesthesia will be used. Regional anesthesia can be "epidural" or "spinal" anesthesia. In Chapter 7, we described how regional anesthesia is administered. In a vaginal delivery, epidural anesthesia is more likely to be used. However, either spinal or epidural anesthesia might be used for cesarean delivery. Each has its advantages and disadvantages.

Since regional anesthesia can lower the blood pressure, it must be avoided in some situations. When regional anesthesia is used, epidural anesthesia may be preferable because it takes effect more slowly. Then, if blood pressure should go down, the change is more gradual and controllable.

A disadvantage of spinal anesthesia is that some women may suffer "spinal headache," which lasts from several hours to several days after the birth. (A more correct term is "postdural puncture headache," because the same headache may occur if an epidural needle accidentally punctures the dura.) Some literature on this subject states that as many as 10% of women who have spinal anesthesia will develop headaches, but recent improvements, including the use of smaller needles, have reduced the incidence of headaches in some hospitals to less than 5%. The headache is caused by a leakage of cerebrospinal fluid through the needle puncture. Sheila commented, "The headache was so bad that I refused the spinal for my second labor. I felt great after the second delivery. I was ready for anything."

Celeste, who had a vaginal delivery, was very dissatisfied with spinal anesthesia: "The baby and I were both sick from medication. I had this dopey baby. I had difficulty urinating after [having] the baby. I decided to go natural with the second one." The small doses of medication used in spinal anesthesia do not make a baby drowsy, but sedatives accompanying them do. Celeste's comment raises a second major concern about analgesics and anesthesia—their effect on the fetus. Medication that is effective against labor pain can cross the placenta and affect the fetus. Numerous studies have shown that, if dosages are kept to a minimum and carefully timed, medications are unlikely to have a long-term effect on the baby. Still, medications can cause the baby to be sleepy and unresponsive at birth, and may temporarily depress its breathing.

While epidural anesthesia is less likely to cause postpartum headache, it is more difficult to administer and slower to take effect. While there may be some leeway in deciding whether to use regional anesthesia, the choice between spinal and epidural anesthesia must depend on the anesthesiologist's expertise.

General anesthesia uses a combination of medications which relax the muscles, block out pain, and make the woman sleepy. Some medications are given intravenously, others are gasses which are breathed in through a special mask.

General anesthesia can be administered quickly and takes effect quickly. It may be necessary to use in emergencies, or for some women whose disabilities prevent the use of regional anesthesia. Heather's unusual experience led to an emergency use of general anesthesia. She explained, "I had an epidural, and I was fine while they made the incision, but just as they took the baby out, it suddenly wore off. I was only numb from the knees down. The pain was terrible—a ripping feeling, like I was being torn in two. They had to put me out so they could finish." (This happened when Heather had her second child. Her experience during her first delivery was quite different: "I was numb—there was no feeling, just a little pressure and a stretching sensation when they lifted the baby out.")

General anesthesia has three main disadvantages. It is more likely to affect the baby, and there is some risk that the mother will vomit and breathe in food or stomach acid, resulting in pneumonia. To balance these disadvantages, surgery is performed as quickly as possible to minimize the baby's exposure to anesthesia, and emergency equipment is available to help the mother or infant if necessary. Still, there is no way to get around the third main disadvantage—the mother will not be awake for the birth of her baby.

The main advantage of regional anesthesia is that the mother is awake to see her baby's birth. Because she and the baby are less likely to feel groggy, they may be able to spend more time together immediately after the birth.

The Surgery

Cesarean delivery usually takes less than an hour. In many hospitals, a woman who has regional anesthesia may be joined by her husband and/or her labor coach after preparations for surgery are completed. They will be wearing sterile caps, masks, and gowns like those worn by the medical team.

She may be surprised to find that the operating table is somewhat tilted to the left; the tilted position helps maintain good blood pressure. The anesthetic will make her numb up to about the level of her nipples. She may not be able to feel her own breathing—a frightening experience for some women. Some women who have had cesarean surgery suggest that a woman who cannot feel her own breathing can say aloud, "I can't feel my breathing." A support person, or the sound of her own voice, can tell her, "If you're talking, you're breathing."

A screen will be placed above the abdomen to help keep the surgical area sterile and to keep the parents from seeing the incision (cut) as it is being made. In some hospitals, the parents can request that the screen be removed while the baby is being delivered. Or, if the umbilical cord is long enough, the doctor can lift the baby high enough for the parents to see. The baby's appearance may be a little startling. It helps to remember that a vaginally born baby might also have some blood smears, and that all newborns look bluish for a few seconds before they start breathing.

The anesthetic blocks out any pain from the incision, but many women feel some pulling or pressure discomfort when the baby is delivered. While Heather recalled feeling "a little pressure and a stretching sensation" during her first cesarean delivery, Leslie "couldn't feel a thing when they lifted the baby out." The change in uterine pressure after the baby is born might make the mother feel dizzy or nauseous. Breathing oxygen through a mask can help with the dizziness.

After the baby is delivered, separate teams will care for mother and baby at the same time. It may be possible to watch as mucus is suctioned from the baby's nose and mouth, the umbilical cord is cut and clamped, and the baby is washed, dried, and wrapped in a warm blanket.

After the baby is removed from the uterus, amniotic fluid will be suctioned out. Any noise the suction equipment makes is nothing to worry about. The placenta will then be removed manually, and the doctor will examine the uterus and ovaries. If the mother has requested it, sterilization can be done at this time.

The most time-consuming part of the surgery begins next. The surgeon carefully sutures (stitches) the uterus, abdominal muscles, and skin, layer by layer, matching the edges of the incisions as closely as possible. The bladder, which was moved out of normal position for the delivery, is also put back into place, and the incisions around it are stitched. The top layer of skin will be closed with self-dissolving stitches or metal clips, and covered with a gauze bandage.

Cesarean Incisions

Many women are concerned about the effect of cesarean delivery on their appearance. They may prefer a "bikini cut" in which the skin incision and the resulting scar are in a horizontal line where the pubic hair begins. The alternative is a vertical incision from just below the navel to just above the pubic hair. The vertical skin incision can overlie more than one type of uterine incision.

By far the most common uterine incision is the "low transverse" incision, a horizontal incision in the lower portion of the uterus. (At times, a low vertical incision is made.) This type of surgery has real advantages: less blood loss and better healing. The incisions are less likely to become infected, and fewer adhesions are likely to form. Also, a woman has a better chance of giving birth vaginally in later pregnancies, because there is less risk that the resulting scar on the uterus will separate during pregnancy or labor.

The other type of incision is known as the "classical" incision because it was most widely used in the past. The incision on the uterus is a vertical cut in the mid-line that is higher than the low transverse incision. The classical incision can be made more quickly, which might be an advantage in some emergencies. In some cases it is also the safer choice. For example, with some malpresentations, a low transverse incision may be too small for delivering the baby. In some cases of placenta previa, there is a risk that a low incision will start placental bleeding. The disadvantages of a classical incision are the possibility of more bleeding and a higher risk that the scar on the uterus will rupture during later pregnancies.

RECOVERY

. . . .

Early Recovery

The mother will spend the first few hours after surgery in the recovery room, where she will stay until the effects of anesthesia have worn off. Nurses will frequently check her breathing, pulse, temperature, and blood pressure. They will also check the incision and watch for excessive vaginal bleeding. The catheter will still be in place, so nurses will measure urine output by checking the level of urine in the bag that catches the flow, and replace full bags. They will also feel her abdomen to make sure her uterus is beginning to *involute*. (The uterus continues to contract after childbirth, and these contractions begin the process of returning the uterus to its pre-pregnant size, a process called "involution." Postnatal contractions also help to stop bleeding at the site where the placenta was attached.)

The IV line will still be in place and the IV solution may include oxytocics to stimulate contractions of the uterus. As the anesthetics wear off, the surgical incisions will become painful, and uterine contractions might make the pain more intense. If these contractions become too painful, and the uterus is involuting well, oxytocic medication may be discontinued.

The nurses will administer pain medications as anesthesia wears off. Women who are nauseous from pain medications should tell their nurses so they can be given additional medication for nausea. Report any sign of nausea immediately. It is important to prevent vomiting because it is painful.

Women who have had regional anesthesia will be watched for return of sensation and motion; their nurses may ask them to wiggle their toes, or to tell whether they can feel a touch on their legs. These signs of returning sensation and motion cannot be used to verify that a spinal-cord-injured woman is recovering from anesthesia. Instead, the muscle tone and reflexes below the level of injury should have been evaluated during her pregnancy, and the anesthesiologist or nurse should watch for the return of the mother's usual spasticity and reflexes during recovery. As sensation returns to numb areas, there may be a tingling feeling like the feeling in a foot that "wakes up" after it was "asleep." Women who have had spinal anesthesia may be instructed to lie flat on their backs, so that they will be less likely to develop headaches. If lying flat is difficult, as it was for Heather, a woman can ask for a pillow for support, or she can ask the anesthesiologist for permission to lie on her side, if she had not done so before surgery.

Women who have had general anesthesia will feel confused when they awake, almost as if they are dreaming. All our interviewees used the word "groggy." Arlene said, "I was groggy. I could hear and remember what was said. They told me I gave birth to a girl. My mouth wasn't working and I couldn't respond." Often, a woman has only sketchy memories of what happened while she was recovering from general anesthesia. Athina, who had given birth at ten o'clock in the morning, said she remembered being told that she had had a girl, but she remembered almost nothing else that happened that day.

If the mother had regional anesthesia, her husband or friend can probably be with her in the recovery room. Sometimes she can have her baby with her; this depends on hospital policy and the baby's condition. (The baby may need special care if it was premature or distressed, or depressed by anesthetics.)

Even people who are not expecting a cesarean delivery might like to plan ahead for the possible separation of mother and baby. Where should the father be? Some couples will feel that it is most important for the mother to have his companionship, while others will feel it is more important for him to be holding and cuddling the baby. When the mother has had general anesthesia, the father cannot see her until she is conscious, but may be able to spend time with the baby. Later, any disappointment the mother feels about the separation from her baby may be eased by knowing that the father and baby were together. Hilary liked knowing the details of what happened: "My husband bonded with her because I was asleep. The hospital staff had him sit in a rocking chair so he could rock her." While Faith was still unconscious, her husband tape-recorded their baby's cry. After she woke up, she still had to wait to see the baby but, she said, "hearing the tape lessened my sadness a little."

When the family can stay together, the mother may still feel too tired or weak to hold the baby. The father or a friend can hold the baby where the mother can see it, or help her support the baby on her chest. Sybil, who could not hold her baby by herself until the third day after the birth, recalled, "I was very grateful to the nurse who helped me hold my baby."

The Hospital Stay

Women who have given birth surgically experience many of the same physical changes as those who give birth vaginally. Changes that all women experience, such as lactation, are discussed in Chapter 9. Here, we concentrate on recovery from the physical and emotional effects of cesarean surgery.

The progress women make during their first few days in the hospital can seem amazing. A woman who has just left the recovery room often needs to be lifted from the gurney to her bed. She still has her IV and catheter in place, and even deep breathing is painful. It seems hard to believe that in just a few days she will be eating, using the bathroom, and walking independently, but she will be.

Pain and discomfort are most intense on the first day, and gradually decrease during the next few days. Not all women react to the pain in the same way. Dawn recalled, "I found it difficult to move. The painkiller only helped a little. I only got painkiller four times a day; I wish it was prescribed for me to take 'as needed.'" Hilary, on the other hand, did not want help moving from her gurney, and used her arms to maneuver into bed. Hilary said, "I didn't want any pain medications. I already felt too groggy from the anesthesia."

Most women are between the extremes that Hilary and Dawn represent. They do find pain medications helpful, particularly in situations that intensify pain. For example, Pam commented that "the painkiller also helped with contractions." Some women may find that pain medications make them dizzy or nauseous. Women who are breast-feeding naturally feel concerned that medications will enter their milk and affect their babies. Faith said, "It was hard to balance the pain medicine and nursing. I took it after nursing so she wouldn't be taking enough drugs to affect her." Women who are breast-feeding need to tell their doctors about their concerns.

Women who simply feel more comfortable with less medication, like Hilary, can always tell their nurses they do not want any. It is also important to tell nurses when pain medication is not helping because unusually severe pain can be a sign of problems. The first sign of an infection in Athina's incision was persistent pain that was not relieved by medication.

Many women find that the same relaxation techniques that are useful in labor help them cope with surgical pain. Their nurses can also give them ideas for keeping comfortable. One of the most useful ways is to gently but firmly press both hands or a pillow against the lower abdomen when moving, coughing or walking. The support and pressure from the pillow counteract the painful pulling on the incision. The pressure of the pillow also lessens the feeling that "things are going to fall out."

Though changing positions can be painful, it is helpful to find more than one comfortable position for resting. Many women find it is most comfortable to lie on their sides, with their backs well supported by pillows and a pillow between their slightly bent legs. This position can also be comfortable for breast feeding.

Athina commented that some of her worst pain was caused by other people moving her since they could not know which movements jostled or pulled on her incision. Hilary had been thinking of the same problem when she decided to move from the gurney by herself. She said, "It wasn't easy but it was worth it. I knew it would hurt a lot more if other people tried to move me."

Here are some ways to avoid or reduce pain when others help you:

- If you are planning a surgical birth, and have a community hospital with a small staff, arrange to visit the maternity floor ahead of time. Discuss your needs with the nursing staff. Perhaps you or your attendant can show them ways of lifting and transferring.
- Even if you are not planning a surgical birth, try to arrange ahead of time to have your spouse, attendant, or a friend who has cared for you avaiable to help in the hospital. Your friend may be able to give the nurse or nurses some tips, demonstrate ways of helping you, or help when the nurse is delayed in coming to your room.
- Try "talking through" a move step by step, telling nurses what works best for you at home. Give feedback about what is most comfortable. This feedback encourages your nurse to offer reassurance. You may need to be reminded, "Don't worry, you can't *really* split open. You have several layers of stitches."
- Use assistive devices. The controls on hospital beds are a real help. Hilary said, "I couldn't use my prostheses, but I rigged up an assistive device in the hospital." She explained, "It's hard for people to help me walk because I'm so short. I walked to the bathroom by myself an hour and a half after I got to my room." Even if you use crutches rather than leaning on another person, have someone with you during your first few walks in case you get dizzy or lose your balance.
- Try to arrange to exercise when you are most comfortable—for example, about half an hour after pain medication is injected.

Whether you move on your own or with help, movement, deep breathing and coughing will increase pain, but they must not be avoided. Breathing exercises help prevent pneumonia, which can be a complication of abdominal surgery. Exercise and walking maintain circulation and help prevent pneumonia and the formation of blood clots in the leg veins. Although breathing and other exercises are painful at first, they do speed recovery. Breathing exercises are so important that women may even be encouraged to get started while they are still in the recovery room.

A good exercise to begin just a few hours after surgery is simply taking the deepest breath possible and holding it briefly. This is also a way to begin gently reconditioning abdominal muscles. Later, begin coughing gently. There is no need to wait for nurses to encourage this exercise, but they will begin soon. Athina was taken to an intensive care unit because she has breathing difficulties, and the nurses there encouraged her to start coughing as soon as she arrived. As coughing and breathing grow deeper, the hospital may provide an exercise device. This device is clear plastic, and blowing through a flexible tube moves a part inside which shows how well you are breathing.

Whole body exercises can also begin in bed. You can gently stretch your limbs, tense and relax one limb at a time, and carefully roll to one side and back. Later, exercise lower abdominal muscles by pulling the heels toward the body, as if to put the feet flat on the bed with the knees making a "tent" under the covers. As the days go by, the feet can be brought closer and closer to the body. Most women take at least one walk by the end of the first day.

For women with disabilities, of course, the exercise may be different, and their experiences may even be different with each birth. While Athina was ready to use her her wheelchair on the first day, Arlene's nurses waited until the second day. Arlene commented, "It felt as though things were going to fall out—I never had internal surgery before." Heather said, "With my first baby, it took me a whole day to get my balance. All I could do on the first day was sit on the edge of the bed. With my second delivery I got up on my crutches the same day as I delivered." Julie said, "Because of my dystonic reaction to the anesthetic, my whole body was sore, even my jaw. They got me up anyway. Within the first 24 hours they lifted me onto a rolling shower bench so I could take a shower. The next day, a nurse made me walk to the bathroom. I remember how cruel I thought she was. I was in a lot of pain and running a high fever. But later I learned from my aunt, who is a nurse, how important it was for me to get up and moving."

Gradually, the walks last a little longer; the first few walks are only as far as the bathroom, then into the hallway, then farther. Each woman learns to find the right balance—just enough exercise to increase her strength, but not so much that she gets exhausted.

Although none of the women we interviewed mentioned problems with blood clots in her legs, it is possible that using a wheelchair will not be sufficient exercise for some women. Women who cannot walk may need to have their doctors prescribe passive exercise or special stockings.

Most women have a urinary catheter in place for the first 24 hours after surgery. Hilary was an exception. She explained: "My first doctor never did use catheters. Near the end of the operation, after he had the bladder in place, he pressed it gently so all the urine ran out. Later, I didn't have any problem going to the bathroom. I never did like catheters, so when I had my second baby and got the on-call doctor, I told him I wanted to go without. He said we could try, but if I had any problems I'd have to have a catheter. I never needed it."

Some women, like Hilary, dislike having a urinary catheter. Faith felt that her catheter caused the stress incontinence that bothered her after her baby was born. Pam said, "I couldn't wait until they took the catheter out." The catheter should not cause any discomfort, but it can get in the way of walking. Most women need a urinary catheter because their bladders do not function well after the trauma of surgery. Also, even if a woman is able to empty her bladder shortly after surgery, she may not be ready to walk to the bathroom, and getting up and down from the toilet or on and off a bed pan will be painful. After about 24 hours, the catheter will be removed, although it may be reinserted if it is still difficult for the woman to empty her bladder.

The IV line also remains in place for about 24 hours. Some women are bothered by it. Pam complained that "the IV made it hard to move my arms." Other women are annoyed because the IV gets in the way when they are walking or holding their babies. If the IV is in a woman's "good" arm, she can ask to have it moved to her other arm. If the IV is actually painful, a nurse should be told because there may be an infection or the needle may have moved out of place. The IV is necessary because after abdominal surgery the intestines stop functioning for about a day. During that time, most women cannot eat or drink, and must receive fluids, nutrients, and some medications by IV. However, some women may be permitted to sip liquids on the same day as surgery.

Near the end of the first day, your nurse or doctor will occasionally put a stethoscope against your abdomen and listen for bowel sounds, and ask whether you have passed any gas—these are signs that the intestines are functioning again. When digestion is functioning, the IV will be removed and you will be allowed to sip clear liquids such as apple juice, broth and gelatin. If clear liquids do not cause vomiting, the next meal may include full liquids like milk and custard. At the same time, some pain injections and other medications will be replaced by oral medications. Some women eat solid foods by the second day, others by the third. Most women welcome solid foods; they are starting to feel hungry and, also, eating "real food" helps them feel that they truly are recovering. Even though it is pleasant to eat solid food, it is still important to drink plenty of liquids. Liquids are important because they provide fluid to replace blood lost in surgery, replace fluid used in milk production, and help to prevent constipation and bladder infection.

As the digestive system begins returning to normal, many women have problems with gas pain and/or constipation. Mild exercise gives some relief from gas pains; some women find it helpful to sit in a rocking chair and rock gently. Lying on the side, slightly curled up, may be most comfortable. Labor breathing and relaxation techniques help many women cope with gas pain and painful bowel movements. It also helps to press a pillow against the abdomen during a bowel movement. Many doctors routinely prescribe stool softeners, but if stools are still hard and dry after the first one or two bowel movements, ask a nurse for one.

If the skin was closed with metal staples, these will be removed by the doctor on the second or third day. There is little or no discomfort in having the staples removed. Many women see their incisions for the first time when stitches are removed. There may be some dry blood caked around the stitches, but these superficial scabs will fall off soon. Bruises around the incision will disappear in a few weeks, like any other bruise. The incision will look red and "angry," and the sight of it may be upsetting, but it can help to remember that the scar will eventually fade to a thin, white line like any other scar from a clean cut.

Some women also develop "spinal headaches." These are very uncomfortable—Laura described hers as "the worst headache I ever had." Drinking plenty of fluids will help, since the ultimate solution to the problem is replacement of the spinal fluid that has leaked through the puncture. Until the headaches stop, the best way to relieve them is to lie down. Unfortunately, it is not possible to lie down all the time. Pain medications also help. Most spinal headaches disappear after a few days, but Laura's lasted 3 months. She said simply, "I used cold compresses and toughed it out."

Recovery at Home

Leaving the Hospital

Before a cesarean mother is sent home, she will have a complete physical examination. There should be no signs of infection in her lungs, her uterus, her bladder, or her incision. Often, this last examination is done the day before she leaves. The time of the last examination is a good time to bring up questions. Here are some issues you might want to discuss with your doctor:

- Ask the doctor about any symptoms that have been bothering you. Ask what can usually be expected as you recover.
- If there has not been a chance earlier, ask the doctor to explain why an unanticipated surgery was necessary. If surgery was planned, but not everything went according to plan, ask why. Ask about any aspect of the surgery that continues to trouble you. Some possible questions are, Why was it necessary for me to have the type of anesthesia I had? Why did I have a vertical incision? I expected my husband to be with me all the time, what happened? Perhaps some of the answers will be unsatisfactory, but others may help you feel better. For example, you may feel that your doctor gave you a vertical incision because it was easier, and may appreciate learning that the incision was necessary because the baby was in transverse presentation.
- Ask the doctor to explain any prescriptions—why the prescription is necessary, how long to continue taking medication, and what side effects to expect. Sometimes a doctor will order a partial prescription from the hospital pharmacy, to be refilled later at a more inexpensive one. If your prescription is not what you expected, call your doctor's office and find out whether it needs to be changed or refilled.

- Discuss whether you will need physical therapy or additional attendant care. Get a written prescription if necessary. You may not be given the prescription until you leave the hospital.
- If you will need a wheelchair or an assistive device such as a cane, and your insurance will help to pay for it, ask for a prescription.
- Ask the doctor if s/he has any special instructions for you, such as restrictions on activity, or danger signs to watch for (we say more about this below). Ask when you can resume restricted activities.
- Find out when you should schedule your next visit to the doctor.

There may be quite a few details to take care of on the last morning: Packing the mother's and baby's possessions, doing some final paperwork, collecting prescriptions and doctor's instructions, getting the baby from the nursery. Usually it works best to have the driver carry luggage to the car, get the baby's car-seat ready, then, when all is ready, drive around to the hospital entrance to pick up mother and baby. Most likely a nurse will take the mother and baby to the exit in a wheelchair. In some hospitals, the mother's identification bracelet is removed just when she is about to leave—a ceremony that may remind her of a ship being launched!

Home Care

Once she is home, it is important for the mother to take good care of herself. Certainly the same is true for any new mother, but remember that a cesarean mother is a new mother who is *also recovering from surgery*. It is especially important for her to balance infant care and mild exercise with plenty of rest.

Many doctors suggest some type of restriction on the mother's activity at least until the first office visit. For example, your doctor may advise you not to drive, not to lift heavy objects, not to climb stairs too often, or to avoid bending and lifting. It is important to follow this advice; the mother who pushes herself too hard will suffer more pain and fatigue in the long run. Different people find different ways to follow this advice. For example, people who live in a two-story house might put an ice chest and hot plate for snacks in the bedroom, or set the mother up on the guest bed in the living room. If you had a low, old-fashioned cradle ready for the baby, you might borrow a friend's bassinet.

There is still a chance that uterine bleeding or infection will occur, although the chance is smaller with each passing day. Watch for these warning signs:

- *Increased lower abdominal pain.*
- *Pain, swelling, or oozing in the area of the incision.* Women who have lost sensation in this area should ask their attendants to inspect the incision when bathing them. Remember that the lower abdominal muscles and the

incision are still uncomfortable. Muscles can get sore from too much work. The incision will hurt more if you bump into a piece of furniture or a toddler jumps into your lap. Remember, too, that the uterus contracts occasionally for a few weeks after the birth, and that these contractions are sometimes stimulated by breastfeeding. You should watch for unexplained or persistent pain, or increased discomfort.

• *Change in vaginal bleeding.* All women have a discharge called *lochia* for several weeks after giving birth. If the amount of discharge increases or its color darkens, you should report the change to your doctor.

• *Fever.* If you feel hot and feverish, take your temperature. If it is higher than 100.0°F, call the doctor or, if you do not have a regular doctor, call an emergency room. Some women have a temperature that is usually lower than the normal 98.6°F. They should call their doctors if their temperature goes higher than what is normal for them.

Some women develop bladder or urinary tract infections even after they leave the hospital. Any of these signs of bladder infection justifies a call to the doctor:

• Fever.
• Frequent urination (urinating more frequently than at the time of discharge from the hospital).
• Often feeling the urge to urinate, then being unable to pass urine or only passing a few drops.
• Painful burning when urinating.

The incision should gradually become less sore and tender during the first few weeks after surgery. Wearing loose, airy clothes, with elastic at waist level (not hip level), will be more comfortable. Many women are uncomfortable with sanitary belts and feel more comfortable with the kind of sanitary napkin that sticks to the inside of the panties. Do not use tampons without your doctor's permission. Occasionally the incision will itch, sometimes intensely, but some itching now and then is a sign of healing. After 4 to 6 weeks have passed, the area around the incision will no longer be sore, but it may be slightly numb.

Drinking plenty of fluids continues to be important, especially if you are breast-feeding. Fluids are important for the same reasons given above: replacing blood lost during surgery, making up for fluids lost in milk production, and preventing bladder infection and constipation. A well-balanced diet also contributes to recovery. Complicated cooking will be too much of a challenge—just remember to eat simple, nutritious foods and to snack on fruits and vegetables instead of junk food. Eating plenty of fruits and vegetables also helps to prevent constipation, which is important because straining in the bathroom continues to be very uncomfortable.

Because the abdominal muscles have been stretched by pregnancy, then injured by surgery, mobility will be affected. Other muscles, particularly the muscles of the lower back, may become sore from the strain of doing the work usually done by the abdominal muscles. Rest and heat are good for any sore muscles, including abdominal muscles. Women with physical disabilities may need to work with an occupational or physical therapist to find alternate ways of moving, transferring, and doing household tasks. Some women may need to use a wheelchair or crutches temporarily. This may be upsetting, but it can help to remember that the change is only temporary.

As strength and mobility improve, beginning some gentle abdominal exercises can help recovery. Your doctor can help decide when it is safe to begin exercising.

EMOTIONAL EFFECTS OF CESAREAN BIRTH

Women respond to cesarean birth with a variety of emotions. The same woman can feel different emotions at different times: at one moment, excited because she has given birth; at another moment, frustrated by her helplessness; and at still another moment, depressed by pain and fatigue. Women may feel upset about having had surgery, or they may be concerned about their babies' welfare.

Some negative feelings are unavoidable. When we describe negative feelings women have had, we do not mean to suggest that anyone *should* have these feelings. We describe these feelings so that women reading about them can recognize that they are not alone. We do not believe that women who have cesarean deliveries are "failures"; we do hope that women can be helped to overcome such feelings by knowing that other women share them.

A number of factors influence women's feelings about cesarean birth: the type of anesthesia used, whether the surgery was anticipated or unanticipated, whether the mother felt she had a part in the decision to use surgery, the presence or absence of a support person, the reactions of people important to the mother, and the physical effects of surgery.

Women who did not anticipate cesarean birth often feel disappointment. They may feel disappointed in themselves for "failing" to give birth vaginally, or because they had looked forward to a certain kind of experience. Women who expected a cesarean birth may not be entirely happy about it, but they have had time to adjust to the idea and prepare for the experience. Faith, who had not expected to give birth surgically, felt "robbed," while Heather said, "I was emotionally prepared." Julie was glad she had attended a C-section class because "they eliminated most of my fears. I was mentally prepared for surgery." Hilary commented that because she took classes, "I knew all along what to expect." Learning about cesarean section beforehand may not be completely reassuring. Athina carefully discussed all of her concerns with her doctor, but still felt anxious just before her surgery.

Even though classes cannot eliminate all fears, they are helpful. We agree with the recommendation that *all* women take such classes, because a woman who knows what to expect during and after surgery is better prepared to cope with an unanticipated cesarean. Support people should also attend these classes, for two reasons:

1. Those hospitals which allow a support person to be present during surgery usually require him or her to take the class.
2. The class will prepare him or her to give the mother the help she needs after surgery.

The cesarean class also prepares women to take part in the decision to have surgery. Stephanie did not feel upset about having had surgery because she felt involved in the decision and, she added, "I am a pragmatic person. Besides, my labor was *very* uncomfortable."

Whether or not surgery was anticipated, concern for their babies' safety may counteract women's negative feelings about surgery. For example, Laura said, "I was disappointed I couldn't go natural, but I was glad the baby was alive." Julie, too, said, "I just thanked God I was alive and the baby was alive."

According to some studies, women who have regional anesthesia feel more positive about cesarean birth than women who have general anesthesia. This result is not surprising, since women who have general anesthesia miss the experience of seeing their babies' births. Hilary and Sybil shared these feelings: Sybil said, "I didn't feel good about the C-section because I wanted to see my baby, like any other mother." Hilary, who had hoped to use hypnosis instead of anesthesia, said, "When I woke up I was frustrated and all I could do was cry. I didn't feel anything negative about having a C-section. It was just that I wanted to see the baby being born." Still, most of the women we interviewed were not very concerned about what kind of anesthesia they had. Eight out of the 14 women had general anesthesia, yet only three said they were disappointed. Some pointed out that general anesthesia was needed for a specific reason, like Stephanie, who explained, "They were unsure how a spinal would react with my spinal cord injury."

Julie was not disappointed, but she wondered whether she could have prevented her adverse reaction to the anesthesia. Julie had taken her cesarean class late and went into labor before she had time to talk to an anesthesiologist. She said, "I experienced a lot of pain, not only in my abdomen—my jaw and muscles were sore and weak. It's really important to find an anesthesiologist prior to surgery so s/he knows your body." Faith, who said, "Next time I would make sure I could get a spinal," added, "I wish I had talked to the right people."

For other women, the physical effects of surgery are upsetting. They may be frustrated by helplessness and immobility, or by feeling more pain than they expected. Pain tends to intensify other negative feelings as well. Some women were also upset by the way pain or loss of mobility affected their ability to care for their babies. Stephanie said, "The pain was so uncomfortable that I didn't want to see my baby. I was not disappointed about the cesarean. I just wanted to feel better to enjoy my baby." Carla said, "I had postpartum depression because I couldn't move or do anything with my body. I had difficulty turning over. I had loss of mobility and couldn't see my baby." (We suspect that Carla simply meant that she was very sad, and that she did not have the syndrome psychiatrists describe as postpartum depression.) Heather compared her feelings about her two birth experiences in terms of her relationship to her baby: "The hospital staff didn't leave me alone with my first baby until I had my balance back. It was very different with my second. I had rooming in within eighteen hours of surgery, so I wasn't as upset."

A woman's feelings about being separated from her baby can be influenced by the attitudes and behavior of the hospital staff. One of Judi's students has never forgotten her annoyance about a nurse who, without asking about her abilities, told her, "We can't let you carry the baby because, if you dropped it and it was hurt, the hospital might get sued." A supportive staff can relieve the mother's frustration and help her cope with practical difficulties. Sybil's painful memories were softened by recalling the nurse who helped her hold her baby. Athina was in intensive care because her disability causes breathing problems and her doctor wanted to make sure that she did not develop pneumonia after surgery. She was able to have her baby brought to her and found that she could nurse lying on her side, supported by pillows.

Although the mother may be separated from her baby for only a few days, that separation can be very painful. It is important for hospital staff to remember that a disabled woman feels as much need to spend time with her baby as an able-bodied woman, and she may be able to do more for her baby than they realize. Flexibility and imagination are important: Perhaps an obstetric nurse can simply ask nursery staff to bring the baby to cuddle with the mother when it is sleeping, and put up the sides of the mother's bed to protect the baby. The baby's father or a friend can help by arranging to be at the hospital to help while the baby visits the mother.

Perhaps the most painful situations are those in which the mother is anxious about her baby's welfare. Carla recalls, "I went crazy when I couldn't see my baby for a whole day because I was too groggy. I needed to know if my baby was normal." For a woman in Carla's situation, reassurance is important. Perhaps the best help a friend can give her is to leave her long enough to check on the baby, if only to look through the nursery window, then come back to tell her, "Your baby is fine."

Julie spoke for many women when she said, "I was concerned because the baby was so drugged that he couldn't respond." It is helpful to remember that a sleepy baby is not necessarily in trouble. The after effects of anesthesia or, later, pain medications in the mother's milk, can make the baby sleepier, but these effects are temporary, just as they are for the mother. Any newborn baby spends a lot of time sleeping, and this normal pattern can contribute to the mother's feeling that the baby is "dopey." If the hospital staff feel comfortable bringing the baby to the mother, she can relax and enjoy the baby—s/he will be waking the parents up during the night soon enough!

Sometimes the mother is anxious because her baby really is ill. For some women, concern about the baby is an incentive to "get it together." Pam's baby was born one month early and, because he was premature, he was depressed by the anesthesia. Pam commented, "I had to keep my wits about me, because I was very concerned about my son." For other women, worry about the baby is overwhelming. Leslie, whose baby was premature, recalled, "I was anxious about the baby. He was transferred to another hospital. It was hard for me to get out of bed because I wasn't motivated."

Again, anything the hospital staff can do to help the mother spend time with her baby can be very helpful. It is important for the mother to know that her relationship with her baby is appreciated, and an effort is being made to help her be with him. When her daughter needed intensive care, Laura could not hold her for 4 days. Still, Laura felt that "the hospital worked in a humanitarian fashion" because "they made sure I saw my child 98% of the time. They made sure I didn't go it alone, especially since I didn't have any husband."

Meanwhile, it is important for the mother to remember that by taking care of herself, she *is* helping her baby. Whether doing breathing exercises, or resting when necessary, everything she does to further her own recovery prepares her to care for her baby. Friends can help in a number of practical ways, such as donating blood if the baby needs transfusions, contacting a La Leche League milk bank to get breast milk for the baby, helping to contact cesarean support groups or support groups for parents of ill children, or finding books about caring for premature babies. The mother feels less helpless when receiving this kind of practical support.

VAGINAL BIRTH AFTER CESAREAN SECTION

For many years, "Once a C-section, always a C-section," was a standing rule. So, for example, Portia had five children born by cesarean surgery. In the early 1950s, the first studies were performed which suggested that vaginal birth after cesarean ("VBAC") can be as safe as repeat cesarean birth. Additional studies in the 1960s and 1970s confirmed this finding. The increasing use of transverse incisions contributed to the safety of VBACs, since the scar from a transverse incision is less likely to rupture during labor than the scar from a classical incision.

While there is still some controversy about the safety of VBAC, more and more doctors and hospitals are willing to discuss it with women who want to try it. That does not mean a hospital or doctor willing to attempt VBAC will automatically agree to try it with any woman who asks. Faith belonged to a prepaid health plan which had a policy of considering every woman who had had a cesarean birth as a candidate for vaginal birth. Yet when Faith wanted a vaginal birth, her doctors were reluctant to agree to a trial of labor.

The three most important factors affecting a decision to allow VBAC are as follows:

1. *The nature of the uterine incision.* As we said above, a classical (high vertical) incision is somewhat more likely to rupture than a low transverse or vertical incision. A decision to try VBAC may be altered during the course of pregnancy, or even after labor begins, if there are signs that the incision could rupture.
2. *The reason for the original surgery.* Perhaps the original indication for surgery is one that is unlikely to be repeated during a later pregnancy. For example, cord prolapse or placenta previa will not necessarily occur again. If the original indication is not present, the mother can try labor and, if no problems occur, she can give birth vaginally. If the indication for surgery was fetopelvic disproportion, a woman interested in VBAC would do well to look for a doctor willing to work with her. Women have been known to give vaginal birth to babies larger than those that had needed surgical delivery.
3. *The mother's current health and current obstetric considerations.* A problem could arise that is completely different from the one that made a previous labor difficult. For example, a woman might need surgery because of cord prolapse during one labor, and because of fetal distress during another.

Clearly, many women with disabilities will not be candidates for VBAC. Many disability indications, such as pelvic deformity or breathing difficulties, will not change from one pregnancy to the next. However, a disabled woman who had surgery for obstetric reasons may want to try VBAC.

Two women interviewed for this book had vaginal birth after cesarean surgery. Their experiences were different, and the contrasts are interesting. Faith had surgery because her first labor was not progressing. She had only labored for 8 hours, and she felt that she might have given birth vaginally if she had been allowed to labor longer. She knows that many women are allowed to labor longer, and had the impression that her doctor overreacted to her disability. She was very interested in vaginal birth because "that's the normal way to have a baby." She added, "The C-section was so awful physically that to me it was worth it to try a vaginal birth."

When doctors at Faith's prepaid health plan expressed their reluctance to try a vaginal birth, she decided "it would be less of a hassle to get my prenatal care there and have the baby someplace else." Faith found a teaching hospital where she could have a trial labor. She said, "The doctors thought I would have a slim chance. They said, 'You're the one who will have to deal with the pain.' However, they didn't think of the pain I would have after surgery." Two weeks before her due date, Faith wrote a letter explaining her reasons for wanting a vaginal birth, and her doctors agreed to try.

Faith succeeded in giving birth vaginally, and was glad she had done so. She explained, "I bounced back in three or four weeks with my second baby—it took three or four *months* after the C-section. With the C-section, the medication affected my balance and gave me a foggy head. Then there was the pain. I was really run down the first month. All that made it quite difficult to take care of the baby."

Leslie's experience was very different from Faith's. She, too, wanted to try VBAC because she felt that it is normal to give birth vaginally. Leslie had needed surgery because her baby was in a transverse presentation, and she knew she was not likely to have that problem again. She had no problem convincing her doctor to allow her to deliver vaginally. Her doctor simply told her, "It's important for me to be around when you're in labor."

When Leslie had her second child, she had a cervical laceration, so, unlike Faith, she felt that vaginal birth was more painful than cesarean birth. For Leslie, recovery from vaginal birth was just as difficult as recovery from surgical birth. She had uterine infections after both births, and blood loss and lupus flare-up made recovery from the second (vaginal) birth difficult. Still, Leslie was glad to give birth vaginally because she felt "it was important to feel a part of the birth process."

CLOSING COMMENTS
· ·

One approach to Cesarean delivery involves evaluating the appropriateness of this procedure in a general sense. This perspective involves asking such questions as, "How often should this procedure be performed?" "Does the increase in the Cesarean birth rate reflect a proper balance of concern for the mother and the baby?" "When should this procedure be used?" These questions sometimes generate controversies that can be rather worrisome to the prospective mother. Yet the search for their answers can develop information that is useful for individualized decision-making.

The second approach is that of the individual, of the woman who wonders, "What should I do, what is the best way for me to give birth?" and the doctor asking, "What is the best way to care for my patient?" From this perspective, one cannot absolutely say that either Cesarean or vaginal delivery is "better." Instead, there must be a choice as to which is most appropriate in a particular situation.

Yet, even when a woman believes that Cesarean delivery was appropriate, even when the circumstances included good communication with her doctor and plenty of time to make a decision—she may feel disappointed. These feelings, too, may depend on a particular perspective. During pregnancy, and just afterward, childbirth does not seem like a beginning, but an end—the climax of nine months of planning, anticipation, and anxiety. Having a "perfect" childbirth experience can seem very important, and to many, Cesarean delivery is a less than ideal ending.

Yet childbirth is only a beginning, and a very brief beginning. The great majority of labors, whether they end in Cesarean or vaginal delivery, last less than a day, while pregnancy lasts about 280 days and parenthood goes on forever. Most women find, as time goes by, that the way they gave birth seems unimportant in comparison to the cares and joys of mothering.

Leslie's final comment on her birth experiences makes the perfect closing to a chapter about Cesarean birth. She said, "I was pleased and excited to have both kids and in the end it didn't matter."

9 BACK TO NORMAL—
THE POSTPARTUM PERIOD

· ·

During the weeks following childbirth, the mother's body returns to its pre-pregnant condition. In a sense, these weeks are the final phase of pregnancy, a phase commonly called the *postpartum period,* meaning after the birth. It is traditionally considered to last 6 weeks, but can last longer for some women.

Many first-time mothers look forward to the end of pregnancy as a time when life goes back to normal. But any woman who has already had a child can tell them that life never goes back to the way it was before you were pregnant. The new mother experiences many changes in her emotions and her relationships during this time. Just as her body gradually changed and adapted during pregnancy, the return to a non-pregnant condition is a gradual process accompanied by a number of physical symptoms. In this chapter, we will discuss the following topics:

- Medical care in the hospital, and postpartum office visits.
- Physical changes, self-care, and postpartum complications.
- Emotional changes, including "postpartum depression."
- Sexuality and birth control.
- Breast feeding: The choice between breast feeding and bottle feeding, suggestions for breast care, the art of breast feeding, and combining breast and bottle feeding
- Suggestions disabled women can use in caring for infants.

311

MEDICAL CARE

Hospital Care

Alternative Birth Center

A woman who gives birth in an alternative birth center (ABC) will leave the hospital in less than a day. In some hospitals she may stay for up to 8 hours; in others, she can stay for as long as 12 hours. If she needs to stay longer, she will be moved to another room in the hospital (and there will be an additional charge).

After giving birth, a woman may want to use her remaining time in the ABC for resting or sleeping. She will not necessarily be asked to exercise, but she will be encouraged to use the bathroom. In fact, she must urinate at least once before she can leave. If she cannot urinate, she may have to be transferred to another part of the hospital. Her nurses will also check her temperature, pulse, and blood pressure at least once before she leaves. They will also check for bleeding, and feel her abdomen to make sure that her uterus has begun to involute. The perineal area may be swollen, even if there was no episiotomy. If there is swelling, the nurses will apply an ice pack to reduce the swelling and keep the area more comfortable. Many nurses also help a new mother with her first attempts to nurse her baby.

A pediatrician will examine the baby, and the obstetrician may visit as well. If the obstetrician visits, take this opportunity to ask any questions you have about self-care, and ask when to schedule your next appointment. Otherwise, call your doctor's office when you get home.

Your nurses can also give you advice before you leave, and they may have written information to give you. The nurses may offer you a kit to take home. You may want to ask what is in it and whether there is an extra charge, because the kit may contain items you already have at home (like a thermometer), and you may prefer not to pay for it. Do take some peri-pads; they are more absorbent than ordinary sanitary napkins, and will be very handy for the first few days after the birth.

Many alternative birth center programs include a home visit by a nurse 3 days after the birth. Usually, the nurse will be the same person who attended the birth. Some pediatricians are willing to make a similar visit. When looking for a pediatrician who will visit the hospital to examine the baby after birth, ask whether s/he is also willing to make home visits.

The Hospital Stay

A postpartum hospital stay usually lasts no more than three days, although women who develop complications, such as infections, may need to stay longer.

During this period, medical staff normally provide routine medical care, assistance with recovery from childbirth, and help with baby care and breast feeding. Since much of what nurses do to assist recovery may also be useful at home (for example, using ice packs to reduce perineal swelling), we will describe this aspect of care in the section describing normal physical changes.

Routine medical care includes checking blood pressure, pulse, and temperature. Changes in these vital signs can be the first indication of infection or other complications. Medical staff will also occasionally check the abdomen to assess the condition of the uterus, and examine the genitals for swelling and signs of bleeding or infection. Nurses will encourage the new mother to urinate, and may ask her to use a bedpan, or a "catcher" on the toilet, to measure the amount of urine produced. While the obstetrician will do an examination and answer any questions during his/her visit, nurses are also a link with the physician. For example, if a woman develops symptoms of infection, a nurse will telephone the doctor, describe the symptoms, and follow the doctor's instructions in giving medications or arranging for tests until the doctor can perform an examination.

Maternity nurses are a good source of advice and help in coping with postpartum physical changes, such as constipation. Nurses will also help with infant care. For example, they will show a first-time mother how to diaper or breast feed her baby. This kind of support and encouragement from the nurses can make a new mother feel much more comfortable about caring for her baby. The emotional support nurses give is important, too. Sibyl recalled, "The nurse in the recovery room was good. She was excited for me. She made me feel really good."

Many women will find that their postpartum hospital stay is different from their other hospital experiences. Rather than give intensive care to a few patients, as rehabilitation nurses do, obstetric nurses give more generalized care to many patients. Maternity nurses are responsible for caring for women who are recovering from cesarean surgery and helping women cope with postpartum discomforts. Their responsibilities do not usually include caring for the particular needs of women with disabilities. For example, helping a paralyzed woman change position several times a day is not within the usual responsibilities of an obstetric nurse.

The difference in nursing care made some women feel they did not have all the help they needed. Looking back on her hospital stay, Celeste said she would advise nurses to "be aware that a disabled woman may need more time and more involvement than other new mothers. Be patient and more understanding. I had trouble with nursing because I was left alone with my baby. Stay around and see if the woman needs extra help, or extra support." On the other hand, some women have felt that their nurses offered more help than necessary. Clara said, "*Ask* the woman if she needs help before you give it, both during labor and postpartum." Clearly, good communication between the disabled mother and the nursing staff is important. If they take time to discuss special concerns, they will have a more cooperative relationship, and nurses will be able to work more efficiently and with a better understanding of your particular needs.

The difference in viewpoints between disabled mothers and their nurses can lead to misunderstandings. One such misunderstanding occurred when Sharon, who had used an indwelling catheter when she was pregnant, began to catheterize herself again in the hospital. Sharon was annoyed when a nurse criticized her technique. She said afterwards, "The nurse was so certain she was right and I didn't know anything. I don't have to use the same sterile technique a nurse uses. I'd probably been cathing myself more years than she was a nurse." Sharon and her nurse were both right: Many rehabilitation units do teach a clean method of self-catheterization which is not sterile but is adequate for use at home. However, in a hospital setting, sterile technique is important in preventing nosocomial infection (infection acquired in the hospital, where there may be germs which are resistant to many antibiotics).

Other misunderstandings can occur when obstetric nurses are not familiar with the particular skills and problems of women with disabilities. These misunderstandings can be quite painful to the disabled mother. A disabled student in Judith's birthing class recalled, "They wouldn't leave my baby alone with me. They told me, 'If you drop your baby, we might get sued.' They could have asked me how I planned to carry the baby." Marsha, who had had problems with incontinence while she was pregnant, continued to have problems after her catheter was removed in the hospital. Marsha said, "Some of my nurses got impatient or angry when I wet the bed. They seemed to think I wasn't bothering to get out of bed, when it was really an MS problem. I wasn't happy about it, either!"

It is important to find ways to improve communication between disabled mothers and their nurses. Some women suggested that, before the disabled woman gives birth, her nurses receive special training. Hilary said, "The obstetrician... [could] have a meeting with the hospital staff to coordinate plans." Jennifer suggested that nurses could "have sensitivity training in dealing with disabled persons."

A rehabilitation nurse could help coordinate planning before birth, or consult with maternity nurses after birth. Besides explaining the kind of special care a disabled mother might need, the rehabilitation nurse can suggest solutions for particular problems. For example, s/he can show nurses how to use a local anesthetic jelly to avoid stimulating hyperreflexia when inserting a catheter, or how to help a patient transfer without incurring back strain. A rehabilitation nurse could have helped Marsha's nurses find ways to cope with her incontinence. They might have given Marsha absorbent underwear, or borrowed a mattress protector from the nursery and placed it under her hips. (A mattress protector is absorbent material with waterproof backing. It will keep sheets dry.) A rehabilitation nurse could also help staff to decide when to "bend the rules," as Laura, Heather, and Jennifer suggested.

Other health professionals might also need to become involved. For example, an occupational therapist can help to find ways the mother can care for her baby. A physical or occupational therapist can help provide passive exercise for the prevention of thrombophlebitis (blood clots in the veins) in women who have spinal cord dysfunctions.

Some women suggest that extra help should be available. Stephanie said, "Make sure the hospital lets the husband room with the mother. They shouldn't just allow it, they should encourage it, because he can be such a big help. Some hospital rules really make life more difficult than it has to be." Since hiring a special-duty nurse, or arranging for a private room where the husband can "room in," are expenses that may not be covered by the mother's insurance, the hospital's social worker may need to participate in planning for special care.

Leaving the Hospital

Before you leave the hospital, your doctor will visit you and do a brief physical examination. It is important to discuss the doctor's recommendations for your care before your first postpartum office visit. Ask about medications your doctor prescribes, and be sure to ask how long you should continue taking them. Sometimes doctors prescribe only a small amount of medication that is dispensed by the hospital pharmacy, so that the mother can refill the prescription at lower cost at her own pharmacy.

It is important to discuss the possibility that you will experience pregnancy complications, or remission or exacerbation of disability symptoms.

The relationship between pregnancy and exacerbation of autoimmune diseases is the subject of a number of studies. Some studies have found a tendency for myasthenia gravis to improve in the postpartum period, others have found a tendency towards exacerbation. An individual woman needs to be aware that she *might* have an exacerbation. While the long-term course of MS does not appear to be affected by pregnancy, women are especially vulnerable to exacerbation postpartum, even more than during pregnancy. Symptoms of SLE may become worse, also. It might be more accurate to say that remission of rheumatoid arthritis ends with pregnancy, than to say that an exacerbation takes place; pain and stiffness do get worse.

Women who have spinal cord dysfunctions usually find that their bladder control returns to whatever was normal for them before pregnancy. However, they are more susceptible to anemia, blood clots, and urinary infections in the postpartum period.

Ask your doctor what signs and symptoms you should watch for, whether to call your obstetrician or your disability specialist when symptoms appear, and what tests might be done to differentiate between disability exacerbation and postpartum complications.

Office Visits

The first office visit takes place 3–6 weeks after the birth. If all is well at this time, it may not be necessary to see the doctor again until it is time for a yearly checkup. During this first visit, the doctor will do a general physical examination, ask a number of questions about how the mother is doing, and answer any questions she may have. If the doctor is a family practitioner, consider scheduling a well-baby visit at the same time as the postpartum office visit. The postpartum office visit is also the best time to discuss birth control. The physical examination will include these procedures:

Routine checkup: The doctor will check blood pressure, temperature, weight, and heart and lungs. While blood pressure measurement is part of every routine examination, it is also important in choosing a birth control method. Since women with high blood pressure should not use hormones (birth-control pills or implants) for birth control, blood pressure must be checked before hormones can be prescribed.

Most women lose 17–20 pounds by the sixth week after giving birth (including a loss of about 10 pounds at the time of birth). Women who feel that they should have lost more weight can use the office visit to talk to their doctors about diet.

Temperature measurement is more than a matter of routine, because a high temperature may be a sign of postpartum infection.

Breast examination: The breasts will be examined for any abnormalities, masses (lumps or cysts), tenderness, or signs of infection. Women who are breast feeding may want to ask questions about breast care at this time.

Examination of vagina and uterus: The size of the uterus is assessed. The uterus should be reducing at a normal rate. It should be close to pre-pregnant size by 6 weeks after the birth. The vagina and cervix will be examined. The cervix should be closing. If there were lacerations of the vagina or cervix, the doctor will inspect them to see that they are healing well. The doctor will assess the type and amount of discharge from the uterus, since discolored lochia, or too much lochia, can indicate infection or a retained placenta. (Lochia is defined in"Normal Physical Changes" below.) If the flow of lochia has stopped (it should have stopped by the fourth week afterbirth), the doctor will do a routine Pap smear.

Perineum: If there was a tear or an episiotomy, the perineum will be examined to assure that it is healing well.

Rectal examination: This examination is done as part of a general health assessment, checking for the presence of hemorrhoids, and, when necessary, checking that lacerations are healing.

Calves: The calves are examined for any signs of thrombophlebitis (blood clots).

Blood test: Some doctors routinely test for anemia during the first postpartum visit. Others test only if the mother is very tired, or if she had been anemic during pregnancy.

Evaluation of special health problems: Any special health problems that occurred during pregnancy are evaluated—for example, varicose veins or diabetes of pregnancy.

The doctor will ask questions about how the mother is feeling, both physically and emotionally. Some answers will help the doctor assess the mother's health, some will help the doctor decide if she needs advice about particular problems, and others will help in choosing the best birth-control method. The conversation will indicate whether the mother is feeling generally happy, has a temporary case of the "baby blues," or has postpartum depression. The doctor will also answer any questions the mother may have. You may want to ask some of the following questions:

When can my husband and I make love again? One family practitioner told us, "That is the most popular question." The doctor's reply will depend on how well the mother is healing. Most women can resume lovemaking within 3–6 weeks after giving birth.

What can I do about discomfort during lovemaking? (This is discussed in the section entitled "Normal Physical Changes.")

What family-planning method should I use? (Birth control is discussed in detail in a later section of this chapter.)

What about my diet? Women who want to lose or gain weight should use the office visit to talk to their doctors about diet. It is important to follow a nutritious diet even while losing weight, especially for women who are breast-feeding or who are anemic. Many people worry that doctors do not know about nutrition, but in recent years this aspect of medical education has been improved. Also, many physicians employ a dietitian or a nurse with special training in nutrition; others will make a referral to a dietitian.

Questions in the following areas are more individual in nature:

Questions about breast care: A common question is, *What can I do about sore nipples?* We give information about breast care in the sections on physical changes and breast feeding, but it is a good idea to discuss any concerns with your doctor. If your doctor is a family practitioner, you can also discuss breast feeding in terms of your baby's needs.

Questions about individual problems: These questions will be different for different women. One woman may be bothered by fatigue, another by constipation. Another may ask, *Now that I've had my baby, shouldn't I update my vaccinations?*

Questions about medication: If medication was stopped during pregnancy, it may be started again after birth. Women who are breast feeding need to discuss this with their doctors, since many medications pass into breast milk. Be sure to discuss all possibilities: Perhaps one medication was substituted for another during pregnancy, and it may be desirable to change back to the original medication. Or, like Sylvia, a woman may find that she is more comfortable with a medication she started during pregnancy, and she may want to ask her doctor about continuing with it. Discuss whether the dose might be changed. Will it be necessary to see the doctor again, or call the doctor to discuss the dosage? Sometimes the dosage is based on a person's weight, so the dose will be changed with the weight loss after pregnancy.

Some women may hope to discontinue medications, but they must consult their doctors first. Many doctors prescribe corticosteroid or other anti-inflammatories to prevent SLE exacerbation, especially if symptoms were severe before pregnancy. Some women who have SLE need immunosuppressive medications during pregnancy, and the dosage should not be lowered abruptly.

Questions about rehabilitation: If disability symptoms worsened during pregnancy, it may be possible to make some improvements after pregnancy is completed. For example, if weakened abdominal muscles have affected mobility, you can discuss an exercise program or consider physical therapy. If your baby was delivered by an obstetrician, you may have to discuss some questions with your family doctor, your disability specialist, or another specialist.

Questions about other prescriptions or referrals: You may need a signed recommendation from your doctor to get some help you need, such as increased attendant care, an assistive device, special medications, or temporary changes in medical or disability benefits. If you are not able to bring forms from your social worker or insurance company when you go to the doctor's office, your doctor may be able to obtain the forms for you, or tell you what you will need.

You may wish to ask the doctor one last time whether there are other issues you need to discuss.

NORMAL PHYSICAL CHANGES

All the body systems that changed during pregnancy, change again after birth. Here we discuss the normal changes and minor problems that women experience, and ways to cope with them. In the next section, "Postpartum Complications," we describe the more severe problems that can develop during the weeks after birth.

Generalized Changes

The two changes that are most noticeable to many new mothers are weight loss and fatigue.

Weight Loss

While a woman who has just given birth often finds that she still *looks* pregnant, the scales tell a different story. When giving birth, she loses approximately 12 pounds in a matter of hours. During the week after birth, she loses another 3–6 pounds as her body sheds extra fluids retained during pregnancy. She may lose a few more pounds during the following weeks. Although many women are pleased to lose some weight after they are pregnant, they should not plan to restrict their diets during the postpartum period, as we will explain below. Women who are concerned that they are losing too much or too little weight should discuss their concerns with their doctors during their postpartum office visit.

Fatigue

Many people feel tired during late pregnancy, but fatigue is often more of a problem during the postpartum period. Ask any woman what she remembers about the weeks after she gave birth, and she is likely to tell you how tired she was. A new mother feels exhausted, and while it may be hard to believe that her exhaustion is normal, it usually is. There are many reasons the new mother feels so tired:

The birth process: Like other kinds of strenuous exercise, the work of giving birth can make a woman feel tired for days afterwards. (The birth process is not called labor without reason.)

The new infant: The effort of caring for a new infant can be tiring.

Emotional stress: Emotional stress causes fatigue. It is important to remember that any life change, even the joy one feels at having a new baby, can be stressful. And there may be painful changes as well, such as coping with a jealous sibling or feeling frustration about unfinished housework. We will say more about emotional changes in a later section.

Sleep loss: Newborn babies have very irregular sleep patterns. Being awakened by the baby several times a night is a major cause of fatigue.

Anemia: Fatigue may be a symptom of anemia. Even minor blood loss associated with birth can lead to anemia. And there is always some bleeding from the site where the placenta was attached, even if there are no other cuts or tears.

Knowing the causes of fatigue suggests some simple solutions: get help, eat well, and get plenty of rest. Many women feel uncomfortable about taking the rest they need. They worry about unfinished chores, or fear that they are babying themselves. It is important to remember that a spot on the bathroom mirror, or some unfolded laundry, cannot make anyone sick, but lack of rest can. Also, someone who is well rested can do her chores more easily and efficiently. Resting after childbirth is just as reasonable as resting after an athletic event.

As we discussed in Chapter 2, many disabled women have learned to cope by forcing themselves to ignore fatigue. Sometimes it is appropriate to cope that way, and sometimes it is not; the postpartum period is a good time to learn to use rest as a way of coping. While adequate exercise is important to postpartum recovery, adequate rest is equally important—each woman will need to find her own way to balance rest and exercise.

Good nutrition in the postpartum period is as important as it was during pregnancy. Women who are breast feeding will need to follow a diet similar to what they ate while pregnant, so that they will get enough nutrients to nourish themselves and to produce milk. Some women will need to eat iron-rich foods as their bodies replace blood lost during childbirth. All women will feel better if they follow a healthy, well-balanced diet. It is a good idea to ask your doctor about a vitamin supplement. If a postpartum blood test shows that you are anemic, your doctor will probably prescribe an iron supplement. Remember, though, while vitamins can *add* to a well-balanced diet, they cannot *replace* the variety of nutritious foods you need.

Often a new mother feels that there is no time to cook and eat the kind of food she needs. Yet, if she only snatches a snack here and an incomplete meal there, she will feel even more tired and more unable to care for herself and her baby. Here are some tips for keeping well nourished:

Make meals a priority: When the baby is napping, it is tempting to take this opportunity to catch up on work. Eat (or rest) *first*, then take time for other tasks.

Take advantage of convenient appliances: If you cannot afford a microwave oven and/or a slow cooker, borrow them, or mention them to anyone who offers to give you a really special gift.

Cook simple meals: Save complicated recipes for a less hectic time.

Shop wisely: Begin in the produce and dairy sections of the store. Make it easy for yourself to have an apple or a tuna sandwich for a snack, rather than a doughnut!

Use some convenience foods: Frozen vegetables may not be as pleasing to some people as fresh vegetables, but frozen peas are better than peas growing moldy in the refrigerator because there is no time to shell them!

Cook ahead of time if possible: When making dishes like stews and casseroles, double the recipe. It takes just a little more time, and some food can be frozen for another day. Stephanie suggested cooking and freezing several meals *before* the baby is born.

Let others help: If asked, "What can I do to help?" tell your friend (or your husband), "Bring food!"

For many women, the help of others makes the difference between bearable fatigue and unbearable exhaustion. When Stacy was asked what advice she would give to other women, one of the first things she said was, "It is important to get help. Exhaustion was the main reason I was so depressed." Stephanie, who said "extra help is essential," paid for professional help with child care and housework. Margie commented, "After my first baby, I was so exhausted my MS got worse. The main problem was blurry vision. After my second baby, I made sure to get plenty of help, and my MS didn't flare up."

When arranging for help, think about your individual needs and the talents of the people offering to help. If someone offers to help with the baby, and you would prefer help with housework, say so. A friend who is good at sewing could adapt baby clothes so a mother with limited hand control can dress her baby; a friend with carpentry skills could lower a changing table to wheelchair height.

Some women may be able to get extra help through private insurance, Medicaid or disability insurance, or a local program providing home health care. A hospital social worker may be able to make arrangements before the new mother leaves for home, or her regular social worker may arrange a change of benefits. If a woman or her advocate checks with social workers before a scheduled visit to her doctor, she can bring the necessary forms to the office when she sees her doctor.

Sometimes fatigue is a sign of a physical or emotional problem. Since it is so common for women to be very tired during the weeks after birth, it is not always easy to tell when fatigue is a sign of other problems. No woman should hesitate to tell her doctor about her concerns. The new mother may simply need a few words of encouragement and a reminder to rest, or she may need tests or medication. If she has MS or myasthenia gravis, her doctor needs to determine that she is not experiencing a disease exacerbation. Her doctor must have complete information to know what she needs.

Preventing fatigue is especially important for women whose disabilities are exacerbated by fatigue (MS, SLE, myasthenia gravis). Mary recalled, "My doctor made a point of telling me to have my mother or my mother-in-law come help out so I wouldn't get too tired." She also decided to bottle-feed her baby, rather than risk getting tired out from breast feeding. Michelle, too, said she would advise women with MS to breast feed "as little as possible." (We will say more about this issue in the section entitled "Breast Feeding.")

Changes in Body Systems

The Uterus

After childbirth, the uterus returns to normal size in a process called involution. The inner surface of the uterus heals and materials left in the uterus after childbirth, such as bits of the amniotic sac, are shed in the discharge of lochia.

Uterine contractions do not end when the baby is born. They become weaker and less frequent, but they continue for up to a week and are felt as "afterpains." Some women feel so much discomfort from afterpains that they need to use the same breathing techniques they used during labor. Women who have had more than one child, or whose uterine muscles were stretched by a very large pregnancy, may feel stronger afterpains. Because oxytocin, the hormone that stimulates uterine contractions, is released when a baby suckles, many women have sharper afterpains while they are breast feeding. Sheila said, "When I nursed my baby I could feel the contractions and it made me feel better." (She felt better because she understood that nursing her baby was helping her uterus to recover.)

The temporary sharp pain of a uterine contraction feels different from the constant pain which is a sign of bleeding or infection. During the first few days after giving birth, a woman who is worried about uterine pain could reassure herself by placing her hand over her uterus to feel it contract, and then relax. A woman who still feels uterine pain more than a week after giving birth should call her doctor, since the pain could be a sign of infection.

During the first 2 days, the uterine fundus involutes to a level between the navel and the pubic hair. After about 6 weeks, the uterus returns to pre-pregnant size.

As the uterus involutes, the muscle contractions squeeze the blood vessels, so involution helps to stop bleeding from the placental wound. This blood, mucus, and other tissues make up the lochia. For the first 2–4 days, the flow of lochia will be dark reddish brown and comparatively heavy, like menstrual flow. There may be some small clots. For the next 4–5 days, the lochia grows paler, a brownish pink color. During the next week or two, it fades to a brownish white, then a yellowish white. The flow of pale yellow fluid may continue on and off for up to 6 weeks.

Always use sanitary napkins to absorb the lochia. Tampons should not be used because the uterus is vulnerable to infection. Unusual changes in the color, odor, or amount of lochia may be signs of renewed bleeding or infection. (The causes of excessive bleeding are discussed in the section entitled "Postpartum Complications.")

The Vagina

The vagina will be sore and stretched from the passage of the baby. Although the vaginal muscles regain some tone with the passage of time, they should be exercised to assure that they will become as firm as they were before pregnancy. Strong vaginal muscles are important not only for sexual satisfaction, but for long-term health. The Kegel exercises we described in Chapter 5 can be started the day after the baby is born. For the first few days, it will be enough to do a few gentle squeezes daily. In the days and weeks that follow, the number of repetitions can gradually increase. Many women cannot even feel their muscles moving at first, but if they keep exercising daily, they will notice the change in a few weeks. Some women find that the best way to make sure they do these exercises is to do them first thing in the morning, even before they open their eyes. Others do a few "Kegels" every time they use the bathroom.

The lining of the vagina will be thinner, drier, and more sensitive. These changes are caused by *prolactin,* a hormone involved in milk production. For most women, the change is not noticeable except during sexual intercourse, which may be uncomfortable. Women who do not breast-feed will find that the problem disappears in a few weeks, possibly before they start making love again. However, women who breast feed will continue to be sensitive for several months. Sometimes, doctors prescribe a cream containing estrogen which can be applied in the vagina. The estrogen (a hormone) causes the vaginal lining to grow thicker, but the amount in the cream is too small to affect breast milk. However, women who are susceptible to blood clots should discuss whether it is better not to use this cream. A water-based lubricant, such as K-Y Jelly, may be used as an alternative to make intercourse more comfortable. The spermicides used for birth control are also lubricating.

If there was an episiotomy or a tear in the perineum, this area will need special care. The perineum will be very sore at first, and there may be some itching as the wound heals. In the hospital or at home, an ice pack can be used for the first 24–36 hours. The ice pack should be waterproof, and wrapped in a clean, dry cloth. The cold will not only feel soothing, it will prevent or reduce swelling.

After the first day or so, heat can promote healing. An infrared heat lamp may be used in the hospital. A heat lamp used at home should have a timer as a safety feature to prevent burns. It can be used for 15 minutes, 3 times a day. Healing and comfort are also promoted by warm soaks, either in a very clean, partially filled bathtub or a sitz bath. (A sitz bath is a shallow pan which holds just enough water to cover the bottom and perineum. Usually it fits over the toilet bowl.) The sitz bath may be used 5–10 minutes at a time, several times a day. Clara recalled, "I always felt better after using the sitz bath." It is best to dry the perineum well after a warm soak.

Urination can be painful, since urine on the episiotomy wound stings. Jennifer said, "Whenever I urinated, I poured water over the episiotomy at the same time." Clara said, "I would put some warm water in the tub before I urinated, then get in the tub right afterward." Stacy said, "Since it was too hard to transfer into a tub the first week, I would turn on the shower. Sitting in the warm shower while I urinated dulled the pain." Many hospitals provide a squeeze bottle that can be used to spray warm water on the perineum during and after urination. Remember to dry the area well as soon as the pain stops.

Bowel movements can be painful if the cut or tear extends into the anus. Most doctors will prescribe a stool softener to prevent constipation so that bowel movements will be less painful. After a bowel movement, rinsing with plenty of warm water will soothe pain, and help to prevent infection by cleaning the wound.

Very few women had trouble sitting or walking after having episiotomies. Clara said, "I think I had more trouble walking after my first delivery, because I tore up to the anus, and it was really sore." Stacy commented, "I had trouble transferring, mostly because I was weak, but also because the episiotomy was sore."

The Urinary Tract

Many women have difficulty urinating after giving birth. The problem may last for a few hours, or several days. The problem can arise for a number of reasons:

- The bladder may be bruised or swollen because of injury during childbirth.
- Urination may be painful because of episiotomy or tears in the vaginal tract.
- Urine may be retained as an aftereffect of oxytocin use.
- Bladder sensation (the "urge" to urinate) may be reduced as an aftereffect of anesthesia.
- There may be a urinary tract infection.

It is important to urinate within a few hours after giving birth, and to continue urinating regularly. Otherwise, the bladder can become distended (over-filled) and then there is an increased risk of urinary infection. If it is not possible to urinate, it may be necessary to use a catheter, as Patricia, Christina, and Marsha did for several days after giving birth. Even when a woman begins to urinate spontaneously after removal of a catheter, her nurse may still catheterize to remove any remaining urine. If too much urine remains in the bladder, a catheter may be left in place for another 12–24 hours. It is true that using a catheter also increases the risk of urinary infection, but this risk is smaller than the risk of not keeping the bladder drained.

Some women may have problems with incontinence (loss of bladder control) after childbirth, or after use of a catheter. If incontinence is normally not a problem, then it should be discussed with the doctor. Some women make sure they are never far from a bathroom until the problem is solved. Others wear special absorbent underwear.

Many women find that they have to urinate frequently from about the second day to the sixth day after giving birth. However, the increased need to urinate is not necessarily a sign of bladder infection. As we mentioned above, 3–6 pounds of extra fluid are lost after childbirth, and much of this fluid is eliminated in the urine. A bladder infection is different: one often feels the need to use the bathroom, but then produces only a few drops of urine.

Since it is common to produce more urine than usual during the first week after giving birth, women who have occasional problems with incontinence may have more trouble at this time. Those with mobility problems may need to arrange for the inconvenience of urinating more frequently, perhaps by keeping a bedpan handy at night or sleeping closer to the bathroom. Women with indwelling catheters may need to empty their urine bags more frequently.

Digestive System

Quite often, women do not have a bowel movement for one or two days after delivery. Many women also experience constipation (hard stools which are difficult to eliminate). The first bowel movements can be so uncomfortable that, like Clara after her first delivery, a woman can feel "scared to go to the bathroom."

Plenty of fluid and fiber in the diet can help prevent constipation. It is also important to use the bathroom as soon as the need is felt; "holding on" until it is convenient to use the bathroom can make the bowel movement more difficult and painful.

Some women find glycerin suppositories helpful, both for stimulating a bowel movement and for reducing strain. Women whose episiotomies make bowel movements painful are likely to find suppositories helpful. Many women find that breathing and relaxation techniques that helped during labor also help during painful bowel movements.

Circulatory Changes

Many people are surprised to learn that two common postpartum changes are actually changes in the circulatory system.

The first is hemorrhoids, which are swollen blood vessels in the area of the anus. They look like blood blisters. They are often painful, and are especially painful during bowel movements. Hemorrhoids are more likely to appear during pregnancy, and to improve after delivery. However, for some women, like Christina, they appear just after delivery.

The second symptom is only indirectly caused by changes in the circulatory system. As the amount of blood diminishes, and the body eliminates excess fluids, some women find that they sweat profusely at times during the 2 weeks after giving birth. Some perspire so heavily that they need to put towels on their pillows at night. Women who are quadriplegic may want to ask their doctors how to tell the difference between postpartum sweating and "quad sweats." Some women might like to buy a home blood pressure kit, and have their blood pressure checked when they start to perspire.

Some women become anemic after giving birth. A woman who is feeling very tired should call her doctor and discuss whether she should take iron supplements.

Breasts

Here we discuss the changes experienced by all women, whether or not they nurse their babies. In the section entitled "Breast Feeding," we will explain the advantages and disadvantages of breast feeding and bottle feeding, and give advice on breast feeding and breast care.

During pregnancy, the breasts start changing in preparation for milk production. Often, the breasts even begin to produce colostrum (a thin, clear "pre-milk") during the last weeks of pregnancy. Every woman will begin to produce colostrum by the second day after giving birth.

The milk comes in about 4 days after the birth. (Milk usually comes in even sooner after a second birth.) Most women will have some problems with engorgement. The breasts become swollen, painful, and hard. Sharon said, "When the milk came in, it felt like I had two stones on my chest." Cheryl said, "It felt like two bricks." Sometimes women with breast engorgement have a slight fever. Some women find that ice packs or cold compresses make their breasts more comfortable; others prefer a hot shower or a hot pad. Wearing a supportive bra also helps. Sometimes expressing a little milk relieves the discomfort, but women who will not breast feed should be careful to express *very little* milk, because if they express too much it will stimulate more milk production. Mild pain relievers are also helpful. Engorgement usually disappears within a day or two.

When the breasts are not stimulated by suckling, milk production gradually stops, often within a week.

Some women may wonder about having their doctors inject medications to stop milk production. Suppressing milk in this way is much less common than it was in the past. Often the injections only delay milk production, rather than suppress it. Also, these medications, like any other, should not be used without discussing possible side effects.

Abdomen

When women imagine returning to their normal physical condition after the baby is born, they assume they will be able to wear the clothes they wore before they were pregnant, and see their own feet again without craning their necks. So it is always something of a shock when the abdomen does not look very different just after childbirth. If stretch marks appeared during pregnancy, they are still visible. The mother looks as if she is 4 or 5 months pregnant because of weight gain and stretched abdominal muscles. However, stretch marks, like scars, will gradually fade during the year or two following pregnancy and the abdomen will begin to look flatter as weight is lost. To some extent, the muscles will regain their tone during normal daily activities such as walking and carrying the baby. However, it is best to use the abdominal exercises described in Chapter 5 to help the muscles recover more quickly, and to strengthen them as much as possible. Strong abdominal muscles will contribute to good posture and help prevent back discomfort. It is important to begin with gentle exercise, then change to more demanding exercise as the muscles grow stronger. For the first few days, a good exercise is to simply take a deep breath and hold it several times a day.

Some women develop a condition called *diastasis recti,* in which some of the abdominal muscles are separated. These vertical muscles are pushed apart by the pressure of the uterus. A mild separation is likely to heal with rest. If abdominal muscles have been separated more, women should not try to exercise them until their doctors say it is safe. When it is safe to exercise, begin with exercises recommended by the doctor or physical therapist.

POSTPARTUM COMPLICATIONS

Sometimes women experience postpartum changes that are not normal. These changes are signs or symptoms of complications. The most common complications are bleeding and infection. (Sometimes thrombophlebitis occurs, but it is more common during pregnancy.)

Bleeding Complications

There are a number of reasons for postpartum bleeding. Sometimes the bleeding is caused by a laceration (cut or tear) in the cervix, vagina, or perineum. If these tissues were injured during birth, the doctor or nurse examining the mother will find bright red discharge, and/or too much bleeding. It may then be necessary to suture the injury to stop the bleeding.

If the uterus does not involute (contract and shrink), there may be too much bleeding in the area where the placenta was attached. (Just as pressure stops bleeding from an ordinary cut, normal involution compresses blood vessels and stops bleeding.) Some of the causes of uterine bleeding are very unusual. Some reasons why the uterus fails to involute include the following:

- The uterine muscles were stretched by a very large fetus or a multiple birth.
- The muscles were stressed by a prolonged or very rapid labor.
- Contractions were affected by general anesthesia.
- The mother has fibroid tumors (a kind of non-cancerous uterine growth).
- The mother has been weakened by illness or other problems.
- A part of the placenta is retained in the uterus. Although the placenta is examined after birth, sometimes it has an extra lobe that is retained. Also, the placenta may be unusually shaped, or part of it may remain attached to the uterine wall.

Uterine bleeding is usually diagnosed easily. The doctor or nurse will find bleeding that is not caused by a laceration, and an examination of the abdomen will reveal that the uterus is not involuting. Often, massage of the fundus (the top of the uterus) will stimulate good contractions. If massage is not effective, the mother may be given oxytocin.

If retained placenta is causing the problem, the placental material will have to be removed (anesthesia may be necessary). Oxytocin may be given afterwards.

Rarely, a piece of retained placenta blocks blood flow—it acts like a stopper in a bottle. When this happens, the first symptoms of bleeding may be weakness from blood loss, or pain from the pressure of the blood in the uterus. Besides the need to have the retained placenta removed, the mother may need to be treated for blood loss with intravenous fluid or blood transfusion.

Leslie and Samantha both had postpartum bleeding complications. Leslie had a laceration, while Samantha had retained a lobe of the placenta. Each of them commented that it took her a long time to regain her strength.

Postpartum Infections

Postpartum infections may occur in the uterus or genital tract, in a cesarean incision (discussed in Chapter 8), or in the breast. Infection may be fairly easy to diagnose when there is pain in the infected area. Sometimes, the first signs of infection are symptoms like fever or fatigue, and the doctor must examine the mother to find the cause of infection.

There are a number of possible causes for uterine infections. Infection may be introduced during examinations after the bag of water breaks, or during manipulation to help with delivery of the baby or removal of the placenta. Local infection may spread from a wound or an incision (for example, an episiotomy). In some cases, the uterine lining does not slough off completely, and becomes a source of infection. The infection may stay in one area (local infection), or it may be carried to other parts of the body (systemic).

Women who breast feed can get infections when germs from the baby's mouth enter the milk ducts. Women whose nipples crack are especially vulnerable to infection during the first weeks of breast feeding. Like uterine infections, breast infections may be localized or systemic.

These are the signs of postpartum infection:

• Fever. Sometimes a woman is not even aware she has a fever. Even though Athina was in pain, she did not think of taking her temperature until she noticed pus from her incision. Any woman should take her temperature if she feels very hot, dizzy, or weak, aches all over, or simply does not feel well. If she has a fever, she should call her doctor (or an emergency room or urgent care clinic if she does not have a doctor). Some women ordinarily have temperatures lower than normal (98.6° F is "normal"), so when they tell a nurse or receptionist what their temperature is, it may seem that they do not really have fevers. It is important to say something like, "My usual temperature is 97.3°, but now it is 99.0°."

- Pain or tenderness in the breast, lower abdomen (uterine infection), or in the area of an incision.
- Oozing, pus, or dampness in an incision.
- Discolored, frothy, or bad-smelling lochia or vaginal discharge. (These are signs of uterine infections.)
- A red, swollen, discolored, or tender area of the breast that is hot to the touch or hard to the touch (this will not feel like engorgement). These are signs of breast infection.

The mother will need antibiotics unless her infection is very localized and minor. She will also need to rest and drink plenty of fluids. Sometimes a woman is advised to keep nursing while she has a breast infection; at other times, she is advised to stop nursing temporarily, and to use a breast pump to keep up milk production. Severe or repeated breast infections can mean that the mother must stop breast-feeding. (Women who feel breast feeding is important could try asking their pediatrician for suggestions about cleaning the baby's mouth.)

Women with very severe infections of the uterus or of surgical incisions may need to return to the hospital for treatment, such as drainage of an infected incision or administration of intravenous fluids.

BREAST FEEDING

Deciding Whether to Breast Feed

Before we compare the advantages and disadvantages of breast feeding and bottle feeding, we want to emphasize that there is no single right choice. In reading about feeding methods, and talking to experienced mothers, you are likely to hear some very strong opinions on the subject. Many people write and speak as though there is only one correct way to feed babies, and the babies' entire lives will be changed by the choice. In fact, both breast-fed and bottle-fed babies grow into healthy children and adults. Also, the mother's needs are as much a part of the choice as the baby's needs. It is also important to remember that it may be possible to combine breast feeding and bottle feeding, and gain some of the advantages of each method.

Advantages of Breast Feeding

During the first few days, the baby receives colostrum. The baby has little appetite, and may only suck 1 or 2 teaspoonsful at each feeding, but colostrum is very nutritious. It has more protein and less sugar than breast milk or formula. Also, the colostrum contains antibodies which help to protect the baby from infection.

Breast milk also contains many of the mother's antibodies and helps to protect the baby from infection, especially intestinal infections. This protection is most helpful during the first 6–12 months after birth, while the baby is developing the ability to resist infection.

Breast milk is more digestible than formula. While some babies adjust to formula easily, others may react with upset stomachs, constipation or diarrhea, or diaper rash. Sometimes it is necessary to try several different formulas in order to find one that does not cause problems. A baby may be allergic to one or more types of formula, but allergies to breast milk are extremely rare (although milk intolerance could be a problem).

The baby's sucking stimulates the release of the hormone oxytocin, which allows the milk to flow more easily and, during the first few weeks after childbirth, stimulates the involution of the uterus. (The mother may experience some uterine pain, such as she would feel during early labor.)

Some studies suggest that breast feeding may lower the mother's risk of developing breast cancer.

Breast feeding saves money. There is no need to buy bottles, nipples, bottle warmers, formula, and brushes for cleaning bottles and nipples. Women with limited hand control do not have to pay an attendant to prepare bottles.

Many women feel that breast feeding is more convenient than bottle feeding. They don't have to sterilize, fill, and heat bottles, or pack bottles and formula whenever they take the baby out of the house. They are glad they don't have to prepare a bottle when the baby wakes up at night. Women with limited hand control may have difficulty preparing bottles.

Many women get psychological satisfaction from breast feeding, and enjoy it for a variety of reasons. Some women feel that breast feeding is a sign that their bodies are working properly. Breast feeding may compensate for disappointment with a difficult pregnancy or delivery, or the feeling that the breasts are working well may compensate for feelings about disability. Some women like breast feeding because they feel that it is the most natural way to feed their babies. Others feel very womanly when they breast feed their babies. Their increased breast size is also very enjoyable to some women, though others feel just the opposite.

The cuddling and interaction with their babies, which is a part of breast feeding, is very rewarding to many women. They know that it is possible to cuddle and play while bottle feeding, but they feel that there is something special about breast feeding.

Some women enjoy the fact that only *they* can nurse their babies. It seems to make their relationship unique.

Disadvantages of Breast Feeding

Many women feel tied down by breast feeding, especially during the first weeks of the baby's life when it must nurse every 2 hours.

Breast feeding is quite demanding, and many women become exhausted when they must wake up for frequent night feedings.

Many fathers (and sometimes other family members) feel left out when they cannot help to feed the baby. However, they may find other ways to feel close, like bathing, dressing, and playing with the baby.

Breast-feeding the baby can affect the mother's diet. Sometimes the baby has an allergic reaction to something the mother has eaten. She has to try eliminating different items from her diet until the baby stops reacting. This process can be frustrating, and it is a real problem if the baby reacts to an important or favorite food.

For some women, it is stressful to plan a diet that includes all the nutrients needed for breast feeding. After 9 months of watching their diets, they want some relief, especially if they are feeling tired or upset.

Others feel very concerned about losing weight. For example, a woman whose knees or ankles became more painful when she gained weight, may want to lose it as quickly as possible. It is possible to lose weight while eating an adequate diet, but it does take careful thought.

Another disadvantage to breast feeding is that the mother must avoid many medications which could enter her milk and affect the baby.

Breast feeding can also interfere with a couple's sexual relationship. Especially during the early weeks, when the baby nurses frequently, the parents may be interrupted when the baby wakes up, or they may feel inhibited because the baby might wake up at any moment. They may be too tired to make love. However, the same problems could arise if a baby wakes up crying because of indigestion or an allergic reaction to formula.

Breast feeding also affects sexuality because prolactin, the hormone which stimulates milk production, causes the vaginal walls to become thinner and drier. The change in the vagina makes intercourse uncomfortable. Lubricants make intercourse less painful, but some couples are not comfortable with this solution.

During the early weeks of breast feeding, most women will develop sore nipples, which can be quite painful. Some also develop painful breast infections. Often these problems are only temporary, but continued breast feeding can be difficult when there are repeated breast infections. We will say more about these problems, and how to cope with them, when we discuss breast care.

Some women are embarrassed when their breasts leak and stain their clothing. Leaking stops after the first 2 or 3 months, but the wait may be too long for people who are easily embarrassed, or who must return to work after 6 weeks. (Breast pads or shields are not always a good solution, since the dampness can make the nipples uncomfortable.)

Some women feel uncomfortable nursing in public. Others must cope with disapproval even when they are very discreet.

While it is possible to continue breast-feeding after returning to work, it is not possible for every woman. Some find that their breasts simply stop producing milk if they wait too long between feedings. Some women are able to pump or manually express milk during breaks at work, but others are not. Not every workplace has a refrigerator where expressed milk can be stored.

Medical Reasons to Avoid Breast Feeding

Breast feeding is not possible in some cases: If the baby must be hospitalized, it can be difficult or impossible to breast feed. The baby may be in isolation, or may be too weak to suck. Sometimes the baby is bottle-fed, and the mother can pump her breast milk for bottle feeding, but the fatigue and stress of having a sick baby interfere with milk production. It might be more important for the mother to rest and keep healthy than for her to try to breast feed.

The baby may have a problem, such as cleft palate, that interferes with sucking.

The baby may have a metabolic problem such as phenylketonuria (PKU). Phenylketonuria is caused by an inability to digest an amino acid called phenylalanine (proteins are chains of amino acids). The baby has a blood test to detect PKU before leaving the hospital. Babies with PKU must go on special diets, or chemicals from the incompletely digested phenylalanine will cause brain damage. Since breast milk contains phenylalanine, these babies cannot nurse.

Some babies develop jaundice in response to a hormone in the mother's milk. Sometimes it is possible to solve this problem by giving babies water every day for several days, but sometimes the only solution is to stop breast feeding.

Women who have myasthenia gravis carry an antibody (anti-acetyl-cholinesterase) that can reach levels high enough to enter their milk and affect their babies. They need to be tested to determine whether it is safe for them to breast-feed.

Bottle Feeding

The main advantages of bottle feeding are related to the disadvantages of breast feeding. The mother will not have any of the discomforts of breast feeding, such as sore nipples and possible breast infections, once engorgement stops. She will have more freedom and flexibility, and will not have to build her schedule around feeding the baby every 2–4 hours, because anyone can feed the baby. This is especially important to women who do not have flexible work schedules.

A final advantage of bottle feeding is that the baby may not wake up as often during the night because formula is digested more slowly. (But if the baby is bothered by indigestion, there is no advantage.) When the baby sleeps better, the parents sleep better.

A disadvantage of bottle feeding is that as the baby grows older, it can be tempting to leave a bottle propped on a pillow in the crib where the baby can suck it. When the baby is able to hold the bottle, it is even more tempting to leave a bottle with the baby. Many babies fall asleep sucking the bottle. With the nipple in the baby's mouth, formula pools against the teeth, and the sugars in the formula cause tooth decay. This problem is avoidable. It is best to hold and cuddle the baby during most feedings. If the bottle is left in the crib at night or during nap time, it can be filled with water.

Factors Related to Disability

Disability can influence a woman's decision about how she will feed her baby. It is not always obvious which choice will be best for a woman with a particular disability. For example, Stacy and Sylvia are both quadriplegic, but they made different choices. Stacy felt breast feeding would be too difficult. Sylvia said, "I was going to nurse come hell or high water. It looked like I might not be able to because I had inverted nipples, but I did!" Women with disabilities need to consider the following factors:

Medication: Remember that not all medications enter breast milk, and medications that do enter breast milk may not become concentrated enough to affect the baby. Research has been done to investigate which medications enter breast milk.

Of those medications which do enter breast milk, some cause only temporary problems. For example, if a woman develops a bladder infection, her doctor may be able to prescribe an antibiotic that is safe for the baby. The baby might have diarrhea temporarily, and giving the baby extra fluids and changing more diapers might be a problem for a severely disabled woman. Other medications are dangerous for the baby. If a safer substitute is unavailable, then the mother will have to bottle feed her baby, as Sybil did.

Physical limitations: For some women with limited hand control, it is too difficult to prepare bottles of formula, or hold the bottle for the baby. For others, breast feeding can be a problem because it is difficult to support the baby's head, or hold the breast away from the baby's nose.

Women with limited mobility have other problems. Clara needed to have her husband bring the baby to her at night, because balance was difficult when she had been sleeping. If Clara had been a single parent, she might have needed to find an alternative to breast feeding at night, perhaps giving the baby formula at bedtime, so it might sleep through the night. Some women will have the same problem as Pam, who said, "It was very difficult to find a position I could nurse in."

Exacerbation of disability: While breast feeding does not directly affect disability, it must be remembered that breast feeding can be very tiring. Women whose disabilities are exacerbated by fatigue (SLE, MS, myasthenia gravis) should be prepared to stop breast feeding if it is too tiring.

Prevention of fatigue: Some women feel that feeding the baby is less demanding if they breast-feed. Night feedings in particular can be easier if they do not have to get a bottle from the kitchen, but keep the baby near the bed, and nurse the baby in bed. For others, night feedings are a major problem. Heather said, "I couldn't lay down and nurse him because I'm not balanced; I could roll over and fall on him. It meant I had to get up and sit with him in the middle of the night."

For some women, the physical demands of milk production, and holding the baby for every feeding, are too wearing. Portia said, "Being disabled, I didn't need the extra burden of nursing a baby. Bottles were much easier."

Women with MS usually feel better if they bottle-feed their babies. Their first concern is to avoid getting tired and risking a flare-up of symptoms. Mary told us, "I didn't even try to nurse. My neurologist didn't think it would be a good idea." Margie said, "I nursed my first, but I bottle fed my second because I needed the rest." She added that if she could make the decision again, she would bottle feed her first child. Michelle suggested a compromise: "When your milk is established, let someone else bottle feed the baby at night so you can sleep. Stop after the first few months—by then the baby has gotten the most benefit." Still, Michelle stressed the need to protect the mother's health. When she was asked how she would advise new mothers, she said, "Minimize breast feeding. I thought it would be easy—a piece of cake. But I would get tired out and my milk supply would drop. I let myself get over-tired, and in the long run that didn't help the baby."

Many women will not be able to choose a feeding method in advance, since the reality of caring for a baby is never the same as what we expect. Celeste commented, "I thought the problem would be with carrying the baby, and nursing would be easier. Nursing turned out to be a problem, too." We would encourage women who are interested in breast feeding, and who are worried only about physical limitations, to try breast feeding; changing from breast to bottle feeding is much easier than changing from bottle to breast feeding.

The Art of Breast Feeding

Once breast feeding is an established pattern for mother and baby, it can be very enjoyable. Feeding time becomes a time for cuddling, affection, and even play: very small babies stare intently at their mothers' faces while they nurse; older babies hold and pat one breast while sucking the other; still older babies play with their mothers' lips, laugh, and do silly things like blow bubbles on the breast. However, nursing does not always begin easily and naturally. It can take several weeks for milk flow to become reliable, and for mother and baby to create a comfortable routine. Getting started may be frustrating at times, but a little patience at the beginning can be the start of a precious experience lasting for months or even years. Here are some tips for successful breast feeding:

Help the baby: The baby needs help in finding the nipple. Gently brush the nipple against the baby's cheek, and s/he will turn toward it. If the baby cannot quite find the nipple, gently place it in the baby's mouth. Not just the nipple, but all of the areola (the dark area around the nipple) should be in the baby's mouth. (Women with unusually large areolas may not be able to get the whole areola into the baby's mouth.) Athina commented, "I think my small breasts were an asset. My baby didn't have any trouble finding the nipple and clamping on by herself." Very young babies need to have their heads supported. You can support the baby's head by holding it in the crook of your arm, or laying the baby on a pillow with the upper end near your breast.

Women with large breasts will need to hold part of the breast away from the baby's face so the baby can breathe. If the baby stops after just a few sucks, it is probably pausing to breathe. In this case, you will want to hold the breast away from the baby's nose. Women who do not have enough hand control to hold the breast can try cutting off the tip of the brassiere cup so that the areola is exposed but the rest of the breast is held away from the baby's face.

Find at least one comfortable position for nursing: Stephanie felt that her difficulty in finding a comfortable position was the most important problem to solve. She explained, "There really wasn't a comfortable position because I was in pain from the C-section and it made me less mobile."

Some women will need help from nurses or attendants. Athina said, "I needed help getting the baby in the right position by placing her on a pillow so she could find the nipple. Sometimes it was difficult to find the right position and that was frustrating." Arlene's nurses also helped her find a way to use pillows to support her child while nursing. Christina's home health worker helped her experiment with different positions.

Clara commented, "It wasn't until I got home from the hospital that I found a really comfortable position for nursing. That was 3 days after delivery. I really needed an armchair with pillows supporting my baby to be successful." Many women find that sitting in an armchair or reclining chair is helpful because the furniture supports their arms while they hold the baby. A footstool or recliner helps in relaxing.

Many women feel it works well to lie on their sides, with their babies lying beside them, possibly supported by pillows. Athina found this position very helpful when she went back to the hospital with an infection in her incision. When her baby came to her room, she could just turn on her side to nurse. Jennifer said it worked well to sleep with her baby because "when he woke up I was able to turn over to give him a breast. It was a real energy saver."

Make sure there is a large glass or even a pitcher of water nearby before settling down to feed the baby: It is common for women to begin feeling very thirsty a few minutes after they start feeding the baby. It is good that they feel thirsty, because it is important for them to drink plenty of fluids. Still, it is very inconvenient to have to get a glass of water in the middle of a feeding.

Releasing the nipple: When the baby is almost finished sucking, place a finger in the corner of the baby's mouth to release the suction on the nipple. If the baby lets go suddenly, or if the mother removes the breast without releasing suction first, the pull is painful.

Alternate breasts: Make sure the baby changes sides after about 10 minutes of sucking, or use a different side with each feeding. Changing sides assures that milk production is stimulated in both breasts.

Consider formula feedings: During the first few days after birth, consider giving the baby a little sugar/water or formula for one feeding if your nipples are very sore, or if you are feeling tired and overwhelmed. But make sure to nurse the baby at the next feeding so that milk production continues to be stimulated. (Women are often strictly advised to avoid giving sugar/water, but we believe that it is more important to be flexible. Some women need an occasional break while they adjust to breast feeding.) The sugar solution you brought home from the hospital is a good choice if you are worried about milk allergies. The sweetness is not a problem because breast milk is very sweet.

Choose a comfortable brassiere: Some women prefer brassieres with flaps that can be lowered (women with limited hand control need flaps that fasten with Velcro rather than hooks). Others prefer elastic athletic bras that can be pulled up and down over the breast. Your preference might change as time passes. An occupational therapist's advice might help you make the best choice.

Breast Care

Engorgement, infections, and sore or cracked nipples can all cause discomfort during the weeks after birth. (Breast infections are discussed above in the section entitled "Postpartum Infections.")

There are two conditions called engorgement. The first is painful swelling caused by changes in the breast when the milk comes in. This type of engorgement is described in the section entitled "Normal Physical Changes." The second type of engorgement is caused when the breasts become over-filled with milk. Sometimes the breasts become over-filled if the baby waits longer than usual between feedings. Engorgement can be relieved by pumping or expressing some milk or feeding the baby. If the breasts are very swollen, it may be hard for the baby to take the nipple. It helps to express a little milk before feeding the baby, and gently tug on the nipple, or roll it between the fingers, so that it takes a shape that fits the baby's mouth. It is perfectly all right to gently awaken a sleeping baby for nursing—it is good for both baby and mother to create a regular schedule. On the other hand, as the baby grows older you may want to lengthen the time between feedings so that it is possible to sleep through the night. Remember to lengthen the time *gradually*, to avoid discomfort.

Even women who are careful to toughen their nipples during pregnancy may get sore or cracked nipples during the first few weeks of breast feeding. Sore nipples are just like dish-pan hands; the skin becomes chapped from the rubbing and moisture of the baby's mouth. Here are some ways to care for sore nipples:

Duration of nursing: Try nursing for a shorter period of time. A baby who is nursing efficiently empties most of the milk from the breast in 5-10 minutes. Nurse for 5 minutes on each side, then gradually increase feeding time as the nipples heal.

Positioning the baby: Change the baby's position slightly at each feeding so that a different part of the nipple gets sucking pressure. (For example, prop the baby's pillow a little higher or lower.)

Alternate breasts: If one nipple is more sore, or only one nipple is cracked, pump milk from the affected breast and let the baby nurse on the other side.

Protective cups: Some women like to wear protective cups over their nipples to keep clothing from rubbing. This also protects clothing from stains until leaking stops naturally. Other women find that cups slow healing by keeping their nipples damp. Cups may be helpful when it is necessary to go out, but at home it is better to wear a nursing bra with the flaps down. Exposing the nipples to the air helps keep them dry and promotes healing. Some women use a heat lamp for *short* periods.

Avoid irritants: Do not put antiseptics, scented creams, or anything that could be irritating, on the nipples. Wash with plain water and do not use soap. If it makes nipples more comfortable, put on a small amount of *unmedicated* lanolin, which is available at drug stores. Any lanolin which clings to the skin will not bother the baby, and the lanolin will not irritate the nipples.

Deep breathing: Sometimes nursing with sore nipples is painful. The worst moment is when the baby "latches on." It helps to take a few deep, relaxing breaths before starting to nurse, and to use the deep breathing of early labor for a minute or so until he pain fades.

Avoiding infection: It is possible to get a breast infection even when the nipples are not sore, but germs enter more easily if nipples are cracked. If nipples are cracked, watch for signs of breast infection and call the doctor if necessary.

Combining Breast and Bottle Feeding

For some women, the best approach is to combine feeding methods in some way. One way to combine methods is to breast feed at first, then change to bottle feeding. This approach gives the baby the benefits of the immunity protection in breast milk, and delays the risk of an allergic reaction to formula. A second approach is to give some breast feedings and some bottle feedings every day. This approach suits the needs of women who want to have the psychological benefits of breast feeding, but need to avoid physical stress.

Sometimes women are advised to wait 6 weeks before introducing the bottle, so the baby will have time to become attached to the breast. However, some babies become so attached to the breast that they will not take a bottle. They seem to be bothered by the unfamiliar taste of the nipple or the formula. Others come to prefer the bottle because it is much easier to suck milk from the bottle. The baby may even start to reject the breast before the mother feels ready to stop nursing! Clara had both experiences: "My first baby was so used to the breast, she just wouldn't take the bottle. It was too much trouble to fight with her and she was completely breast fed till she started solid foods. With my second baby it was the opposite. I thought I'd try him with a bottle so my husband or baby sitter could feed him. After that, it was a struggle to get him to take the breast."

There is another reason that women who want to combine feeding methods should wait about a month before introducing the bottle. If they start bottle feeding too soon, it may be more difficult for them to start regular milk production. They could have problems with engorgement, or have trouble producing enough milk. It is easier to wait a few weeks, then use a bottle for one feeding. Wait a few days before replacing another feeding, so the breasts have time to adapt. Many women will begin the change by using a bottle for night feedings, so that they can sleep while someone else feeds the baby.

If a woman wants very much to continue breast feeding, she should think carefully before trying bottle feeding. She must be comfortable with the possibility that her breasts will stop producing milk if she nurses less often, or that the baby will strongly prefer the bottle.

EMOTIONAL CHANGES

· ·

The birth of a child is a major change in the life of the family. Relationships between the parents, and among parents, grandparents, and other family members all change with the birth. Relationships with friends also change. Friends who already have children welcome the new parents to the club, while childless friends worry that the new parents will talk about nothing but diapers and formula. The parents must adjust to a new identity and new responsibilities.

We will focus on two emotional changes of the postpartum period— mood changes and changes in the sexual relationship.

Mood Changes

Quite often, the first few weeks after birth are like an emotional roller coaster. There are times when the new mother is filled with love and joy over the birth of her baby, and times when she is tired, frustrated, and depressed. Stacy recalled, "I felt so overwhelmed that I cried for the first 6 weeks. Then I felt better." It is so common for women to feel weepy and frustrated during the postpartum period that there is even a nickname for this feeling—the "baby blues."

It is important to remember that there are physical reasons for many of the sad, let-down feelings that occur in the postpartum period. Women really are tired in the aftermath of giving birth, and they often lose a lot of sleep when their babies wake up at night. They may be worn down by a variety of discomforts like sore nipples or strong afterpains. Their hormones are changing too, and the change in various hormone levels causes unpredictable mood changes.

It can help to know that upsetting feelings are shared. It is a good idea to find ways of meeting with other new parents, perhaps by staying in touch with friends from birthing class, joining a parents' group at a community center, or starting a play group. Talking with other parents, you will find people who share your feelings, and you may be able to help each other with suggestions for handling problems. Many of the feelings we describe will be familiar to our readers; all of them are common among new parents, and especially new mothers.

Physician T. Berry Brazelton has pointed out one problem that is all the more painful because it may be hard for parents to admit what they are feeling: disappointment in the baby. Parents who visualized a soft, cuddly baby can feel disappointed in a wriggly live-wire. On the other hand, high-energy parents may feel irritated by a placid, sleepy baby. They may worry, or feel guilty about their reaction, until they have had time to learn to appreciate their baby.

Some people, like Patricia and Heather, are disappointed by their first experiences of motherhood. Patricia said, "It wasn't exactly what it was cracked up to be." No matter how hard people try to be realistic before the baby is born, it may come as a shock that it can be weeks before the baby seems to recognize his/her parents—parents who have spent those weeks working hard to take care of the baby. This problem, too, is likely to diminish as time passes.

Marsha and Sharon were troubled by changes in their relationships. Marsha said, "I found it difficult to relate to my husband as a lover and then to relate in my new role as a mother. It was hard to switch between the two. It took several months to fuse both roles." Sharon was not married, and her child's father was not sure he wanted to continue the relationship. Sharon said, "It was nerve-racking thinking about it." Parent support groups may also be helpful for couples whose relationships are troubled. Some parents find that professional counseling helps them adjust to their new situation.

Sometimes the new parents fear that the responsibility will be more than they can handle. Christina said, "I got overwhelmed at the hospital. The staff taught me to take care of the baby, so when I went home I wasn't really depressed." Other women feel comfortable in the hospital, where they have help, but become overwhelmed when they go home and they are alone with the baby. Often, having someone come into the home to help with the baby makes the transition easier. The emotional support is as important as the practical support. Sharon recalled, "My mother came and stayed for a month. It really lifted my spirits and helped me in an all-around, general way."

New mothers may feel sad about changes in their lives. They can miss the freedom they had before they had to worry about baby sitters and feeding schedules. They may even miss the way they looked before childbirth changed their bodies.

Sometimes people feel guilty about negative feelings. They feel as though it is wrong to resent the baby for waking them up at night. Talking with other parents can be very helpful in coping with guilt feelings. It helps to hear other parents, who obviously love their children, say that they get angry too.

Finally, parents may be upset by worries about their baby. Even the healthiest baby can catch a cold, develop a rash, or cry for long periods no matter what the parents do to comfort it. First-time parents can be the most upset. Cheryl said, "It was worst with the first one, because I didn't know what to expect. With the second one I was too busy to even stop to think and feel." Women with disabilities may be even more frightened by any hint that something is wrong, like Carla, who said that she worried unnecessarily that minor symptoms were signs of disability.

Some women with disabilities do have babies with health problems, and their concern for their babies adds to the emotional and physical pressures they feel. Their doctors and some hospital staff (for example, the hospital social worker) can help them contact organizations that provide information and support for parents of ill children. It is important for women whose babies are disabled or ill to accept help from friends, relatives, and others, so that they themselves do not become ill from fatigue and stress.

For most women, the "baby blues" gradually disappear. Their hormones return to normal, they start getting more sleep, and they find ways of handling the changes in their lives. Some women, however, develop more serious problems. They do not experience the kind of depression people ordinarily talk about, but have postpartum depression.

It is important to know about postpartum depression because it is not always easy to recognize. Clara told us, "Some years after I had my first child, I read about postpartum depression and many of the symptoms were just what I went through. At the same time, I learned I had a thyroid problem, and I know hormonal problems can cause postpartum depression. I think I had postpartum depression and nobody recognized it at the time."

Still, no one can look at a list and diagnose herself. One woman can have one or two symptoms on the list below, and not have postpartum depression. Another woman might experience symptoms that are not included in this list. However, a woman who is experiencing many of these symptoms, or other disturbing feelings, needs to describe her problems to a doctor. We would also suggest that every woman ask her husband or a close friend to read this information with her. Someone who has postpartum depression may have trouble recognizing symptoms, or may not be able to bring herself to see her doctor. It is important to have someone close to her encourage her, or even insist that she seeks help.

The most important symptom is sleep disturbance which is *not* caused by the baby waking up at night. One type is *initial insomnia.* In this case, you are not able to fall asleep when you first go to bed. If it takes more than half an hour to fall asleep, and the problem lasts longer than a month, or gets worse over time, it is insomnia. *Middle insomnia* is more difficult to recognize because new mothers are so often awakened by their babies. However, if the baby is sleeping through the night, and you often wake up for no reason, then take more than half an hour to go back to sleep, middle insomnia may be the problem. Again, this would not happen just once or twice; it would be insomnia if the problem goes on for more than a month or grows worse over time. *Early insomnia* is insomnia that occurs early in the morning, before your usual time for awakening.

It is a good idea to call the doctor if sleep disturbances are a problem either alone, or in combination with any of these symptoms:

- A feeling of being flooded with too many thoughts, as if your mind is going all the time and cannot stop.
- Any of these feelings: A sense of foreboding, that is, a constant feeling

that something bad is about to happen. Feeling extremely depressed or wishing you were dead. A sense of hopelessness. Feelings of extreme shame—either feeling ashamed for no reason, or feeling very ashamed about something that is usually just slightly embarrassing.

- Feeling unreasonably anxious or fearful about the baby. Clara said, "One of the reasons I think I had postpartum depression is that I worried much too much about my baby. I kept waking up at night to check my baby's breathing. I was sure I'd find her dead of SIDS."

- Excessive euphoria—exaggerated feelings of happiness. Extreme euphoria is not the usual joy people feel the first time the baby laughs or sits up. With extreme euphoria, the mother is so excited that she is too disorganized to take care of the baby, forgetting to feed him or her or change the diapers.

- Hearing a voice no one else hears, or seeing something no one else sees. If this happens *even once*, it is important to see a doctor.

- An urge to hurt yourself or your baby. Many new parents will say something like, "When the baby wakes me up at night for the fifth time, I want to throw it out the window." But they know they do not really mean what they are saying. If you feel as though you really might hurt yourself or the baby, and it seems that you cannot control the feeling, call your doctor right away.

If you or someone close to you notices some worrisome change in your usual behavior, and this change seems connected with other problems, it may be worth discussing this with your doctor.

A woman with symptoms of postpartum depression may need to see a psychiatrist. Some of the symptoms are more obvious than others. At first the woman and her doctor may think she simply has ordinary "baby blues." However, if a woman cannot feel comforted by her doctor's reassurances, if she is not helped by her doctor's suggestions for coping with her problems, or if she has severe symptoms (such as hearing voices), she should see a psychiatrist. Her doctor can suggest one or she can make an appointment herself. It is important to see a psychiatrist rather than a psychologist or a counselor, because the psychiatrist is also a medical doctor, and there may be a physical cause for the problem.

The psychiatrist may need to work with other specialists. Laura told us she suffered a "severe depression" after she gave birth. She assumed her depression was caused by SLE and it may have been. However, a psychiatrist might have worked with Laura's rheumatologist to determine whether she was suffering from SLE symptoms or postpartum depression.

The Sexual Relationship

While some couples feel that their sexual relationship begins to change during pregnancy, others feel that change begins with the birth of their child. Since many couples continue making love even during the last weeks of pregnancy, the need to avoid intercourse during the weeks after birth is a dramatic change.

For some couples, waiting to make love is not difficult, at least for the first few weeks. Often the parents are very tired from taking care of the baby, or from being awakened at night, so they are more interested in sleep than sex.

Sometimes people unconsciously believe that their sex lives will go back to normal after a certain date. For example, if the mother's doctor tells her to wait for 6 weeks, she and her husband may believe that after exactly 42 days they will start making love as freely as ever. Then they are very disappointed when problems occur.

Like other aspects of a marriage relationship, the sexual relationship must change when children are added to the family. The change can be positive if the new parents work together to solve their problems with creativity and patience.

Some common difficulties have very simple solutions:

- One or both partners may feel deprived of affection when they cannot make love. It is important to find time to express affection in other ways, such as cuddling, kissing, and setting aside time to talk to each other.
- Reduce sexual frustration by caressing each other without having intercourse.
- Be aware that intercourse may be painful for the woman. When a woman has had an episiotomy, the first attempts at intercourse must be slow and gentle. If she is too sore, wait a few days and try again. Marsha commented that "my episiotomy interfered with lovemaking at first because it wasn't healed enough," but when enough time passed, there was no problem.
- Many women find that kissing and caressing for a long time before beginning intercourse helps because it increases natural lubrication. Lubricants like K-Y Jelly are also helpful. Breast-feeding women may also find that intercourse is uncomfortable. As we explained, their discomfort is caused by hormonal changes. They, too, will enjoy intercourse more if they use lubricants.
- Often women who are breast-feeding do not want their husbands to kiss or caress their breasts. Even when their nipples are no longer sore, they may feel that, after having their breasts handled by the baby all day, they just want to be left alone. Try to have a positive outlook and take the opportunity to look for sensitive areas you have not discovered before—perhaps the ear lobes, the nape of the neck, or the inner thighs.
- If one partner—usually the new mother—feels too tired to be interested in sex, it is all too easy for resentment to develop. The wife may feel that her husband is making unreasonable demands, or the husband may feel

rejected. Try to work together to solve the underlying problem. Perhaps the husband can take over night feedings or some chores, or a friend or neighbor can help. Perhaps the couple can decide together that it is better for them to let some tasks wait so they will have more energy for their relationship.

- Many people feel inhibited because the baby may wake up and interrupt them. They need to find a baby sitter. Some people leave the baby at the home of a relative or sitter. Others leave the baby at home and go to a motel as a special treat.
- Sexual contact may be less satisfying because the couple do not "fit" as well. If the mother does her Kegel exercises regularly, the muscle tone in her vagina will improve and lovemaking will be more satisfying. Meanwhile, the couple can experiment with different positions and caresses to find satisfaction.

Many problems are solved very naturally as time passes. For example, when the baby begins to sleep through the night, the parents begin to feel more relaxed about lovemaking.

Remember that changes in the sexual relationship may in fact be a reflection of changes in the overall relationship. For example, a woman whose parents avoided expressing affection in front of their children may feel that, since she has become a mother, sex is inappropriate. A man who complains about not making love often enough may be feeling jealous of having to share his wife's affection with their baby. When the couple are able to discuss their feelings openly and cooperatively, the changes in their sexual relationship are an opportunity for their friendship to grow deeper.

One area of communication for new parents is the choice of birth control methods. Many people enjoy pregnancy because it is the one time that they do not have to worry about birth control. After their child is born, they may want to consider trying a new method. Many women with disabilities assume that they cannot get pregnant, so after they give birth, they must choose a birth control method for the first time.

BIRTH CONTROL METHODS

When a woman is ready to start making love again, it is time to choose a birth control method. Although people traditionally think that the postpartum phase ends at 6 weeks after birth, there are many good reasons to delay a repeat pregnancy until at least a year after giving birth.

Few of the women interviewed described the birth control method they used after giving birth. The only clear pattern was a tendency to use the same method that they had used before pregnancy. However, some women may need to change methods after giving birth. For example, a woman who was using birth control pills will need a different method if she decides to breast feed her baby.

The reliability of a birth control method is measured by the percentage of women who do not become pregnant during a 1-year period. For example, if a particular birth control method is said to be 95% reliable, this means that 95% of the women in a study group did not become pregnant while using this method for 1 year. A range of reliability (for example, 80%–99% reliable) often reflects variations in the way people use their chosen methods. For any given method, some study groups have better results than other study groups; the higher number (e.g., 99%) indicates a group which probably used the method more consistently. (For example, *always* using spermicide with a diaphragm, or *never* forgetting to take a birth control pill.) Each method of birth control has advantages and disadvantages. As we discuss these advantages and disadvantages, we will include the comments of the women we interviewed.

Women who are choosing a birth control method and feel strongly about certain advantages or disadvantages need to discuss their concerns with a doctor or family planning practitioner. S/he will have the most recent information on the reliability and safety of each method. There are five types of birth control methods available. Four methods are reversible, which means that a woman can become pregnant if she stops using them. The reversible methods include the so-called natural methods, barrier methods, intrauterine devices, and contraceptive hormones. The fifth birth control method, sterilization, is difficult to reverse and can be permanent.

Natural Methods

The natural methods are lactation, the rhythm method, and the sympto-thermal method, a variation of the rhythm method.

Lactation

Christina voiced a common misconception about lactation when she said, "I thought I couldn't get pregnant while I was nursing. I was sure I read it somewhere." It is true that during the first few months of lactation, the hormones that encourage milk production may prevent ovulation (release of an egg which is mature and ready to be fertilized). However, even women who are breast feeding begin to menstruate again about 6 months after giving birth. For some women, the first ovulation occurs earlier. Since a woman becomes fertile shortly before she starts menstruating again, no one can be sure that she is safe just because she has not had her period. Breast feeding is not a good method of birth control.

The Rhythm Method

The rhythm method is a form of birth control in which a woman avoids sexual intercourse near the estimated time of ovulation. Many women choose this method because they dislike using other birth control methods. Others choose it because of their religious beliefs. A disadvantage of the rhythm method is that it interferes with spontaneity—many people dislike making love by the calendar. This disadvantage is likely to be felt more strongly after a baby is born, since a new baby may also interfere with spontaneity (for example, by waking up at night).

More important is the fact that the rhythm method, as it is currently practiced, is not reliable. No matter how "regular" a woman is, her time of ovulation can be affected by such factors as illness and stress. After she gives birth, the rhythm method will be useless until menstruation has resumed. Also, her menstrual cycle may be different from what it was before she was pregnant. It could be many months before the menstrual cycle becomes predictable. If a woman miscalculates and makes love shortly before ovulation, sperm deposited in her vagina could survive until she ovulates, and she could get pregnant. Sperm can survive in the woman for more than 3 days. As a result of these factors, the reliability of the rhythm method can be as low as 47%. (In other words, some women who practice the simplest form of the rhythm method might as well flip a coin to decide if it is safe to make love.)

The simplest—and least reliable—form of the rhythm method involves keeping a record of the dates of menstruation and estimating the time of ovulation as 14 days before the expected start of the next period. For example, if a woman menstruates every 28 days, she counts the first day of menstruation as Day 1, and would expect to ovulate on Day 14. In this case, she should avoid intercourse from about a week before the estimated date of ovulation to a few days after.

Symptothermal Method

An improved form of the rhythm method is the symptothermal method, also known as natural family planning or fertility awareness. For this method, a woman keeps a daily record of her temperature when she wakes up in the morning, by using a special thermometer. (The basal body temperature thermometer makes it easier to read smaller temperature changes than an ordinary thermometer.) The recorded temperature is charted on a graph. When a woman ovulates, her temperature suddenly rises as much as one degree Fahrenheit, and continues to rise until her next period. She also watches for changes in the mucus on her cervix. When the mucus becomes thinner and clearer, it is a sign that she is about to ovulate. These changes can be subtle, and women who want to use the symptothermal method need to take a class at a family planning clinic.

While the symptothermal method is more reliable than the simpler form of the rhythm method, it has similar disadvantages. A woman can make a mistake in calculating her time of ovulation if her temperature is affected by stress or illness, or if the texture of her cervical mucus is changed by a local infection. Besides the loss of spontaneity in lovemaking, many women dislike the routine of taking their temperature and checking their mucus. In addition, women with limited hand control may have difficulty taking their temperature, reaching into the vagina to collect mucus, or keeping records. Reliability of the symptothermal method can be as low as 80%.

Contraceptive Hormones

Hormonal birth control methods use synthetic imitations of hormones naturally produced in the body. These hormones prevent ovulation, and may also make it more difficult for a fertilized ovum to implant in the uterine lining. They may be taken in pill or implant form.

Birth Control Pills

Some types of pills are taken every day. Other types are taken daily for 3 weeks, are stopped for 1 week and then resumed again. Some women prefer taking a pill without interruption because they worry that if they must stop, then start again, they will forget to start when they should. Some women prefer pills which have very small doses of hormones. These women feel it is important to have a small dose because they want to reduce side effects. Others dislike low-dosage pills because these pills may need to be taken at the same time each day, thereby giving the woman less flexibility.

Hormone Implants

As of this writing, hormone implants are about to be approved for general use. Implants work the same way as birth control pills, but the hormone is delivered directly into the blood stream. Time-release capsules of the hormone are placed under the skin (usually in the upper arm), and the hormones are released into the blood stream slowly for many months. The implant contains a progesterone-like hormone, but not the estrogen used in some birth control pills.

Some women may prefer pills to implants because they can stop taking them at any time. Some women prefer implants because they do not need to renew prescriptions, or remember to take a pill every day or pack their pills when they travel.

The major advantage of using the hormone method is its effectiveness. This method can be more than 99% reliable when properly used. Some women also like this method because they know when they will menstruate. Another advantage is that, unlike barrier methods and natural methods, the hormone method does not interfere with lovemaking in any way. Those women who are not troubled by side effects may find this method very convenient. Women whose disabilities make barrier methods awkward for them might also prefer the hormone method.

However, women who are breast-feeding cannot use hormones. Birth control hormones can interfere with milk production, and they can enter the mother's milk. So, some women base their choice of a birth control method on their decision about breast feeding. Pam commented, "I chose the pill because I wasn't going to nurse."

Hormones can have both positive and negative side effects. One of the positive side effects is that, since menstrual flow may be reduced, a woman is less likely to develop anemia with a lighter menstrual flow. Women who use hormones are also less vulnerable to certain types of pelvic infections (but hormones *do not* protect against sexually transmitted diseases such as herpes and gonorrhea).

Not all women experience negative side effects. Some women may have some side effects and not others. Possible negative side effects include weight gain, fluid retention, nausea, fatigue, and breakthrough bleeding (slight bleeding at unexpected times in her cycle). The only way a woman can know whether she will experience side effects is by trying hormones. If she used them before she was pregnant, she can expect them to affect her in the same way after she gives birth, unless she changes to another kind of hormone.

Women with the following health problems should avoid birth control hormones:

- Liver, kidney, or heart disease
- Family or personal history of stroke
- Smoking
- Diabetes
- High blood pressure
- Sickle cell disease
- Other health problems as determined by your physician

Because these hormones can sometimes cause high blood pressure and blood clots, women who have spinal cord injuries that have caused such problems should consult with a doctor familiar with their health histories when considering this method of birth control. If they do choose to use hormones, they should know the signs and symptoms of circulatory problems:

- Tenderness and swelling of the calves
- Severe abdominal or chest pain
- Shortness of breath
- Severe leg pain
- Severe headaches
- Eye problems such as blurred vision or flashing lights

Also, women who have SLE are advised not to use birth control hormones because they may exacerbate their symptoms. If they must use hormones, pills containing only progestogen are considered the safest (estrogen can cause lupus flares).

A woman usually does not start taking birth control pills until after her postpartum visit.

Barrier Methods

Barrier methods involve the placement of an obstacle between the sperm and the cervix. Barrier methods include the diaphragm, cervical cap, sponge, condoms, and foam. These methods are most effective when a physical barrier is combined with a spermicide (a chemical which destroys or inactivates sperm). Diaphragms are used with a spermicidal cream or jelly that is applied separately. Sponges combine a physical and chemical barrier in one device. Different studies rate the reliability of barrier methods from 75% to 97% effective. Those who use the barrier methods correctly and regularly achieve higher reliability.

An advantage of barrier methods is that they do not have any of the side effects of birth control hormones. They are a good choice for women who are breast feeding and women who must avoid hormones for health reasons (including women who have SLE). Some people find that the chemicals in spermicide preparations are irritating. They can try using different brands, but they may have to choose another method if all brands are irritating.

Condoms

The best-known barrier method is the condom, a special sheathe which fits over the man's penis and catches sperm so it cannot be deposited in the vagina. The condom's reliability can be as low as 75%. However, condoms are more reliable when they are used in combination with a spermicide. Here are some tips for proper condom use:

- Use latex condoms, not condoms made from animal membranes. They are more reliable and offer better protection against sexually transmitted diseases. Some research has been done to compare the reliability of different brands of condoms (they have been tested for leakage). Ask a family planning practitioner or clinic for a list of reliable brands. If your usual brand is unavailable, use another brand on the list.
- If one brand of condom seems to reduce pleasure, try another reliable brand. There is no point in buying condoms if there is a temptation not to use them.
- The man should be wearing the condom throughout intercourse. Some people wait until he is close to orgasm (ready to "come") before putting on the condom. This is a mistake because some sperm leave the penis before the man ejaculates (comes).
- Do not use lubricants containing oils, since oils cause latex to disintegrate. Many people mistakenly use lubricants which contain oil. Read the ingredient list or, better yet, ask your family planning practitioner to recommend

a good water-based lubricant (one popular brand is K-Y Jelly). Spermicidal creams and jellies can also be good lubricants.

- Use a spermicidal cream or jelly with the condom. Besides being good lubricants, they contain spermicides which make condoms more reliable. (We will say more about these spermicides when we discuss diaphragms.)
- When putting on the condom, leave about a half-inch of space between the tip of the condom and the tip of the penis. This space catches sperm, so the condom is less likely to leak when the man ejaculates.
- Do not let sperm spill from the condom into the vagina after orgasm. Before the man loses his erection, he should withdraw while holding the condom to the base of his penis.

There are several advantages to using condoms. They are easily available and no prescription is needed. It was not long ago that one had to ask a pharmacist for condoms kept behind the counter, but now most drugstores and some supermarkets display condoms on open shelves. Condoms prevent transmission of venereal diseases and minor genital infections. For some people, it is easier to remember to use a condom than to remember to take a pill, since condoms are directly associated with lovemaking. Some women prefer condoms because they want their partners to share the responsibility for birth control.

One disadvantage of the condom method is that it can be easy to make a mistake. Sometimes people are tempted to have intercourse when no condom is available. This accounts for many condom "failures." Many men feel that condoms interfere with pleasure, others feel they do not. Some people feel that stopping to put on a condom makes lovemaking less pleasant, while others enjoy putting on the condom as part of lovemaking. The unpleasant taste of spermicides discourages some people from using the condom method properly. For disabled couples with limited hand control, it may be difficult to open the wrapper or put on the condom. Some women solve the problem by putting the condom on their husbands with their mouths. Jennifer and her husband, who are both disabled, are very satisfied with the condom method.

Diaphragms

The diaphragm is a dome-shaped piece of rubber with a spring rim. A woman puts some spermicidal cream or jelly in the diaphragm, and inserts the diaphragm into her vagina in such a way that it covers the cervix. Then she uses a special applicator to put more spermicide in her vagina. The diaphragm method is 80%–95% reliable. Diaphragm users, like condom users, must be careful to use them properly. Here are some tips for using the diaphragm properly:

- The diaphragm must be fitted to the individual user. Be sure to have a new diaphragm fitted at a postpartum examination. The size and shape of the vagina change after childbirth, so a diaphragm that was used before pregnancy will not be reliable after pregnancy.

- Do not use the diaphragm without spermicidal cream. One application of cream is only enough for one male climax. Reapply cream with each intercourse.
- Do not remove the diaphragm for at least 8 hours after intercourse. (This is easy to do if one makes love at night—just sleep with the diaphragm in place.)
- After removing the diaphragm, wash and dry it carefully. Do not dust it with scented powders (a little cornstarch is all right). Store it in its case in a cool, dark place.
- Diaphragms should be inspected before each use for obvious tears. Periodically, hold the diaphragm up to the light and check for pin-sized holes. Replace if necessary.
- Replace the diaphragm every year. In addition, make an appointment to have the diaphragm checked for fit after a weight gain or loss of 10 pounds or more.
- When the diaphragm is fitted, make sure it is comfortable and easy to insert. Diaphragms have different types of rims. Try both kinds to see which feels better and which is easier to insert. Practice inserting and removing the diaphragm when it is prescribed, so your family planning practitioner can make sure you are inserting it properly. If your partner will be inserting or removing your diaphragm for you (see below), have him practice in the office.
- If it is difficult to insert. or remove the diaphragm while lying down, try crouching, sitting with one foot propped up, or sitting on a toilet.
- If the diaphragm is unavailable (perhaps because it was not packed before a trip), substitute a condom or sponge.

Some women prefer using diaphragms because they like to be in charge of their birth control method. Diaphragms are a good choice for people who dislike condoms. Some women feel that lovemaking is more pleasant when a diaphragm has been inserted ahead of time, and there is no need to stop to put on a condom. Others prefer having their partners insert the diaphragm as part of lovemaking.

For some women, inserting or removing a diaphragm is difficult and awkward. Sometimes the difficulty is caused by the position of the uterus. This method can be difficult for some women with spine or pelvic deformities, and those with limited hand control. Hilary solved the problem by having her husband insert the diaphragm during lovemaking, then removing it herself while sitting on the toilet. Some women feel that the possibility of having their partner insert the diaphragm is an advantage, while others feel that relying on help is a disadvantage.

Women with weak pelvic muscles may not be able to use a diaphragm because of the possibility that it will slip out of position. Women who must empty their bladders by the Crede method (abdominal pressure) could dislodge their diaphragms.

Some women feel that diaphragms make lovemaking during menstruation more pleasant, because they often prevent menstrual fluid from staining the sheets.

Some people feel that an advantage of spermicides is that they are also lubricants. Others dislike them because they feel they are messy, especially when the diaphragm is removed. Some women remove it while sitting on the toilet so that the melted spermicide does not run down their legs. Some women remove their diaphragms just before getting in the shower, and others remove them in the shower. People avoid the unpleasant taste of spermicides by applying them at the last possible moment.

Cervical Caps

Cervical caps are an alternative to diaphragms. The cap is smaller than a diaphragm, and fits more closely over the cervix. Some women feel it is more comfortable. However, a woman who has difficulty inserting a diaphragm, would also have difficulty inserting a cervical cap.

Contraceptive Sponges

Contraceptive sponges are made of a synthetic, sponge-like material impregnated (soaked) with spermicide. The spongy material acts as a physical barrier. The advantage of a sponge is that there is no need for a prescription—the same size fits any woman. But like a diaphragm, the sponge may be difficult for some women to insert or remove. Women who can insert the sponge themselves may feel that lovemaking is more spontaneous than with a condom, because the sponge can be inserted well ahead of time. (It is recommended that the sponge never be left in place longer than a total of 30 hours.) No additional spermicide is needed with the sponge, so lovemaking seems more spontaneous and less messy. However, the sponge irritates some women.

Contraceptive Foams

Contraceptive foams, because of their texture, may act as a physical barrier as well as a spermicide. Women who are considering this method should ask their family planning practitioner for recent information about its reliability. Women who want to use a barrier method, but have difficulty inserting a diaphragm or a sponge, may prefer foam.

Intrauterine Devices

Intrauterine devices, commonly known as IUDs, are small objects made of plastic or a combination of plastic and metal that are inserted into the uterus by a doctor. Because of concerns about the safety of IUDs, only two types are currently available in the United States. The IUD is 94%–99% reliable.

Usually it is easier to insert an IUD in a woman who has had at least one child, so someone who has not used an IUD might want to consider it after giving birth. The IUD can be inserted during a postpartum office visit, from 3 to 8 weeks after birth.

The advantage of an IUD is that it is almost as reliable as hormones, without having their side effects. Women who want to breast feed, and/or have difficulty with barrier methods, might consider using an IUD.

An important disadvantage of using an IUD is that it increases the risk of pelvic infection. Other disadvantages are that IUD use can cause heavier or more painful periods, and that the IUD may be expelled. (A string attached to the IUD protrudes from the cervix, so that one can check whether it is in place, but this may be difficult for some women.)

Women with certain health problems should not use the IUD:

- Women who do not have a normally shaped uterus (this will include some disabled women).
- Women who have had "PID" (pelvic inflammatory disease) or ectopic pregnancy.
- Women with more than one sex partner (because they have a greater risk for infection).
- Women who have heavy periods.
- Women who have cardiac disease, a history of strokes, or problems with emboli (blood clots).

Women with disabilities that would make it difficult for them to watch for signs and symptoms of pelvic infection should not choose an IUD. Women with disabilities that make them more susceptible to infections (for example, women with SLE) should use another method of birth control.

Sterilization

Sterilization is a surgical procedure that makes a person infertile. It is difficult—sometimes impossible—to reverse sterilization. Some researchers are working to develop surgical procedures for reversing sterilization, and some are working to develop reversible sterilization procedures. However, even if such procedures become widely available, reversing sterilization will not always be reliable. Sterilization should be seen as permanent, and should only be chosen by people who are sure they do not want any more children. For these people, sterilization may be ideal. Sheila commented, "I'm really glad I did it. It gave me real peace of mind."

The advantages of sterilization are that it is more than 99% reliable, and that there are none of the risks or inconveniences of other birth control methods. Either partner can be sterilized.

Vasectomy

Sterilization of a man is called vasectomy, and the procedure can be done in a doctor's office with a local anesthetic. An incision is made in the scrotum (the skin over the testicles or "balls"). Inside the scrotum are a pair of tubes, the vas deferens. Each tube carries sperm from a testicle to the penis. The doctor removes a small section of the tube, seals the open ends, then closes the incision. For a few days after surgery, the area around the incision will be uncomfortable. Some sperm may have been left in the part of the tube closest to the penis, so the couple will need to use another birth control method for a few weeks after surgery, until a sperm count shows that the husband really is sterile.

It is very rare for uncomfortable scar tissue to form after vasectomy, but men who are worried should discuss their concerns with their doctors. Some men feel that somehow surgery makes them less masculine. They, too, should discuss their concerns with their wives and doctors before having surgery.

Tubal Ligation

Sterilization of women is called tubal ligation. The procedure is done on the fallopian tubes, the tubes that carry ova (eggs) from the ovaries to the uterus. A section of each fallopian tube is either removed or clamped.

The two most common procedures are laparoscopic tubal ligation and mini-laparotomy. They are done in the hospital, but the woman enters and leaves the hospital on the same day the surgery is performed (sometimes she may stay one night). The surgery is comparatively minor, but it usually requires general anesthesia. Women who are considering this method need to read about anesthesia in Chapters 7 and 8, and discuss what they have learned with their doctors.

In the first procedure, a tiny incision is made just below the navel. Some gas is injected into the abdomen so that internal organs are gently pushed apart. The doctor inserts instruments which make it possible to see into the abdomen, and seals the fallopian tubes. Then the instruments are removed, the gas is removed, and the incision is sutured.

After surgery, the woman experiences the usual after effects of anesthetics. Her incision is so tiny that it is covered with an ordinary band-aid. When the incision heals, the scar is barely visible. However, the shape of the navel may be changed slightly. Sometimes not all gas is removed from the abdomen, so some women may experience sharp pains for a few days as the gas is absorbed. Women should ask their doctors about these pains so they will know what to expect.

A mini-laparotomy can be done immediately after delivery or after the postpartum visit. If it is done just after delivery, the skin incision is made under the navel, since the uterine fundus and fallopian tubes are in that area. If it is done after the postpartum visit, the skin incision is made in the same area as the bikini cut for cesarean surgery, since the uterus and tubes have shrunk back into the pelvis. In either case, the tubes are elevated out of the incision, each tube is tied in two places, and a section of tube between the ties is removed. The tubes are replaced, and the skin incision is sutured. Like the incision made for a laparoscopic ligation, this incision is so small that it can be covered with a band-aid.

A tubal ligation can be performed during cesarean surgery. Arlene chose to be sterilized at the time she gave birth because "I was too old. I was sure I didn't want to get pregnant again." It is not a good idea to make a last-minute decision about sterilization during cesarean birth, because it is important to take enough time to feel completely comfortable with the decision. Sybil made such a last-minute decision. She felt she had been pressured into the decision, and she regretted her choice.

Women who have been sterilized continue to menstruate. Some women's periods become heavier. Also, 10% of women who have tubal ligations by any method develop irregular, painful periods within 3 years after the procedure. This post-tubal ligation syndrome may be due to partial impairment of the blood supply to the ovaries, caused by the cutting of some blood vessels during surgery.

INFANT CARE

Caring for her baby begins a new chapter in a woman's life. However, in this book, a discussion of baby care is limited to a few words at the end of the last chapter. In our directory of resources, we will list some of the many good books about baby care. Here, we will simply offer a few helpful suggestions drawn from the experiences of the women we interviewed.

Women's feelings about the task of child care have changed over time. Many women said that when their children were first born, they felt overwhelmed by the new responsibility. Stacy said, "I was scared to change diapers, dress the baby, nurse him, even to hold him."

Yet when they were interviewed weeks, months, or years after giving birth, all the women said that they were glad to be mothers, that they would make the same choice again, and that they would encourage other disabled women to have children. Although they remembered the postpartum period as a time of tears and frustration, their comments revealed that it was also a time of learning. This section describes some of the general lessons they learned and offers their practical suggestions about caring for small babies.

Many women emphasized that babies learn to adapt to the mother's disability, and that women can take advantage of that adaptability. Hilary commented, "As soon as my children were able to sit, they moved to me." Sheila said, "I taught my babies from birth to help me when I picked them up. I would put one hand underneath their bodies and put one hand gently around the baby's wrist and pull gently. I would wait, because they were eager to be held and they were able to help. I discovered that by even 5 months old they can help a lot. I would take care of someone else's baby—these women weren't disabled—and their babies didn't respond as my children did. I couldn't lift them up. As my children got older, they were able to help more."

There are some women whose babies will take longer to adapt to the mother's disability. This may include women with involuntary movement in their arms. A good technique to help in this situation is to stop during the activity and talk to the baby.

Women who were not able to give their children much physical care arranged to have help. Athina said that at first she had attendants available around the clock.

Many women commented that it is important to find ways to simplify housework and baby care. Hilary gave a favorite example: "I stacked all the clean sheets right under the crib so I wouldn't have to run around getting sheets every time the baby wet the bed."

Furniture and Equipment

Many women found that they could have baby-care furniture and equipment modified to meet their needs, or that they could use generally available equipment in new ways. Hilary said, "Before my children could move to me, I used a portacrib, because I could reach all around the crib easily." (Hilary was describing a crib which is meant to be used for travel and is smaller than a standard crib.) Some people use specially designed cribs with a side that swings out rather than one that slides up and down (See Figure 9.1); a woman who uses a wheelchair can open the door, then roll her wheelchair under the crib so she can reach her baby.

Heather and Stephanie shopped carefully for well-designed changing tables. Stephanie "made sure the changing table was the correct height for me to get my wheelchair under." Heather said, "I needed something sturdy, one that wouldn't be wobbly so I could lean up against it. The one that worked best was wooden." Some women prefer a table that has a built-in belt that holds the baby in place so a parent has both hands free for changing the diaper and cleaning the baby.

Stephanie found a new use for a harness that parents use so their toddlers will not run away. She said, "I dressed my baby in the harness and took off the straps. When I wanted to take her out of her walker, I could get a good grip on the harness and lift her up by it."

Carrying and Moving the Baby

Each woman seemed to invent her own clever way of carrying her baby. Hilary said, "I would carry my babies on my shoulder like a sack of potatoes, with one arm holding onto the baby's trunk. Since they were small, I could use the same hand to support their heads. Then I'd use my other hand to hold onto a crutch, a piece of furniture, or the wall for support." Heather, who uses two crutches, also managed to carry her baby. She explained, "I used my upper arm and elbow to hold the crutch, then used my forearm to support my baby against my body, with my hand hooked in his armpit."

Clara does not use crutches, but has some difficulty with balance. She felt she could carry her babies most securely when she hugged them against the front of her body. She said, "That way my chest and tummy supported the baby's back and head, and they could look around because they were facing forward."

Many of the women who used wheelchairs held their babies on their laps. Celeste said, "I would hold the baby on my lap with one hand, and push the chair with the other." Sheila said, "When I used the footrest I had more of a lap for my babies, and I would also use receiving blankets to pad around them. When they got to be about 4 months old and began to get some sitting balance, I made a spot beside me where they could ride." A friend of Judi's who recently became disabled developed a unique way to

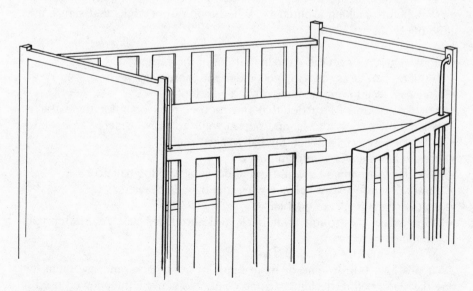

FIGURE 9.1. Breakfront crib.

carry her newborn baby in her wheelchair. Janet used an infant carseat, a luggage strap, and a padded board. The cushion is made out of a piece of foam and mat board. Janet then places the padded side of the board on her lap and rests the carseat sideways on the board. The luggage strap is used to attach the carseat to her chair.

Some women preferred not to hold their babies on their laps. Pam said, "I felt he could fall off." Athina said, "I would carry her on my lap in the house, but when I went outside it was just too precarious. I'd put the baby in the stroller, and my attendant would push the stroller and I'd push my own chair." Pam solved the problem by strapping her baby to her body, commenting, "That way my hands were free." Dawn put her baby in a front pack.

Women who could walk, often used strollers or front packs to carry their babies. Heather found difficulties with these methods. She said, "The front pack didn't work because it felt like the baby was just hanging there. I just didn't like the sensation. Using my prosthesis didn't work either. I also tried to use a stroller but it was difficult to bend down and lift the baby up. My crutches got in my way. The heavier stroller was more secure, but the lightweight stroller would go right out from under me." However, several women liked using front packs and strollers. Some even used wheeled bassinets or strollers to move their babies from room to room at home. Christina said, "Using an umbrella stroller was easier because my balance is a problem."

Be sure to experiment with several types of front packs, baby slings, and strollers before making a purchase. When trying front packs and slings, ask these questions:

- How easy is it to get the baby in and out of the carrier?
- Will it be harder as the baby gets older and more wiggly?
- How easy is it to put the pack on and take it off?
- If it is the kind of carrier that the mother puts on after the baby is inside, how easy is it to lift and put on with the baby inside?
- Will it be just as easy when the baby gains weight?
- Are the fasteners easy to manipulate?
- How does carrying a baby in front affect your walking balance?
- How will it affect your balance when the baby is heavier?
- Do the straps feel comfortable?
- Does it feel as though your back and shoulders will ache after you use the carrier?

If possible, borrow one or more kinds of front packs and use them for one day each before deciding. (None of the women we interviewed used a backpack. A woman who is considering a backpack should also try several models.)

These are the questions to ask when choosing a stroller:

- If you need to lean on it for support, is it heavy enough to support your weight without starting to roll away?
- Is it light enough to push easily?
- Does it have a brake you can use while putting the baby in or taking him out?
- How easy is it to use the brake?
- How easy is it to place the baby in the stroller or take her out? (Is it hard to bend, or do crutches get in the way?)
- How well does the stroller turn, and how well does it roll on uneven surfaces?
- Is it easy to store?
- If it is collapsible, how easy is it to collapse and set up again?
- Can it be used to carry packages? (Some strollers are so light that, if a carrying bag is hanging from the handles, the whole stroller tilts over when the baby is lifted out.)

Hilary pointed out that the idea of getting the children to help applies to the problem of getting them from place to place. She said, "I never carried either of them once they began to crawl. Sometimes I would have to coax them, other times I needed more patience. I even got them to crawl to me when I wanted to change their diapers. After a while they would follow me wherever I wanted them to go."

Changing Diapers

Women offered several suggestions on how to change diapers. As we said before, Stephanie and Heather were careful to find changing tables that were easy to use. Sheila found a way to change her baby in any room she happened to be in. She said, "I would use the bed, the bassinet, or the kitchen table. It just depended on where I was." Christina liked to sit down on her bed when she changed her baby. She explained, "That way I didn't have to worry about my balance."

Most of the women felt that paper diapers worked best, because it is easier to use tape than pins. Women who strongly prefer cloth diapers could look for diaper covers which are designed to hold the diaper in place without pins. Sheila commented, "Sometimes it was hard to get the diapers tight enough. I used one hand, but sometimes I needed to use my teeth."

Some women may need help with caring for the baby's navel while it is healing during the first 4–7 days after birth. Occasionally, the area must be cleaned by gently dabbing with a swab dipped in alcohol. If the mother does not have sufficient hand control, her husband or attendant can do the job. Also, the baby's diaper must be changed by someone who can be sure it is kept below the navel, since it is important to keep the area dry to prevent infection.

Bathing Babies

Several women who were comfortable with other tasks preferred not to bathe their babies. Sheila, who found ways to carry her babies and change their diapers, would ask her mother to bathe them. Clara explained, "I really have good control of only one hand and arm, so I was scared the baby would slip away. Until my babies were able to sit on their own, I would have my husband bathe them, or at least make sure he was there to help. I would get in the bathtub and he would give me the baby and then take it back. I finished my bath while he dried the baby."

Hilary used a baby seat. She explained, "I kept the baby in the seat while I got settled in the tub. Then I took the baby in the tub with me while I ran the water. Then I did the whole thing in reverse—I'd let the water out, then put the baby in the seat, then get out of the tub."

Women who shop for bathing equipment will need to think very carefully about whether the equipment will really work for them. For example, is there a secure surface in the kitchen or bathroom for an infant tub? If not, is it really practical to carry the water-filled tub, or carry water to the tub? Will the sides of the tub allow women with limited hand control to reach in comfortably to bathe and support the baby? Some stores have floating seats that can be used for bathing babies (see Figure 9.2). These seats can only be

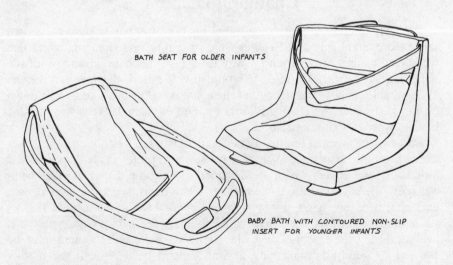

BATH SEAT FOR OLDER INFANTS

BABY BATH WITH CONTOURED NON-SLIP INSERT FOR YOUNGER INFANTS

FIGURE 9.2. Bath seats.

used after the baby is able to sit independently. When choosing a seat, try to see whether it will be easy to get the baby in and out. Once the baby is in the seat, how easy will it be to lift the seat into the tub and out again? Perhaps someone else can put the seat in the tub, and then the mother can bathe the baby. Is the seat designed so that the baby cannot slip out easily? Is it well balanced, so that it will not tilt over if the baby moves vigorously?

CLOSING COMMENTS

Portia commented that pregnancy is just a step on the way to motherhood. In the same way, infancy is just a step on the way to childhood. Newborn babies are very dependent, and the responsibility for their care can be frightening. It helps to remember that they adapt quickly, adjusting their movements to their mother's so that she can lift and carry them more easily. Most babies will sit independently by 8 months of age, walk and spoon-feed themselves by 14 months of age, and help dress themselves when they are about 2 years old. The frustration of bathing a slippery, wriggly baby will become a laughable memory. The baby's adaptability and independence, and the mother's flexibility and creativity, will combine to make parenthood a joyous experience.

APPENDIX A—DIET PLAN AND SUGGESTED FOOD LISTS

The following meal plan is adapted from the Dietary Guidelines and Daily Food Guide in *Nutrition During Pregnancy and the Postpartum Period: A Manual for Health Care Professionals,* published by the California Department of Health Services. A woman who uses this plan will meet all her nutritional requirements. It is different in some respects from other diet plans you may have seen. A short explanation should help you feel comfortable with this plan and use it wisely.

Rather than making suggestions for what you should eat at each meal, we have provided information on the food groups and serving sizes (Table A) to allow you greater flexibility in planning meals according to your individual needs. For example, if you are eating small, frequent meals to cope with indigestion (as we suggest in Chapter 6), you might want to include some suggested servings in between-meal snacks. You might prefer to have more protein servings at breakfast, and fewer at dinner, to avoid getting heartburn from a heavy evening meal. If you are troubled with muscle cramps at night, you might eat some calcium-rich foods as a bedtime snack, to see if the calcium alleviates the cramping.

Another difference from many diet plans is that the number of portions may seem high. That is because the portion sizes given in this meal plan are smaller than in others. Using smaller portions adds flexibility and variety to your diet, which is especially helpful during the first trimester when food is

363

so often unappealing. The smaller portions also help you in planning several small meals a day, which can help prevent many pregnancy discomforts.

The amount of protein provided in this meal plan is greater than the minimum daily requirement. Eating the additional protein is the only way to obtain enough vitamin B_6, iron, and zinc from food.

Tables B–H list a variety of foods in each food group. Enough choices are listed to help you plan interesting, enjoyable meals. If you have allergies, these lists will help you safely meet all your nutritional needs. They also make it possible to plan meals that are relatively high or low in calories. The key difference is in how well you follow the advice to limit fats and sweets. For example, if you choose to eat cooked yams because they are rich in vitamin A, canned, candied yams will supply more calories than a plain, baked yam. If you choose lean meat, fish, and vegetable proteins, and avoid fried foods and sugary foods, you probably will not consume too many calories. If you need to gain weight, do not eat more fatty or sweet foods, but more breads and cereals. Your doctor or nutritionist can advise you.

Because fiber is now known to be an important part of your diet, fiber-rich foods are marked accordingly. The inclusion of several ethnic foods, such as tortillas, chitterlings, and tofu, should help make sensible eating enjoyable eating.

We have eliminated charts listing foods rich in some nutrients, such as magnesium, because they contain foods which are included on other lists, and have expanded the list of sweeteners to include names that are frequently included on food labels (for example, "sucrose" for sugar).

TABLE A
DAILY FOOD GUIDE FOR WOMEN

Food Group	Minimum Number of Servings		
	Nonpregnant Adolescent Female	Nonpregnant Adult Female	Pregnant/Lactating Adolescent/Adult Female
Protein foods	6[a]	6[a]	8[b]
Milk products	3	2	4
Breads, cereals, grains	6[c]	6[c]	6[c]
Fruits and vegetables			
Vitamin C-rich	1	1	2
Vitamin A-rich	1	1	1
Other	3	3	3
Fats and sweets		Use sparingly	
Water[d]			

[a]Equivalent in protein to 6 oz of animal protein; at least one of these servings should be from the vegetable protein list.
[b]Equivalent in protein to 8 oz of animal protein; at least two of these servings should be from the vegetable protein list.
[c]At least four of these servings should be from whole grains.
[d]Eight 8-oz servings per day are recommended for all groups.

TABLE B
PROTEIN FOODS

Type of Protein	Serving Size[a]
Animal: Low in Fat (< 5 g/serving)	
Beef: lean cuts (round, sirloin, flank steak)	1 oz cooked
Chicken	1 oz cooked
Clams	3 medium raw or 1/4 cup canned, drained
Crab	1 1/2 oz or 1/3 cup
Duck	1 oz cooked
Fish: fresh or frozen	1 oz cooked
Fish, canned: salmon, tuna	1 oz or 1/8 cup
Fish, canned: sardines	3 medium or 1 oz drained
Hogmaws (pork stomach)	1 1/2 oz cooked
Lobster	1 1/2 oz cooked
Organ meats: heart, kidney, liver	1 oz cooked
Oysters	6 medium, 3 oz, or 1/3 cup raw or canned
Pork: ham roast	1 oz cooked
Pork: loin, roast, chop	1 oz cooked
Rabbit	1 oz cooked
Scallops	2 medium or 1 oz cooked
Shrimp	2 large, 1 oz cooked, or 1/3 cup breaded
Turkey	1 oz cooked
Tripe (cow stomach)	1 oz cooked
Veal: ground, cube, roast, chop	1 oz cooked
Animal: High in Fat (≥ 5 g/serving)	
Beef: ground, cube, roast, steak, chuck	1 oz cooked
Beef: short rib	1 small
Chitterlings (hog intestines)	3 oz cooked
Eggs	1 large
Fish sticks, breaded	2 medium
Frankfurters	2 medium
Lamb: ground, cube, roast, chop	1 oz cooked

[a]Each serving provides a minimum of 6 g of protein.
Abbreviations: F, Moderately rich in fiber (1 to 3.9 g/serving); FF, rich in fiber (≥ 4 g/serving).

TABLE B *(CONTINUED)*

Type of Protein	Serving Size[a]
Animal: High in Fat (≥5 g/serving)	
Luncheon meat: bologna, ham, liverwurst	2 slices or 2 oz
Organ meats: sweetbreads	1 oz cooked
Oysters, fried	7 medium
Pig feet	2 oz cooked
Pork: ground, roast, chop	1 oz cooked
Pork: spareribs	2 small ribs
Sausage	3 small links or 2 oz cooked
Tongue	1 oz cooked
Vegetable: Low in Fat (<5 g/serving)	
Beans: garbanzo, kidney, navy, pinto, baked, pork and beans (FF)	1/2 cup cooked
Lentils (F)	1/2 cup cooked or 3/4 cup lentil soup
Peas, split (FF)	1/2 cup cooked or 3/4 cup split pea soup
Soybeans	1/4 cup cooked
Soybeans, roasted	2 1/2 tbsp
Soybeans, fermented (tempeh)	1/4 cup or 2 oz
Soybean curd (tofu) (F)	3 oz
Yeast, nutritional	tbsp
Vegetable: High in Fat (≥5 g/serving)	
Baked beans with franks (FF)	1/2 cup
Chile con carne (FF)	1/2 cup
Falafel (garbanzo croquette)	3 patties
Hummus (garbanzo-sesame dip) (F)	1/2 cup
Nuts: almonds, mixed nuts, walnuts (F)	1 1/2 oz or 1/3 cup
Nut butter: cashew, sesame	3 tbsp
Nut butter: peanut	2 tbsp
Peanuts (F)	1 oz or 1/4 cup
Seeds: pumpkin, sunflower	1 oz or 1/4 cup

TABLE C
CALCIUM-RICH FOODS: MILK PRODUCTS

Milk Products	Serving Size
Low in Fat (< 5 g/serving)	
Milk: nonfat dry milk powder	1/3 cup
Milk: nonfat or nonfat dry reconstituted	1 cup
Milk: nonfat, evaporated	1/2 cup
Milk: buttermilk or lowfat	1 cup
Yogurt: nonfat or lowfat, plain or fruit-flavored	6 oz
High in Fat (≥ 5 g/serving)	
Cheese: brick-type or semi-soft (except bleu, Camembert, cream)	1 1/2 oz or 1/3 cup grated
Cheese: cottage (creamed or lowfat)	2 cups
Cheese: hard, grated (e.g., Parmesan, Romano)	4 tbsp
Cheese: ricotta (from whole or part-skim milk)	1/2 cup
Cheese: spread or cheese food (e.g., Velveeta)	2 oz
Cream soups made with milk	1 1/2 cups
Custard (flan)	1 cup
Ice cream	1 1/2 cups
Ice milk	1 1/2 cups
Milk: whole or chocolate	1 cup
Milk: whole, evaporated	1/2 cup
Milkshake	1 cup homemade or 1 average commercial
Pudding	1 cup
Yogurt: whole (plain or fruit-flavored)	8 oz
Yogurt: frozen	1 1/2 cups

TABLE D
CALCIUM-RICH FOODS: NONDAIRY PRODUCTS[a]

5 medium sardines (2 1/2 oz)
1/2 cup canned salmon (with bones)
9 oz tofu (must be processed with a calcium salt)
4 oz almonds
1/4 cup tahini (sesame butter)
2 cups baked beans or pork and beans
7 corn tortillas (treated with lime or calcium carbonate, as is masa
  harina)
5 medium oranges
1 1/2 cups broccoli, fresh cooked
1 1/2 cups turnip, cooked
2 cups bok choy, collard or dandelion greens, cooked
3 cups kale or mustard greens, cooked
2 tbsp blackstrap molasses

[a]Each serving is approximately equivalent in calcium to one serving from
the milk products group (250–300 mg calcium) in Table C.

Note: Other dark, leafy greens, such as spinach, are not good sources of calcium
because they contain a chemical that binds the calcium and makes it unavailable.

TABLE E
BREADS, CEREALS, AND GRAINS

Whole-Grain	Serving Size
Bread: whole-wheat, cracked wheat, pumpernickel (F)	1 slice
Bran, unprocessed (FF)	1/2 cup
Bran cereals, flaked	1 oz or 3/4 cup
Bulgur, cooked (FF)	1/2 cup
Cereals, cooked: oatmeal, Wheatena, Malt-O-Meal, Roman Meal (F)	1/2 cup
Cereals, ready-to-eat:	
Cheerios, Wheaties (F)	1 oz or 3/4 cup
Cereals, puffed (F)	1 oz or 2 cups
Crackers, fat added: Triscuits (F)	1 oz or 8
Crackers, fat added: Wheat Thins (F)	1 oz or 12
Crackers, no fat added: Kavali, Wasa (F)	3/4 oz or 2–4 slices
Grapenuts (F)	1 oz or 1/4 cup
Granola	1/2 cup
Muffin: bran or whole-wheat (F)	1
Pasta, whole-wheat: macaroni, noodles, spaghetti (F)	1/2 cup cooked
Popcorn (F)	2 cups
Rice, brown (F)	1/2 cup cooked
Rice cake	3
Rye Crisp (F)	4 (2" x 3 1/2" crackers)
Shredded Wheat (F)	1 oz, 1 biscuit, or 3/4 cup
Tortilla, corn	1 small (6" diameter)
Wheat germ (FF)	1 oz or 4 tbsp

Abbreviations: F, Moderately rich in fiber (1 to 3.9 g/serving); FF, rich in fiber (≥ 4 g/serving).

Note: Brand names are cited as examples only and do not imply endorsement or superiority over products with similar nutrient characteristics.

TABLE E *(CONTINUED)*

Enriched	Serving Size
Bagel	1/2
Bread	1 slice
Bread sticks, crisp	2 (4" x 1/2")
Bun: frankfurter or hamburger	1/2
Cereals, cooked: Cream of Rice, Cream of Wheat, Maypo	1/2 cup
Cereals, ready-to-eat	1 oz or 3/4 cup
Cornbread (F)	1 piece (2" square)
Crackers, fat added: Ritz	1 oz or 8
Crackers, no fat added: soda crackers	1 oz or 8
Croutons	1/2 cup
Dumpling	1 small
Grits	1/2 cup cooked
Graham crackers (FF)	4 (2 1/2" squares)
Muffin, biscuit, dumpling	1
Muffin, English	1/2
Pancake	1 medium
Pasta: macaroni, noodles, spaghetti	1/2 cup cooked
Pita	1/2 (6" diameter)
Rice, white	1/2 cup cooked
Roll, dinner	1 small
Stuffing	1/4 cup
Tortilla, flour	1 small or 1/2 large
Waffle	1 (4 1/2" x 4 1/2")

TABLE F
VITAMIN C-RICH FRUITS AND VEGETABLES

Product	Serving Size[a]
Juices	
Orange	6 oz
Grapefruit, lemon	6 oz
Fruit juices enriched with vitamin C	6 oz
Tomato Juice	6 oz
Vegetable juice cocktail	6 oz
Fruits	
Cantaloupe (F)	1/4 medium or 1/2 cup cubed
Grapefruit (F)	1/2 medium
Guava	1 medium
Kiwi	1 medium
Lemon	1 medium
Mango (F)	1 medium
Orange (F)	1 medium
Papaya	1/4 medium
Strawberries (F)	1/2 cup
Tangerine (FF)	2 medium
Vegetables	
Broccoli (F)	1/2 cup raw or cooked
Brussels sprouts (F)	3 medium or 1/2 cup cooked
Cabbage (F)	1 cup raw or 1/2 cup cooked
Cauliflower (F)	1/2 cup raw or cooked
Peppers: hot, chili	2 tbsp raw or 1/2 cup canned/bottled
Peppers: sweet	1/2 raw or 1/2 cup cooked
Snow peas	1/2 cup raw or cooked
Tomatoes: green, red (FF)	2 medium raw
Tomato paste	1/2 cup
Tomato puree	1/2 cup

[a]Each serving provides a minimum of 30 mg of vitamin C.
Abbreviations: F, Moderately rich in fiber (1 to 3.9 g/serving); FF, rich in fiber (≥ 4 g/serving).

Note: While fresh, frozen, or canned fruits and vegetables may be eaten, fresh is preferable.

TABLE G
VITAMIN A-RICH FRUITS AND VEGETABLES

Product	Serving Size [a]
Juices	
Apricot nectar	6 oz
Vegetable juice cocktail	6 oz
Fruits	
Apricots (F)	3 medium raw or 1/4 cup dried
Cantaloupe (F)	1/4 medium or 1/2 cup cubed
Mango (F)	1/4 medium or 1/2 cup cubed
Papaya	1/2 medium or 3/4 cup cubed
Vegetables	
Bok Choy	1/2 cup cooked
Beet greens	1/2 cup cooked
Carrots (F)	1/2 cup or 1 small
Chard, swiss	1/2 cup cooked
Collards (F)	1/2 cup cooked
Dandelion greens (F)	1/2 cup cooked
Kale (F)	1/2 cup cooked
Mustard greens (F)	1/2 cup cooked
Parsley (F)	1 cup raw or 1/2 cup cooked
Peppers: hot, chili	2 tbsp raw or cooked
Pumpkin (F)	1/2 cup cooked
Onions, green	1/2 cup chopped
Spinach (F)	1 cup raw or 1/2 cup cooked
Squash, winter (F)	1/2 cup cooked
Sweet potato (F)	1/2 cup cooked
Tomatoes, red (F)	2 medium raw
Yams (see note below) (F)	1/2 cup cooked

[a]Each serving provides a minimum of 2,000 IU of vitamin A.
Abbreviations: F, Moderately rich in fiber (1 to 3.9 g/serving).

Note: Yams commonly available in U.S. markets are actually sweet potatoes and thus rich in vitamin A. True tropical yams are not deep yellow or orange and are not rich in vitamin A.

TABLE H
OTHER FRUITS AND VEGETABLES[a]

Products	Serving Size
Juices	
Apple	6 oz
Cranberry	6 oz
Grape	6 oz
Pineapple	6 oz
Prune	6 oz
Fruits	
Apple (F)	1 medium or 1/4 cup dried
Applesauce (F)	1/2 cup
Avocado	1/2 medium
Banana (F)	1 medium
Blackberries (FF)	1/2 cup
Blueberries (F)	1/2 cup
Cherries (F)	1/2 cup
Dates (F)	4
Figs (F)	1/2 cup fresh or 1/4 cup dried
Fruit cocktail	1/2 cup
Grapes	1/2 cup or 15 small
Kumquats	1 medium
Nectarine (F)	1 medium
Peach (F)	1 medium or 1/2 cup sliced or canned
Pear (F)	1 medium or 1/2 cup sliced or canned
Persimmon	1 medium
Pineapple (F)	1/2 cup
Plums (F)	2 medium
Pomegranate	1 medium
Prunes (FF)	1/2 cup cooked or 1/4 cup dried
Raisins (F)	1/4 cup

[a]Foods in this group contribute varying amounts of fiber and other nutrients.

Abbreviations: F, Moderately rich in fiber (1 to 3.9 g/serving); FF, rich in fiber (≥ 4 g/serving).

TABLE H *(CONTINUED)*

Products	Serving Size
Fruits *(continued)*	
Raspberries (FF)	1/2 cup
Watermelon	1/2 cup
Vegetables	
Artichoke (FF)	1/2 medium
Asparagus (F)	6 medium stalks or 1/2 cup cooked
Bamboo shoots	1/2 cup
Bean sprouts: alfalfa, mung (F)	1 cup raw or 1/2 cup cooked
Beans: green, wax (F)	1/2 cup
Beans: lima (FF)	1/2 cup
Beets (F)	1/2 cup
Celery (F)	1/2 cup
Corn (F)	1/2 cup or 6" cob
Cucumber	1/2 cup
Eggplant (F)	1/2 cup
Hominy	1/2 cup
Jicama	1/2 cup
Kale (F)	1/2 cup
Lettuce	1 cup raw
Mushrooms	1/2 cup
Okra (F)	1/2 cup
Onion (F)	1/2 cup
Parsnip (F)	1/2 cup
Peas: green (FF)	1/2 cup
Potatoes: red, white, russet (F)	1/2 cup
Radishes	1/2 cup
Seaweed	1/2 cup
Summer squash (F)	1/2 cup
Tomatillos	1/2 cup
Turnip (F)	1/2 cup
Zucchini (F)	1/2 cup

TABLE I
FATS, SWEETS, AND OTHER FOODS WHICH
SHOULD BE LIMITED

Unsaturated Fats

   Margarine (listing liquid oil as first ingredient on label)
   Mayonnaise
   Oils, vegetable (except palm and coconut)
   Olives
   Salad dressing (oil-based)

Saturated Fats

   Butter
   Bacon
   Coconut
   Coconut oil
   Coffee whitener
   Cream, coffee
   Cream, sour
   Cream, whipping
   Cream cheese
   Lard
   Margarine (not listing liquid oil as first ingredient on label)
   Palm oil
   Salad dressing
   Salt pork
   Shortening

Sweeteners

Corn syrup	Sucrose	Fructose
Honey	Dextrose	High-fructose corn sweetener
Molasses	Levulose	
Sugar	Maltose	

Sweets

   Candy
   Cake
   Cookies
   Doughnuts, sweet rolls
   Pie
   Soft drinks (e.g., sodas, sweetened fruit drinks, punch, Kool-Aid)

Other Foods

   Chips
   Pork rinds
   Fruit leather

APPENDIX B—
RESOURCE DIRECTORY

. . . .

There are literally hundreds of organizations providing direct and indirect services to people with disabilities, and only a partial selection is given here. The list of organizations assisting pregnant women is also partial. Many organizations provide more services than are mentioned here; this guide emphasizes services that would be helpful for women who are pregnant, or considering pregnancy.

If you cannot find the resource you need in this directory, it is likely that one of the organizations listed here can give you an appropriate referral. Another excellent resource is the reference librarian at your public library; librarians are trained to locate such information, always eager to help, and usually able to answer questions by telephone. If your local telephone directory does not list a local chapter of an organization listed below, the national headquarters may be able to give you a referral. Sometimes local chapters vary; if yours does not meet your needs, the national affiliate may be able to refer you to a chapter in a neighboring community, or to another organization. Your State Department of Rehabilitation, among the other services it provides, can refer you to the nearest independent living center.

AMERICAN RESOURCE CENTERS

. . . .

Organizations Serving All Disabilities

AT&T National Special Needs Center
2001 Route 46, Suite 310
Parsippany, NJ 07054-1315
(800) 233-1222 (Voice)/(800) 833-3232

Answering the telephone quickly is always a problem for new mothers, who cannot leave the baby unattended. Mobility impairment makes the problem worse. It may be possible to install special telephone equipment, such as speakerphones, and the Special Needs Center can advise you.

Epilepsy Foundation of America
4351 Garden City Drive
Landover, Maryland 20785
(301) 459-3700/(800) EFA-1000/(800) 322-4050 library service

Information for people with epilepsy, their families, and the general public. Library service—medical library for health care professionals contains information on clinical and psychosocial aspects of epilepsy.

National Easter Seal Society
2023 West Ogden Avenue
Chicago, IL 60612
(312) 243-8400/(800) 221-6827

Distributes a wide variety of information on rehabilitation issues for children and adults. Referrals to local chapters throughout the country for information, rehabilitation, transportation, treatment, and other services.

National Health Information Center
ODPHP National Health Information Center
P.O. Box 1133
Washington, DC 20013-1133
(301) 565-4167/(800) 336-4797
Identifies health information resources and provides referrals to more than 1,000 health-related information organizations. Provides directories, bibliographies and resource guides on health-related topics.

National Library Service for the Blind and Physically Handicapped
Library of Congress
Washington, DC 20542
(202) 287-5100/(800) 424-9100

A free national library program for individuals who cannot use standard printed materials. The national service also develops information packets, many of which are related to technology. The library may be able to refer you to a regional library near you which provides disability-related information.

National Rehabilitation Information Center
8455 Colesville Road, Suite 935
Silver Spring, MD 20910-33-19
(301) 588-9284/(800) 346-2742

The National Rehabilitation Information Center (NARIC) is funded by the National Institute on Disability and Rehabilitation Research of the U.S. Department of Education (NIDRR). Its library facilitates access to NIDRR and Rehabilitation Services Administration (RSA) reports, and disseminates other rehabilitation related information. NARIC's database, REHABDATA, lists over 19,000 documents including NIDRR and RSA reports, journal articles, and commercial publications. The data base and the library are open to the public, and information seraches and referrals may be requested.

Through the Looking Glass
c/o Megan Kirschbaum
801 Peralta Avenue
Berkeley, CA 94707
(415) 525-8138

Counseling project to assist parents with disabilities with infant and child care.

World Institute on Disability
510 16th Street
Oakland, CA 94612
(415) 763-4100/FAX (415) 763-4109

WID is a public policy and research institute specializing in independent living, personal assistant services, aging technology and international affairs, which provides limited international fellowships for study in the area of disability. If necessary, WID can provide referrals to local independent living programs.

Organizations Serving Individuals with Specific Disabilities

American Paralysis Association
500 Morris Avenue
Springfield, NJ 07081
(201) 379-2690/(800) 225-0292
FAX (201) 912-9433

Supports research for cure of spinal cord injuries. Maintains computerized database. Sponsors information and referral hotline (see APA Spinal Cord Injury Hotline).

Avenues, National Support Group for Arthrogryposis Multiplex Congenita

c/o Mary Ann Schmidt
P.O. Box 5192
Sonora, CA 95370
(209) 928-3688

Information exchange for individuals with AMC, their families and interested professionals. Newsletter, bibliography of research articles, pamphlet. Self-help orientation.

Lupus Foundation of America, Inc.

11921-A Olive Boulevard
St. Louis, MO 63141
(800) 558-0121

Services include referrals.

Muscular Dystrophy Association

810 Seventh Avenue
New York, NY 10019
(212) 586-0808

Sponsors research on a number of disorders including dystrophies, myotonias, Friedreich's ataxia. Referrals to local chapters which may provide services including consultation, medical follow-up and physical therapy.

Myasthenia Gravis Foundation

53 W. Jackson Boulevard, Suite 1352
Chicago, IL 60604
(312) 427-6252/(800) 541-5454

Research and education in MG, support for individuals and their families. For women who are pregnant or considering pregnancy, will provide referrals to physicians with expertise in MG, and information on MG and pregnancy and effects of MG on the newborn baby. Ask for education director.

National Arthritis and Musculoskeletal and Skin Diseases Information Clearinghouse

P.O. Box 9782
Arlington, VA 22209
(703) 554-4999

Information and referral center. Information exchange for those involved in public and patient education. Locates relevant research and literature.

National Multiple Sclerosis Society
205 E. 42nd Street
New York, NY 10017
(212) 986-3240/(800) 624-8236

Services include resource center with 10,000 reprints, computer searching of biomedical databases, informational publications, and referrals to 124 local chapters for direct services.

National Spinal Cord Injury Association
600 West Cummings Park, #2000
Woburn, MA 01801
(800) 962-9629

Comprehensive services include development of regional systems for treatment and rehabilitation; consultation and education for individuals with SCI, their families, and professionals; advocacy; publications including newsletter. Encourages development of network of local chapters offering information or peer assistance programs. Call toll-free hotline for information and referral service.

National Stroke Information Service Referral Clearinghouse
1255 23rd Street NW, Suite 275
Washington, DC 20013-1133
(202) 429-9091/(800) 336-4797

Health information clearinghouse. Answers information requests; publishes fact sheets; offers referrals to a variety of health-related organizations.

Parkinson's Disease Foundation
William Black Medical Research Bldg.
Columbia Presbyterian Medical Center
640 W. 168th Street
New York, NY 10032
(212) 923-4700/(800) 457-6676

Although Parkinson's rarely occurs in women of child-bearing age, it does happen. Women who are pregnant or considering pregnancy can call the Foundation for information, advice, and referrals. Maintains list of clinics and patient self-help groups.

Polio Information Center
510 Main Street, Suite A446
Roosevelt Island, NY 10044

(212) 223-0353

Information on post polio research; referral services.

P.R.I.D.E. Foundation
Box 1293
71 Plaza Court
Groton, CT 06340
(203) 445-1448

Helps people find or adapt attractive, convenient clothing. Publications include resource directory and information on adapting ready-made clothing for adults and children (including adaptations of infant clothing). For specific information, inquiries are welcome.

Spina Bifida Association
1700 Rockville Pike, Suite 540
Rockville, MD 20852
(301) 770-SBAA/(800) 621-3141

Numerous programs include information and referral service; publishes newsletter and informational pamphlets.

APA Spinal Cord Injury Hotline
2201 Argonne Drive
Baltimore, MD 21218
(800) 226-0292

Information and referral service for individuals with spinal cord injuries (SCI) and their families. Hours are Monday–Friday, 9 A.M. to 5 P.M. Eastern Standard Time, but volunteers answer emergency questions 24 hours a day. Referrals for peer support (nationwide network), expert advice, other SCI support and service organizations, rehabilitation facilties, and SCI literature. Helps with problems ranging from finding rehabilitation facilities to designing an accessible home or choosing a wheelchair. The Hotline is sponsored by the American Paralysis Association.

United Cerebral Palsy Associations
66 E. 34th Street
New York, NY 10016
(212) 481-6300/(800) USA-1UCP

National federation of state and local affiliates assisting individuals with CP and their families. The national organization can refer to local affiliates. Some of the local affiliates may offer medical, therapeutic and social services, advocacy, assistance with independent living.

CANADIAN RESOURCE CENTERS

. . . .

Canadian Rehabilitation Council for the Disabled
45 Sheppard Avenue East, Suite 801
Willowdale, Ontario M2N 5W9, Canada

CRCD provides information on issues related to disability and rehabilitation to member organizations, professionals, and the disabled community. Publications include quarterly newsletter.

Disabled Living Resource Centre
Kinsman Rehabilitation Foundation
2256 West 12th Avenue
Vancouver, British Columbia V6K 2N5, Canada
(604) 736-8841

Lending library and computer database on resources and adaptive equipment, and evaluation and demonstration of equipment.

INTERNATIONAL RESOURCE CENTERS

. . . .

Disabled Living Foundation Equipment Centre
380-384 Harrow Road
London W9 2HU, England
01-289-6111

Provides information on technical devices for the disabled. Includes an equipment demonstration center open to professionals and the disabled community.

European Technical Aids Information System
Patrick Daunt
Bureau for Action in Favor of Disabled People
A1 613 200
Rue de la Loi
B-1049 Brussels Belgium

The European Economic Community is developing "Handynet," a new technical aids system for disabled persons. So far there are two components: Handyaids, which lists information on technical aids available in the EEC and Scandinavia; and "Handywho," which has information on professionals and organizations that develop or provide such aids. Future components include

"Handysearch," an inventory of research in the field of technical aids; "Handyce," information on EEC documents and legislation concerning the disabled; and "Handynews," which will report new developments, meetings, and conferences in the field.

SEXUALITY, FAMILY PLANNING, PREGNANCY, AND CHILDBIRTH

American Academy of Husband-Coached Childbirth
P.O. Box 5224
Sherman Oaks, CA 91413
(818)768-6662/(800) 422-4784

Promotes the "Bradley method." Training programs for childbirth educators, referrals to local teachers.

ASPO/Lamaze
1840 Wilson Boulevard, Suite 204
Arlington, VA 22201
(703)524-7802/(800) 368-4404

The American Society for Psychoprophylaxis in Obstetrics (ASPO) promotes the Lamaze Method, trains childbirth educators, and provides referrals to local teachers.

C/SEC
22 Forest Rd.
Framingham, MA 01701
(617) 877-8266

Goal is to "make the Cesarean delivery a good and meaningful experience for each couple." Provides information on Cesarean birth and VBAC, referrals to local support groups, help in developing support groups for parents who expect a Cesarean birth, or have already experienced it.

International Childbirth Education Association (ICEA)
P.O. Box 20048
Minneapolis, MN 55420
(612) 854-8680/(800) 624-4934

Among other services, ICEA offers a wide variety of publications about pregnancy, childbirth, and breastfeeding. Also operates a mail-order bookstore. For information or catalogs, call toll-free.

National Birth Defects Center
Kennedy Memorial Hospital

30 Warren Street
Brighton, MA 02135
(617) 787-4957/(800) 322-5014 (in Massachusetts)

For those outside Massachusetts, provides referrals to agencies which can give your or your physicians information about how medications and other chemicals taken during pregnancy will affect your baby. Provides this information directly to Massachusetts residents.

Planned Parenthood

380 Second Avenue
New York, NY 10010
(212) 777-2002

Family planning and fertility information; referrals to local service providers.

SIECUS

84 Fifth Avenue, Suite 407
New York, NY 10011
(212) 819-9970

SIECUS stands for Sex Information and Educational Council of the United States. Services include sexuality information and advice, including special materials for individuals with disabilities.

Tokos Medical Corporation

1821 E. Dyer Rd., #200
Santa Ana, CA 92705
1-800-678-6567

Referrals to branch offices around the country for home uterine monitoring services for women at risk of giving birth prematurely. Not only can this service prevent the need for early admission to the hopital, but the nurses providing the service can be an important source of information and support for the mother to be.

DATABASES AND COMPUTER NETWORKS

If you do not have access to a computer, a disability-related service agency may be able to conduct an information search for you.

ABLEDATA (BRS ABLE) Adaptive Equipment Center

Newington Children's Hospital 181 East Cedar Street
Newington, CT 06111

(203) 667-5405/(800) 344-5405

Lists commercially available rehabilitation and adaptive equipment from over 1900 companies. List is updated monthly and includes manufacturer, product description, price, and, sometimes, comments. A Macintosh computer version, using Hypercard software, is available form the Trace Center, University of Wisconsin, Madison, Wisconsin.

HEALTH CARE FACILITY DATABASE (STSC/ONLINE)
Urban Decision Systems, Inc.
P.O. Box 2593
2040 Armacost Avenue
Los Angeles, CA 90025
(213) 820-8931

Listing of hospital facilities including type of hospital, facilities available, patient admissions, and other data. Updated quarterly. May be helpful in locating nearby hospital best able to serve special needs.

REHABDATA (BRS/NRIC)
Access to the NARIC database, updated monthly (see NARIC above).

CompuServe
5000 Arlington Center Boulevard
P.O. Box 20212
Columbus, OH 43220
(614) 457-8600/(800) 818-8199

Network with numerous bulletin boards and databases, includes information on everything from national news to childcare. Has a Mutual Aid Self-Help secton (MASH). The magazine *Disability Rag* is available through the disability Special Interest Group (SIG). To access Handicapped Users Database, type [GO HUD].

DISC
Walter Dinsdale Centre
839 5th Avenue, Suite 610
Calgary, Alberta T2P 3C8
Canada
(403) 266-0095

A national telecommunications network for exchange of information among persons with disabilities and those who work on disability issues. Includes electronic mail, bulletin boards, database access, and computer conferences. DISC is decentralized, with four regional representatives responsible for member contact and service.

GLOSSARY

....

This glossary does not list every pregnancy or disability term used, but those which are not defined in the text or are frequently used after they have been defined. To find definitions of terms not listed here, see the index.

Alpha fetoprotein   A chemical secreted by the fetus; amounts in the amnionic fluid and/or the mother's blood may be measured for diagnostic purposes.

Amniocentesis   Removal of a sample of amnionic fluid through a puncture in the abdominal wall, usually for diagnostic purposes.

Amniotic fluid; amniotic membrane   Fluid surrounding fetus in the uterus; the membrane containing the fetus and amnionic fluid.

Anemia   Refers to deficiency of red blood cells, hemoglobin, or iron in the blood. Anemia reduces the blood's ability to transport oxygen, resulting in fatigue and other symptoms.

Areola   The area of darker skin surrounding the nipple.

Atrophy (of a muscle or limb)   Wasting away from lack of adequate exercise or nutrition.

"Bag of water"   The amnionic membrane and fluid. The "bag breaking" refers to rupture of the amnionic membrane early in labor.

Braxton–Hicks Contractions   "Practice contractions" that do not result in cervical dilation.

Cervix   The "neck" of the uterus. Closed and firm during pregnancy, so that the fetus is retained in the uterus. During labor, the cervix softens, thins, and dilates, becoming continuous with the uterus so that delivery is possible.

Clonus   Involuntary, spasmodic movements.

Colostrum   A clear, sticky breast secretion that begins before milk secretion begins—often during the last weeks of pregnancy.

Cramps   Strong, painful involuntary muscle contractions. (Calf muscle cramps are commonly called "Charley horses.")

Dysreflexia (autonomic)   A potentially dangerous condition occurring in people with spinal lesions at or above T6. A reflex response to stimuli including bowel or bladder fullness and labor contractions that is not modulated by higher nerve centers, so that high blood pressure results. Symptoms include perspiration, anxiety, flushing and goose bumps above the level of injury, faintness, and a pounding headache.

Distress, fetal   Response to stresses of labor including hypoxia, signs include extreme activity, changes in heart rate, and/or passing of meconium; prolonged distress is dangerous.

Due date   Expected date of birth, 40 weeks after estimated date of conception.

Ectopic pregnancy   Pregnancy in which the fetus is located outside the uterus (includes "tubal pregnancy").

Edema   Swelling caused by fluid build-up in tissues.

Episiotomy   Incision in the perineum (the tissues between the vagina and the anus); made to prevent tearing or ease delivery.

Fetal monitoring   Electronic measurement and recording of fetal movement and heart activity, done to assess fetal health or response to stress.

Fetus   Used here to mean fetus or embryo—that is, all stages of development before birth.

Full-term pregnancy/labor   Pregnancy lasting 37–42 weeks/labor occurring after 37–42 weeks of pregnancy

Fundus   Top of the uterus. Height of the fundus indicates length of pregnancy; after birth, fundal height indicates how well the uterus is recovering.

HCG, human chorionic gonadotropin   A hormone whose presence in blood or urine is a sign of pregnancy.

Hyperreflexia (autonomic)   Same as dysreflexia.

Hypoxia   Lack of oxygen.

Induction   Stimulation of labor, usually by administration of a synthetic hormone.

Involution   Return of uterus to pre-pregnant size.

Kyphoscoliosis   Scoliosis of the upper spine.

Lochia   A discharge resembling menstrual fluid, in which uterine tissues are eliminated during the postpartum period.

Meconium   A thick, sticky substance eliminated as the baby's first bowel movement; passage of meconium during labor is a sign of fetal distress.

Miscarriage; threatened miscarriage   Expulsion of the fetus from the uterus before the twenty-eighth week of pregnancy; presence of signs or symptoms of a possible miscarriage (such as uterine pain or bleeding)

"Morning sickness"   Nausea caused by pregnancy; may occur any time of day.

Oxytocin   A naturally occurring hormone that stimulates labor contractions. (Also called Pitocin or a "pit drip.")

Phantom pain   The impression that pain is occurring in a missing body part, such as an amputated limb.

Phlebitis   Inflammation of a vein.

Pitocin   Proprietary name for oxytocin. When Pitocin is prescribed, it may be called a "pit drip."

Placenta   An organ which is attached to the fetus by the umbilical cord, and embedded in the uterine wall; it transfers oxygen and nutrients from the mother's blood to the fetal blood.

Position (of the fetus)   Refers to direction the fetus is facing.

Presentation (of the fetus)   Refers to the part of the fetus that is closest to the cervix, and which would emerge first at birth. The vertex (crown of the head) presentation is most advantageous. "Breech" presentations are feet or buttocks first. "Transverse" presentations are sideways—the length of the fetus' body is at right angles to the length of the mother's body.

Pressure sore (decubitus ulcer)   A sore (raw area) caused by prolonged pressure on the skin.

Proteinuria   Presence of protein in the urine.

Quad sweats   A common term for mild dysreflexia symptoms, especially when symptoms stop without special treatment; for example, perspiration and dizziness which stop after urination.

Respiration; respiratory difficulties   Breathing; breathing difficulties.

Scoliosis   Abnormal lateral (sideways) curvature of the spine.

Sign   A physical change or appearance which can be used in diagnosing a change in one's physical condition. The change may not be felt as such, but can be found on examination. For example, softening of the cervix is a sign of pregnancy.

Sonography (ultrasound)   A procedure using sound waves to obtain an image of the fetus in the uterus.

Speculum   An instrument that is inserted into the vagina to separate the vaginal walls, making it easier to examine the vagina and cervix.

Spasms   Can refer to muscle cramps or clonus.

Symptom   A physical sensation that reflects a change in one's health or physical condition. For example, nausea and breast tenderness are sometimes symptoms of pregnancy.

Thromboembolism   Blockage of a blood vessel by a blood clot (thrombus).

Thrombophlebitis   Phlebitis caused by a blood clot (thrombus).

Ultrasound   *see* Sonography.

Vaginitis   Local infection of the vagina, accompanied by discomfort and/or discharge.

BIBLIOGRAPHY

....

SUGGESTED READING

....

Directories

Assistive Technology Sourcebook, A. Enders and M. Hall, editors. This 576 page book, published in 1990, is a comprehensive directory of products, publications, and services providing assistance for independent living. It is available for $60.00 from RESNA, 1101 Connecticut Avenue, NW, Suite 700, Washington, DC 20036, (202)857-1199. If you cannot afford it, try requesting its purchase by your public library or independent living center.

Directory of Independent Living Programs (*see* ILRU).

Directory of National Information Sources on Handicapping Conditions and Related Services. A comprehensive listing, and another must for your local library or independent living center. Published in June, 1986, by the National Institute on Disability and Rehabilitation Research. Available from Government Printing Office Public Office, Public Documents Department, Washington, DC 20402–9325; order must be accompanied by check for $17.00, payable to Superintendent of Documents. Or order by telephone, using Visa or MasterCard, by calling (202)783-3238. Also available for $25.00 from Harold Russell Associates, 8 Winchester Place, Suite 304, Winchester, MA 01890.

Useful Books and Articles

Allied Health Profession Section, Arthritis Foundation, *Guide to Independent Living for People with Arthritis.* Pages 211–227 are about child care for parents with disabilities. Available through local chapters or from the Arthritis Foundation, 1314 Spring Street, Atlanta, GA 30309.

Brown, Judith, *Nutrition for Your Pregnancy: The University of Minnesota Guide* (Minneapolis: University of Minnesota Press, 1983). For those who want more information, a comprehensive, well-researched guide.

Elvenstar, Diane C. *Children: To Have or Have Not? A Guide to Making and Living with Your Decision* (San Francisco: Harbor, 1982). This book is available in many libraries. It thoroughly explores most emotional and practical aspects of the decision, with examples from the author's counseling experience, and lists of questions to help you explore your own feelings.

Ferreyra, Susan, and Hughes, Katrine, *Table Manners: A Guide to the Pelvic Examination for Disabled Women and Health Care Providers* (San Francisco: Sex Education for Disabled People, Planned Parenthood Alameda/San Francisco, 1982). Contains excellent illustrations of alternate positions for pelvic examinations; some of these positions could be adapted for delivery.

Ford, Jack R., and Duckworth, Bridget, *Physical Management for the Quadriplegic Patient* (Philadelphia: F.A. Davis Co., 1982). Excellent illustrated advice on managing daily activities, including a chapter on "Sexual Management."

Harrison, Helen (with Kositsky, Ann, R.N.). *The Premature Baby Book* (New York: St. Martin's Press, 1983). Information and advice on care of the premature infant, treatment options, emotional considerations, resources. Very comprehensive—even has patterns for "premie" clothing. Helpful advance reading for women at risk for premature labor.

Hoye, P., Spinal Cord Injured Mothers: I'm Having a Baby, *Mainstream,* February, 1986. A recent, first-person account which may still be obtainable. The organization serving your disability may also have such information; for example, the Multiple Sclerosis Foundation has a leaflet containing an interview with three mothers with MS.

Hutkins, Laura, R.N., M.S., A.C.C.E., TENS: An Innovative Approach to Labor, *Genesis,* June/July, 1988, 10(3). This consumer-oriented article tells how to get more information about use of TENS for pain relief in labor, and is accompanied by references to research articles about use of the method. (*Genesis* is published by ASPO/Lamaze, *see* Glossary.)

Lodge, Mary Marlborough, Parents with Disabilities, *Equipment for Disabled*

People Series. Available for 12 pounds from Nuffield Orthopaedic Centre, Headington, Oxford OX3 7LD, England (telephone: 0865 750103). Published in 1989. 96 pages.

May, Elizabeth and Waggoner, Neva R., *Work Simplification in the Area of Childcare for Physically Handicapped Women.* Originally sponsored and published through the Office of Vocational Rehabilitation, this is now available through NARIC.

May, Elizabeth; Waggoner, Neva R., and Hotte, Eleanor B. *Homemaking for the Handicapped.* Published in 1966, but still available through NARIC (*see* Glossary). Chapter 4, "Work Simplification in the Physical Care of Children," contains suggestions that are still useful.

Neville, Helen, and Halaby, Mona, *No Fault Parenting* (New York: Facts on File, 1986) This book is highly recommended because it contains many practical childcare suggestions drawn from interviews with parents, some of whom were disabled. Describes an approach that can be consistently applied to any family conflict.

Noble, Elizabeth, R.P.T. *Essential Exercises for the Childbearing Year* (Boston, Houghton Mifflin Co., 1982). Excellent, safe pregnancy exercises for those who want additional suggestions. Illustrated.

Robertson, Laurel; Flinders, Carol; Ruppenthal, Brian. *The New Laurel's Kitchen: A Handbook for Vegetarian Cookery and Nutrition* (Berkeley, CA: Ten Speed Press, 1986). The recipes and information in this book will help vegetarians obtain a complete, balanced diet; recommended by nutritionists.

SELECTED BIBLIOGRAPHY

Disability and Pregnancy

Asrael, Wilma, O.T.R., An Approach to Motherhood for Disabled Women. *Rehabilitation Literature,* July/August, 1982, 43(7–8).

Asrael, Wilma, B.S.O.T., M.H.D.L., Bolding, Mary, R.N., B.A., Eckard, Paula, B.S.N., M.H.D.L., Childbirth Preparation for the Pregnant, Quadriplegic Woman. Paper presented at the Third Annual National Symposium on Sexuality and Disability, New York University, June 20, 1981.

Belfrage, P., Fernstrom, I., Hallenberg, G., Routine or selective ultrasound examinations in early pregnancy. *Obstetrics and Gynecology,* 1987, 69.

Carty, Elaina A., MSN, RN, CNM, Conine, Tali A., MA, DHSc, RPT, Disability and Pregnancy: A Double Dose of Disequilibrium. *Rehabilitation Nursing,* March/April, 1988, 2(13).

Conine, Tali A., BSC, MA, DHSC, RPT, Carty, Elaine A., BN, MSN, CNM, Wood-Johnson, Faith, BPT, MSC, MCPA, Nature and Source of Information Received by Primiparas with Rheumatoid Arthritis on Preventive Maternal and Child Care. *Canadian Journal of Public Health,* November/December, 1987, 78.

Duffy, Yvonne, . . . *all things are possible* (Ann Arbor: A.J. Garvin & Associates, 1981).

Ferreyra, Susan, and Hughes, Katrine, *Table Manners: A Guide to the Pelvic Examination for Disabled Women and Health Care Providers* (San Francisco: Sex Education for Disabled People, Planned Parenthood Alameda/San Francisco, 1982)

Lamki, H., Handicapped Patients, *Clinics in Obstetrics and Gynaecology,* April, 1982, 9(1).

Lindheimer, Marshall D., M.D., and Barron, William, M.D. (guest eds.), Symposium on Medical Disorders During Pregnancy, *Clinics in Perinatology,* October, 1985, 12(3).

Shaul, Susan, Ph.D., Dowling, Pamela, Laden, Bernice F., B.S., Like Other Women: Perspectives of Mothers With Physical Disabilities. *Journal of Sociology and Social Welfare,* July, 1981.

Shaul, Susan, Bogle, Jane, Hale-Harbaugh, Julia, Norman, Ann Duecy, *Toward Intimacy: Family Planning and Sexuality Concerns of Physically Disabled Women* (New York/London: Human Sciences Press, 1980).

Stierman, Elizabeth D., MS, Emotional Aspects of Perinatal Death. *Clinical Obstetrics and Gynecology,* June, 1987, 30(2).

The Task Force on Physically Disabled Women (Shaul, Susan, Bogle, Jane, Hale-Harbaugh, Norman, Julia, Duecy, Ann), *Toward Intimacy: Family Planning and Sexuality Concerns of Physically Disabled Women* (New York/London: Human Sciences Press, 1980).

Tomita, Ann, R.P.T., What is TENS? *Genesis,* June/July 1988, 10(3).

Verduyn, W.H., M.D., Health Care For Disabled Women: A Physician's View-Point. (Personal communication of a paper originally presented October 9, 1989).

Autoimmune Disorders and Pregnancy

Baguley, E., MacLachlan, N., Hughes, G.R., SLE and Pregnancy. *Clinical and Experimental Rheumatology,* April/June, 1988, 6(2).

Bobrie, G., M.D., Liote, F., M.D., Houillier, P., M.D., Grunfeld, J.P., M.D., and Jungers, P., M.D., Pregnancy in Lupus Nephritis and Related Disorders. *American Journal of Kidney Disease,* April 1987, 9(4).

Branch, D. Ware, M.D., Immunologic Disease and Fetal Death. *Clinical Obstetrics and Gynecology*, June, 1987, 30(2)

Branch, D. Ware, M.D., Scott, James R., M.D., Kochenour, Neil K., M.D., and Hershgold, Edward, M.D., Obstetric Complications Associated with the Lupus Anticoagulant, *New England Journal of Medicine*, 1985, 313 (21).

De Swiet, M., Maternal autoimmune disease and the fetus. *Archives of Disease in Childhood*, 1986, 60(9).

Druzin, Maurice L., M.D., Lockshin, Michael, M.D., Edersheim, Terri G., M.D., Hutson, J.M., M.D., Krauss, A.L., M.D., and Kogut, Elizabeth, RNC, Second-trimester fetal monitoring and preterm delivery in pregnancies with systemic lupus erythematosus and/or circulating anticoagulant. *American Journal of Obstetrics and Gynecology*, December, 1987, 157.

El-Roeiy, Albert, and Shoenfeld, Yehuda, Autoimmunity and Pregnancy. *American Journal of Reproductive Immunology and Microbiology*, 1985, 9.

Fennell, Dan F., and Ringel, Steven P., Myasthenia Gravis and Pregnancy. *Obstetrical and Gynecological Survey*, 1987, 41(7)

Gleicher, Norbert, Pregnancy and Autoimmunity. *Acta Haematologica*, 1986, 76.

Hatada, Y., Munemura, M., Matsuo, I., Fujisaki, S., Okamura, H., Yamanaka, N., Myasthenic crisis in the puerperium: the possible importance of alpha fetoprotein. Case Report. *British Journal of Obstetrics and Gynaecology*, May, 1987, 94.

Howard, Paul F., Hochberg, Marc C., Bias, Wilma B., Arnett, Jr., Franc C., and McLean, Robert H., Relationship Between C4 Null Genes, HLA-D Region Antigens, and Genetic Susceptibility to Systemic Lupus Erythematosus in Caucasian and Black Americans, *American Journal of Medicine*, August, 1986, 81(2).

Klipple, Gary L., M.D., and Cecere, Fred A., M.D., Rheumatoid Arthritis and Pregnancy. *Rheumatic Disease Clinics of North America*, May, 1989, 15(2).

Lubbe, Wilhelm F., M.D., and Liggins, Graham C., M.B., Ph.D., Lupus anticoagulant and pregnancy, *American Journal of Obstetrics and Gynecology*, 1985, 153(3).

Mintz, Gregorio, M.D., FACP, and Rodriguez-Alvarez, Encarnacion, M.D., Systemic Lupus Erythematosus. *Rheumatic Disease Clinics of North America* 15(2) May, 1989.

Parke, Ann Leslie, Antimalarial Drugs, Systemic Lupus Erythematosus and Pregnancy. *The Journal of Rheumatology*, 1988, 15(4).

Parke, Ann, Maier, Donald, Haki, Christopher, Randolph, John, and Andreoli, John, Subclinical Autoimmune Disease and Recurrent Spontaneous Abortion. *The Journal of Rheumatology,* 1986, 13(6).

Plauche, Warren C., M.D., Myasthenia gravis in pregnancy: An update. *American Journal of Obstetrics and Gynecology,* 1979, 135.

Plauche, Warren C., M.D., Myasthenia Gravis. *Clinical Obstetrics and Gynecology,* September, 1983, 26(3).

Poser, Sigrid, M.D., and Poser, Wolfgang, M.D., Multiple sclerosis and gestation. *Neurology,* November, 1983.

Poser, Sigrid, Raun, H.E., Wikstrom, J., and Poser, W., Pregnancy, oral contraceptives and multiple sclerosis. *Acta Neurologica Scandinavica,* 1979, 59.

Ramsey-Goldman, Rosalind, M.D., Pregnancy in Systemic Lupus Erythematosus. *Rheumatic Disease Clinics of North America,* April, 1988 14(1).

Rogers, Malcolm P., M.D., Psychologic Aspects of Pregnancy in Patients with Rheumatic Diseases. *Rheumatic Disease Clinics of North America,* May, 1989, 15(2).

Rolbin, Shephen H., M.D.CM, FRCP, Levinson, Gershon, M.D., Shnider, Sol M., M.D., Wright, Richard G., M.D., Anesthetic Considerations for Myasthenia Gravis and Pregnancy. *Anesthesia and Analgesia,* 1978, 57.

Samuels, Philip, M.D., and Pfeifer, Samantha M., M.D., Autoimmune Diseases in Pregnancy—The Obstetrician's View. *Rheumatic Disease Clinics of North America,* May, 1989, 15(2).

Syrop, Craig H., M.D. and Varner, Michael W., M.D., Systemic Lupus Erythematosus. *Clinical Obstetrics and Gynecology,* September, 1983, 26(3)

Thompson, David S., M.D., Nelson, Lorene M., MS, Burns, Arlene, BA, Burks, Jack S., M.D., and Franklin, M.D., M.P.H., The effects of pregnancy in multiple sclerosis: A retrospective study. *Neurology,* 1986, 36.

Thurnau, Gary R., M.D., Rheumatoid Arthritis. *Clinical Obstetrics and Gynecology,* September, 1983, 26(3).

Scoliosis and Pregnancy

Berman, Arnold T., The Effects of Pregnancy on Idiopathic Scoliosis: A Preliminary Report on Eight Cases and a Review of the Literature. *Spine,* 1982, 7(2).

Cochran, T., and Nachemson, A., Long-Term Anatomic and Functional

Changes in Patients with Adolescent Idiopathic Scoliosis Treated with the Milwaukee Brace. *Spine,* 1985, 10(2)

Sawicka, E.H., Spencer, G.T., and Branthwaite, M.A., Management of Respiratory Failure Complicating Pregnancy in Severe Kyphoscoliosis: A New Use For an Old Technique? *British Journal of Diseases of the Chest,* 1986, 80.

Visscher, W., Lonstein, J.E., Hoffman, D.A., Mandel, J.S., Harris, B.S., III, Reproductive outcomes in scoliosis patients. *Spine,* 1988, 13(10).

Spinal Cord Dysfunction and Pregnancy

DeLoach, Charlene, *Adjustment To Severe Physical Disability: A Metamorphosis.* (New York: McGraw-Hill, 1981).

Francois, N., Maury, M., Sexual aspects in paraplegic patients. *Paraplegia,* June 1987, 25(3).

Greenspoon, Jeffrey S., M.D., and Paul, Richard H., M.D., Paraplegia and quadriplegia: Special considerations during pregnancy and labor and delivery. *American Journal of Obstetrics and Gynecology,* 1986, 155.

McGregor, James A., M.D., C.M., and Meeuswen, James, M.D., Autonomic hyperreflexia: A mortal danger for spinal cord-damaged women in labor, *American Journal of Obstetrics and Gynecology,* 1985, 151.

Ohry, Abraham, Peleg, Dan, Goldman, Jack, David, Amnon, and Rozin, Raphael, Sexual Function, Pregnancy and Delivery in Spinal Cord Injured Women. *Gynecologic and Obstetric Investigation,* 1978, 9.

Richmond, David, Zaharievski, I.V., Bond, Andrew, Management of pregnancy in mothers with spina bifida. *European Journal of Obstetrics, Gynecology, and Reproductive Biology,* 1987, 25.

Robertson, D. N. Struan, MB, FRCOG, and Guttman, L., CBE, FRCP, FRCS, The Paraplegic Patient in Pregnancy and Labor. *Proceedings of the Royal Society of Medicine,* 1963, 56.

Rossier, A.B., Ruffieux, M., and Ziegler, W.H., Pregnancy and Labor in High Traumatic Spinal Cord Lesions. *Paraplegia,* November, 1969, 7.

Verduyn, W.H., M.D., Spinal Cord Injured Women, Pregnancy and Delivery. *Paraplegia,* 1986, 24.

Verduyn, W.H., M.D., A Deadly Combination: Induction of Labor with Oxytocin/Pitocin in Spinal Cord Injured Women, T6 and Above. (Personal communication of paper in progress, April, 1989)

Verduyn, W.H., M.D., "Health Care For Disabled Women: A Physician's View-Point." (Personal communication of a paper presented October 9, 1989.)

Wanner, M.B., M.D., Rageth, C.J., M.D., Zach, G.A., M.D., Pregnancy and Autonomic Hyperreflexia in Patients with Spinal Cord Lesions. *Paraplegia,* 1987, 25.

Young, Bruce K., M.D., Katz, Miriam, M.D., and Klein, Steven A., M.D., Pregnancy After Spinal Cord Injury: Altered Maternal and Fetal Response to Labor. *Obstetrics and Gynecology,* July, 1983, 62(1).

Cesarean Birth

Meyers, Stephen A., and Gleicher, Norbert, A Successful Program to Lower Cesarean-Section Rates. *New England Journal of Medicine,* 1988, 319(23).

National Institute of Child Health and Human Development, National Center for Health Care Technology, Office for Medical Applications of Research (Consensus Development Conference), Cesarean Childbirth (U.S. Department of Health and Human Services, Public Health Service, National Institutes of Health, NIH Publication No. 82-2067, October, 1981).

Wainer, Nancy Cohen, and Estner, Lois J., *Silent Knife: Vaginal Birth After Cesarean and Cesarean Prevention* (Westport, Connecticut: Bergin & Garvey, 1983).

Deciding Whether to Have Children

Dowrick, Stephanie, and Grundberg, S. (eds.), *Why Children?* (New York: Harcourt, Brace, Jovanovich, 1980).

Elvenstar, Diane C., *Children: To Have or Have Not? A Guide to Making and Living with Your Decision* (San Francisco: Harbor, 1982)

Figley, Charles R., and McCubbin, Hamilton I., *Stress and the Family,* Vol. 2 (New York: Brunner, Mazel, Inc., 1983).

Frames, Robin, Should I Have a Baby? *Inside MS,* Fall, 1984.

Genevie, Louis, Ph.D., and Margolies, Eva, *The Motherhood Report* (New York: Macmillian Publishing Co., 1987).

Miller, Warren B., and Newman, Lucile F. (eds.), *The First Child and Family Formation* (Chapel Hill, NC: Carolina Population Center, 1978).

Waxman, Barbara Faye, So You Want To Be A Parent? *Mainstream,* January, 1984.

Genetic Counseling

Beeson, Diane, PH.D., Douglas, Rita, M.A., Lunsford, Terry F., J.D., Ph.D., Prenatal Diagnosis of Fetal Disorders, Part II: Issues and Implications.

Birth, Winter 1983, 10(4).

Emery, Alan E.H., M.D., Ph.D., D.C., FRCP(E), FRS(E), Rimoin, David L., M.D., Ph.D.,(eds.) (Sofaer, Jeffrey A., B.D.S., Ph.D., assistant ed., Garber, A.P., M.S., editorial assistant), *Principles and Practice of Medical Genetics,* Vol. 1 (New York: Churchill Livingstone, 1983).

Wapner, R.J., M.D., and Jackson, L., M.D., Chorionic Villus Sampling. *Clinical Obstetrics and Gynecology,* June, 1988, 31(2).

Diagnostic Procedures

Burton, Barbara K., M.D., Elevated Maternal Serum Alpha-Fetoprotein (MSAFP): Interpretation and Follow-up. *Clinical Obstetrics and Gynecology,* June, 1988, 31(2).

Buyon, Jill P.,M.D., Cronstein, Bruce N., M.D., Morris, Mitchell, M.D., Tanner, Martin, BA, and Weissmann, Gerald, M.D., Serum Complement Values C3 and C4 to Differentiate between Systemic Lupus Activity and Pre-Eclampsia. *The American Journal of Medicine,* August, 1986, 81.

Exercise

Amercian College of Obstetrics and Gynecology: *ACOG Home Exercise Programs: Exercise During Pregnancy and the Postnatal Period.* Washington, D.C., 1985.

Casper, Ursula Hodge, *Joy and Comfort Through Stretching and Relaxing: For Those Who Are Unable to Exercise* (New York: The Seabury Press, 1982).

Freyder, Susan Connelly, Exercising While Pregnant. *Journal of Orthopedic Sports and Physical Therapy,* March, 1989.

Noble, Elizabeth, R.P.T., *Essential Exercises for the Childbearing Year* (Boston: Houghton Mifflin Co., 1982).

Nutrition

Abel, Ernest L., *Marihuana, Tobacco, Alcohol, and Reproduction* (Boca Raton: CRC Press, Inc., 1983).

Brown, Judith E., *Nutrition for Your Pregnancy* (Minneapolis: University of Minnesota, 1983).

California Department of Health Services, Maternal and Child Health and WIC Supplemental Foods Branches. *Dietary Guidelines and Daily Food Guide in Nutrition During Pregnancy and the Postpartum Period: A*

Manual for Health Care Professionals (Sacramento, CA: Department of Health Services, 6/7/89 draft).

Hurley, Lucille S., *Developmental Nutrition* (Englewood Cliffs, NJ: Prentice-Hall, Inc., 1980).

National Research Council—Committee on Maternal Nutrition/Food and Nutrition Board, Maternal Nutrition and the Course of Pregnancy: Summary Report (Washington, D.C.: National Academy of Sciences, 1970).

National Research Council—Committee on Nutrition of the Mother and Preschool Child, Food and Nutrition Board, Commission on Life Sciences, Alternative Dietary Practices and Nutritional Abuses in Pregnancy: Proceedings of a Workshop (Washington, D.C.: National Academy Press, 1982).

Watt, Bernice K., and Merrill, Annabel L. (with the assistance of Pecot, Reecca K., Adams, Catherine F., Orr, Martha Louise, and Miller, Donald F.), *Handbook of the Nutritional Contents of Foods,* (New York: Dover Publications, Inc., 1975) Originally prepared for the U.S. Department of Agriculture.

Worthington-Roberts, Bonnie S., Ph.D, Vermeersch, Joyce, R.D., Dr.P.H., Williams, Sue Rodwell, M.P.H., M.R.Ed., Ph.D., R.D., *Nutrition in Pregnancy and Lactation,* 3rd ed. (St. Louis: Times Mirror/Mosby, 1985).

Child Development and Child Care

Bernstein, Anne, Talking about Handicaps. *Parents,* December, 1984.

Brown, Geni, Parents with Special Needs. *Independent Living,* Summer, 1986.

Buck, Francis Marks, and Hohmann, George W., Personality, Behavior, Values and Family Relations of Children of Fathers with Spinal Cord Injury. *Archives of Physical Medicine and Rehabilitation,* September, 1981, 62.

Caplan, Frank (ed.), *The First Twelve Months of Life* (New York: Perigee Books, 1982).

Friday, Nancy, *My Mother, Myself* (New York: Delacorte Press, 1977).

May, Elizabeth Eckhardt, and Waggoner, Neva, Work Simplification in the Area of Child Care for Physically Handicapped Women, O.V.R. Special Project 37, Summary of Final Report, June 15, 1955—December 31, 1960. Research conducted by School of Home Economics, University of Connecticut, in cooperation with the Connecticut Team Approach Committee on Research, Demonstrations and Workshops Concerning

Physically Handicapped Homemakers. Issued by Division of Research and Demonstrations, Office of Vocational Rehabilitation, Washington, D.C.

Neville, Helen, and Halaby, Mona, *No Fault Parenting* (Tucson: The Body Press, 1984).

Shaul, Susan, Ph.D., Dowling, Pamela, Laden, Bernice F., B.S., Like Other Women: Perspectives of Mothers With Physical Disabilities. *Journal of Sociology and Social Welfare,* July, 1981.

Turk, R., M.D., Turk, M., M.D., and Assejev, V., The Female Paraplegic and Mother–Child Relations. *Paraplegia,* 1983, 21.

INDEX